FREE STUFF FOR WOMEN'S HEALTH, FITNESS AND NUTRITION

by

MATTHEW LESKO

and

MARY ANN MARTELLO

Researchers
Laura Difore, Allison Mays, Marcelle McCarthy
Cindy Owens, Bradley Sowash, Emily Subler, Jennifer Maier

Production
Cynthia D. Wade

Marketing
Kim McCoy

Support
Mercedes Sundeen

Cover
Steve Bonham

FIRST EDITION

Library of Congress Cataloging-in-Publication date
    Lesko, Matthew
    Martello, Mary Ann

Free Stuff for Women's Health, Fitness and Nutrition

ISBN # 1-878346-50-4

Table of Contents

Lots of Freebies To Keep Your Life Healthy (cont.)

Free Money and Help for People With Disabilities 207

Free Mammograms / Free Tests For Breast and Cervical Cancer 419

Special Help For Cancer Patients..448

How to Help the Underserved With Health Care 467

The Best Health Care Is Free

Of course it is! But people in our society still believe that you get what you pay for. It's not true with health care.

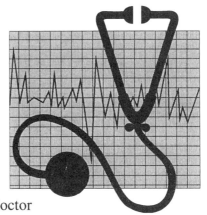

Why pay for an office visit to get medical advice from your local doctor when you can contact the best medical experts in the world for free?

Why spend money on the latest fad diet because some pretty face on television says it's good, when you can find out whether the program works from the best nutrition experts for free?

Why pay for medical treatment by a local doctor who rarely handles your problem when the best doctors in the world get grants to treat your condition for free?

Why have an operation recommended by your doctor when you can obtain a free report showing that 50% of the people who had the surgery really didn't need it?

You can also get:

- Free Prescription Drugs

- Free Mammograms

- Free OB/GYN Exams

- Free Breast Cancer Treatment

- Free Dentures

- Free Plastic Surgery

- Free Health Books

- Free Airfare for Health Treatments

- Free Long Term Care

- Free Health Insurance Counseling

- Free Hearing Aids

- Free Equipment for Disabilities

- Free Eye Care

- Free Health Insurance

- Free Money to Finance Adoptions

- Free Speech Therapy for Kids

- Free Legal Help to Fight Your HMO

- Free Immunizations

Doctors and Congress Don't Know About Free Stuff

You will never see signs at hospitals or in doctors offices saying "Free Care — Come and Get It." Most health professionals are trying to make a living in the health care system, so they're not going to give it away. And they are such busy people they are not going to spend the time figuring out where the free stuff is. They're not the ones who need it.

We did an undercover survey of doctors around the country to see if they were aware of free health care services and here is what we found:

★ 91% of the doctors had no idea where to turn for help if a patient did not have complete insurance coverage.

We also did an undercover survey of Congresspeople and Senators to see if they are aware of these free health care programs. Here's what we found:

★ over 83% of the members of Congress were unaware of the current programs that offer free hospitalization, free care by the best doctors in the world, and free prescription drugs.

The lawmakers who wrote the laws that created these programs didn't even know that they exist!

The same is true for health information. Health professionals can't keep up on all the latest developments in health care. Doctors are busy people, spending most of their time treating patients. They are not sitting in their offices studying new treatments or researching new free health services. When was the last time you spent more than 10 minutes with a doctor when he did not have his hand on the doorknob waiting to get out of the room?

Every day the headlines are filled with news about new discoveries in treatments and cures. It's impossible for doctors to be aware of all this information. But you, as a health consumer, can keep up-to-date with the help of the resources in this book. Now you can contact free health researchers who spend their lives researching your health problem. They can tell you the results of research that isn't even published yet. They can send you free studies that you can take to your doctor and discuss the results with them. Or these experts can tell you where the best doctors are who can treat you. As an informed patient you become the most critical part of your own health care.

In our information society you can't trust the experts anymore. The answers are changing too fast for the health professionals to keep up. But you, as a consumer in the information society, can now get better information than your doctor. And you can start by looking in this book.

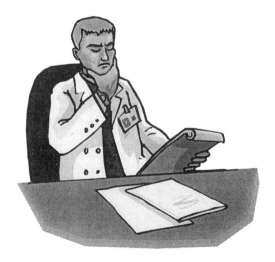

Services For Rich, Poor And Everyone In Between

Sam Donaldson had his cancer surgery done for free, thanks to a government program listed on page 106. A founder of H & R Block raves about the free treatment he received from the government. I'm not eligible for welfare and even I had experts from all over the country look at my son's arm for free because a fracture was not healing properly.

People with money find out about the good stuff and use it, while everyone else pays for it in their tax dollars, and would rather complain about the government than take advantage of it.

Many of the programs in this book have no income requirements but some of them do. Remember, however, that what you and the government consider to be "poor and in need of assistance" may well be two different things. Look:

✔ A single person making $45,000 a year is considered indigent and can receive free prescription drugs;

✔ A family making $32,000 is considered poor and can receive all free health services; and

✔ A business is considered disadvantaged by the government if it has only $750,000 in the bank. (That's almost a million!).

So even if there are income limitations for some of the programs in this book, it is important to ask if you qualify. You may be one of the country's disadvantaged millionaires who are in need of help.

Also remember that the system is always set up for exceptions. Even though you may not meet the income eligibility requirements, persistence and a real need can convince a bureaucrat to bend the system. There have been bureaucrats who told me that they can make exceptions. And you can be one of them.

Does "No" Mean No?

It may for sexual harassment, but it's not necessarily the case in the health care system. Too many times I've personally found that after an expert told me "No," persistence got me to someone who said "Yes."

I was helping a woman whose cancer treatments were stopped at one of the most prestigious hospitals in the country. She had no insurance and everyone in the hospital was telling me that there was no way anyone could help her. The doctor couldn't help her. Two social workers at the hospital couldn't help her. I talked to dozens of people in the director's offices, admissions, accounting, and even personnel, and they all said that she couldn't be helped. But after 4 weeks of calling, a woman in the hospital's accounting division called me back and told me about a little-known program that they have that covers unusual situations like this. Within a week the woman was back in the hospital receiving her free treatment.

A young woman we know was complaining about her roommate's recent liver transplant and how her HMO would not pay for the medications she needed after the operations. The drugs cost $2,000 a month and are absolutely necessary to prevent her body from rejecting her

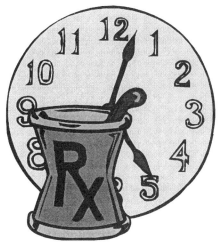

new liver. The doctors who performed the operation offered no help. This surprised me. How can they perform the surgery without knowing the patient can get the necessary drugs to fight rejection? The hospital where the operation was performed also offered no suggestions. It wasn't until she found through one of our books that she was able to get $25,000 worth of free prescriptions with one 10-minute phone call. That's after being told "No" by some of the world's best experts at a first rate hospital in the USA.

Remember, very few people in the world know everything. And they may only know what works for most people. Don't think of yourself as "most people"! You want something special and it is out there just for you. But you have to be willing to go get it. This is a book that will help you do that.

This Book Is Out Of Date

Everything in our country is out of date by the time it's published. Your phone book is out of date as soon as your get it. Your newspaper is even out of date when it hits the street.

We live in a fast changing world, and there is no way any of us in publishing can always have only the latest information in print. So please be patient (no pun intended). Although we updated and verified each listing right before printing, you may contact one of the offices identified in this book and find that the telephone number or program has changed.

For a wrong number you can always call the information operator in the city where the office is located and get a new listing. And, if you happen to contact an agency where the program has changed, be sure to ask the office if they know of any additional programs that may also satisfy your request. New programs are always being added, changed, or transferred to a local level. Use an old source as a lead to a new better source.

Here's to your health!

Matthew Lesko

Lots of Freebies To Keep Your Life Healthy

TEENS CAN GET CONFIDENTIAL GYN EXAMS FOR $5.00

In Montgomery County, MD, teenage girls can get gynecological exams, breast exams and even birth control counseling at the local Planned Parenthood Clinic for only $5.00. All they need to have is a note from the school nurse.

Planned Parenthood has 900 clinics around the country and services vary according to local laws and funding sources. To investigate what your local clinic offers, call 1-800-230-PLAN.

H-E-A-L-T-H-F-I-N-D-E-R

This is a gateway consumer health information web site from the U.S. government that can lead you to online publications, clearinghouses, databases, web sites, and support and self-help groups, as well as government agencies and non-profit organizations that produce reliable information for the public: {www.healthfinder.org}.

Contact: Planned Parenthood Federation of American, 810 Seventh Avenue, New York, NY 10019; 212-261-4647; Fax: 212-261-4560; {www.plannedparenthood.org}.

Abortions Starting At $250

Some of the 900 Planned Parenthood clinics offer abortions during the first 11 weeks of pregnancy starting at $250 for those not covered by health insurance. In some cases they even have special funds to help women pay for services.

To investigate what your local clinic offers, call 1-800-230-PLAN. You can also contact Planned Parenthood Federation of America, 810 Seventh Avenue, New York, NY 10019; 212-261-4647; Fax: 212-261-4560; {www.plannedparenthood.org}.

There is another consumer hotline that can also handle your abortion related questions. Contact: The National Abortion Federation, 1755 Massachusetts Ave., NW, Washington, DC 20036; 800-772-9100 or in Canada 800-424-2282, weekdays from 9:00 to 7:00 EST; {www.prochoice.org/index.html}.

Grants Up To $2,500 and Loans To Finance Adoptions

The National Adoption Foundation helps arrange loans and provides limited grants for parents to cover expenses before and after adoption. They also provide information on sources of other financial help like the 325 Fortune 500 companies who offer an average cash reimbursement of $4,000 for their employees who adopt, or the new adoption expense tax credit that is available from the IRS. Contact: National Adoption Foundation, 100 Mill Plain Rd, Danbury, CT 06811; 203-791-3811.

The following organizations also provide free publications, referral services and advice on adoption and searching for birth relatives:

★ **National Adoption Information Clearinghouse**, 330 C Street, NW, Washington, DC 20447; 888-2551-0075; 703-352-3488; {www.calib.com/naic}.
★ **National Adoption Center**, 1500 Walnut St, Suite 701, Philadelphia, PA, 19102; Answer Line: 215-735-9988; {www.adopt.org}.
★ **National Council For Adoption**, 1930 17th Street, NW, Washigton, DC 20009; 202-328-8072; Fax: 202-332-0935; {www.ncfa-usa.org}.

AN EXTRA $6,OOO A YEAR
IF YOU CAN'T WORK

Is your check too small to live on? If so, don't be discouraged. If you don't qualify for Social Security, or if your benefits are very low, you may qualify for Supplemental Security Income (SSI).

This program was established to help poor seniors over 65, as well as the blind and disabled, meet basic living needs. To qualify, you must meet a maximum monthly income

Free Plastic Surgery For Children

Austin Smiles provides free reconstructive plastic surgery, mainly to repair cleft lip and palate, to the children around Austin, Texas. They do about 75 surgeries a year. Austin Plastic Surgery Foundation, P.O. Box 26694, Austin, TX 78755-0694; 512-451-9300; Fax: 512-451-9312; {www.main.org/smiles/}.

To see if similar services are available anywhere near you contact Cleft Palate Foundation, 104 S. Estes Dr., Suite 204, Chapel Hill, NC 27514; 800-24-CLEFT; 919-933-9044; {www.cleft.com/cpf.htm}.

test. Some of the income and services you receive are excluded when they calculate your monthly income in relation to your personal expenses.

Those who meet SSI's eligibility usually automatically qualify for Medicaid coverage and food stamp benefits. Studies have found that only between 40 and 60 percent of those who qualify for SSI actually receive benefits under the program. To find out if you qualify, contact your local Social Security office or call the Social Security Hotline at 800-772-1213.

Free Speech Therapy For Toddlers

It doesn't matter how much money you earn. You can have your child tested to see if any speech problems are developing and even get free speech therapy.

It's part of the U.S. Individuals with Disabilities Education Act (IDEA) to make sure that children in need receive special education beginning on their third birthday, and in some states, like Virginia, it starts at age 2.

The program is run through your local school district, so check with them first, or your state Department of Education listed in the Appendix. You can also contact Division of Educational Services, Office of Special Education Programs, U.S. Department of Education, 330 C St., SW, Washington, DC 20202; 202-205-9172; {www.ed.gov/offices/OSERS/OSEP/osep.html}.

Emergency Help From Domestic Violence

If you or someone you know is being emotionally or physically abused, call the National Domestic Violence Hotline. This hotline is supported with funds from the Violence Against Women Act, which also gives money for local governments to hire more prosecutors to enforce domestic violence laws, and to improve domestic violence training among prosecutors, police officers, and health and social services professionals.

A Woman's Chance of Violence

- 18% of all women will be a victim of rape or attempted rape
- 54% of rapes occur to women under 17
- over 50% of women will be physically assaulted during their lives
- 76 % of rapes occur by a current or former husband, a cohabiting partner, or a date

Source: U.S. Center for Disease Control, National Center for Injury Prevention and Control; {www.hhs.gov/press/1998pres/98117a.html}

Contact: National Domestic Violence Hotline, P.O. Box 161810, Austin, TX 78716; 800-799-SAFE; TTY 800-787-3224; {www.ndvh.org}.

Kids Get Free Expert Care At 22 Hospitals

Children suffering from orthopedic injuries, diseases of the bones, joint and muscles, or burns can get free treatment from one of the 22 Shriners Hospitals. The requirements for admission are that the child is under the age of 18, and there is a reasonable possibility the condition can be helped.

For more information, contact Shriners Hospitals, P.O. Box 31356, Tampa, FL 33631; 800-237-5055 (in Canada 800-361-7256); {www.shrinershq.org}.

Find Out How Long You'll Live & Save $50

A free, personalized, confidential Health Risk Assessment is available online from a health care consulting firm called Greenstone Healthcare Solutions in Kalamazoo, Michigan. From the information you provide through a questionnaire, they process the data instantly against a database of statistics showing what kind of behavior shortens your life. Your instant report shows you how many years you can add by changing your behavior.

I took the test and it showed that my health is six years younger than my age, but I can still add two years to my life. Such assessments usually cost from $10 to $50. But here, it's free. Contact Greenstone Healthcare Solutions at {www.youfirst.com}.

Free Private Eye and Mediation For Missing Children

Besides location and investigative services, as well as mediation services for families estranged by parental abduction, you can also get free kidnapping prevention programs and referral and support services.

Contact Find-A-Child of America, Inc., P.O. Box 277, New Paltz, NY 12561; 800-I-AM-LOST; 914-255-1848; 800-A-WAY-OUT (for mediation and support); {www.childfindamerica.org}.

Head Lice Hotline

Anywhere from 6 to 10 million kids a year get head lice. That's one of the reasons why the U.S. Federal Trade Commission made three large producers of head lice treatment shampoos change their false advertising claims. They claimed that their shampoos eliminated head lice 100% of the time. They don't.

To get the facts about head lice treatments or to report outbreaks, treatment failures, or adverse reactions to treatments, contact The National Pediculosis Association, P.O. Box 610189, Newton, MA 02161; 800-446-4672; 781-449-6487; Fax: 781-449-8129; {www.headlice.org}.

Law Gives Kids With ADD Free Special Classes

The nonprofit organization, *Children and Adults with Attention Deficit Disorder (CHADD),* identifies a number of federal laws that require the government to provide children with this disorder special educational services. It is only recently that these children became eligible for such

HOTLINE LOCATES WANDERING ALZHEIMER'S PATIENTS

Alzheimer's patients are known to wander away and even wind up in other cities. My father, in his later years, went for a drive that took him into someone's back yard.

Safe Return is a national clearinghouse that helps police and private citizens locate and return lost Alzheimer's patients. Contact The Alzheimer's Association, 919 N. Michigan Ave., Suite 1000, Chicago, IL 60611; 800-272-3900; {www.alz.org}.

Finding A Doctor In A Hay Stack

650,000 doctor practices are online at {www. ama-assn.org}. You can search by name, specialty, and get reference info on all major diseases and conditions.

services, so many eligible children may not be receiving what they deserve.

To learn more about these free educational services, or to find out more and how to treat a child with ADD, or what's good and bad about available treatments, contact: CHADD, 8181 Professional Place, Suite 201, Landover, MD 20785; 800-233-4050; Fax: 301-306-7090; {www.chadd.org}.

Grant Money For Parents of Children With Hearing Loss

If your child is under 6 and has a moderate to profound hearing loss, you can apply for money to pay for intervention, educational and/or rehabilitation services. There is also money available for children with hearing loss between the ages of 5 and 19 to attend art or science courses during the summer, weekends, or even after school.

Contact: Alexander Graham Bell Association for the Deaf, 3417 Volta Place, NW, Washington, DC 20007; 202-337-5220 (voice and TTY); {www.agbell.org}.

Alcohol and Drug Abuse Counseling & Treatment

Georgia provides outpatient counseling services, short-term residential programs, and even school student assistance programs. Florida provides substance abuse treatment programs through a partnership with 102 public and private not-for-profit community providers. Delaware contracts with private organizations around the state to provide screening, outpatient counseling, and detoxification, as well as short term and long term treatment. Contact your state Department of Health, listed in the Appendix, to see what your state has to offer.

There are also nonprofit organizations who, by themselves, offer free treatment to people, like the Center for Drug-Free Living in Orlando, Florida (5029 N. Lane, Suite 8, Orlando, FL 32808; 407-245-0012; {www.cfdfl.com}).

If your state can't help you get the information or treatment you need, one or both of the following hotlines should be able to help:

■ *National Drug and Treatment Routing Service*, Center for Substance Abuse Treatment, National Institute on Alcohol Abuse and Alcoholism (NIAAA), 600

Executive Blvd, Willco Bldg., Bethesda, MD 20892;
800-662-HELP; {www.niaaa.nih.gov}.

■ *The National Clearinghouse for Alcohol and Drug
Information*, 11426 Rockville Pike, Suite 200,
Rockville, MD20852; 800-729-6686 24 hours a day;
301-468-2600 TDD; {www.health.org}.

FREE WHEELCHAIRS

Easter Seals, the American Cancer Society and other
helpful organizations provide free
wheelchairs and other medical related
equipment, like walkers, commodes,
bathtub rails, bathtub chairs, crutches,
transfer benches, electric wheelchairs
and scooters, on a short- or long-term
basis. Some programs require
deposits that are completely refundable.

Check with your local office of Easter Seals and the
American Cancer Society. You can also contact your state
Department of Health listed in the Appendix.

- *American Cancer Society, Inc.*, 1599 Clifton Road,
  NE, Atlanta, GA 30329; 800-ACS-2345;
  {www.cancer.org}.

- *Easter Seals*, 230 West Monroe Street, Suite 1800,
  Chicago, IL 60606; 800-221-6825; 312-726-6200; fax:
  312-726-1494; {www.seals.com}.

Morning After Hotline: Eliminate A Pregnancy Within Three Days After Unprotected Intercourse

When all else fails, the Emergency Contraceptive Pills (ECP) taken within 72 hours after having unprotected intercourse, with a second dose 12 hours after the first, increases your chances of NOT getting pregnant by 75%.

The hotline describes the procedures and will direct you to four local offices and clinics that offer these pills. For

Over-the-Counter Birth Control Made Easy

Find out the cost and what's good and bad about using over-the-counter products like foam, suppositories, vaginal film, sponge, and the male and female condom for birth control. Check out the web page of the Feminist Women's Health Center at {www.fwhc.org}.

women who already have birth control pills, the clinic will instruct her on how to use them correctly as emergency contraception. If you don't already have pills, you can get a prescription for emergency contraception.

Call the hotline operated by the Office of Population Research at Princeton University at 800-584-9911; {http://opr.princeton.edu/ec/}.

Emergency Contraceptive Pill Available Without A Prescription

Call **1-888-NOT-2-LATE** in the state of Washington and you can find a local pharmacist who can directly prescribe Emergency Contraceptive Pills (ECP).

Going directly to a pharmacist allows women to skip the process of going to a clinic or doctor or a prescription and provides access to pharmacies on evenings, weekends and holidays. The use of such pills within 72 hours after unprotected intercourse reduces the risk of pregnancy by about 75%.

Normally 8 in 100 women who have unprotected intercourse once during the second or third week of their menstrual cycle will become pregnant. Taking ECPs will reduce this to 2 out of 100.

For more information about the programs, contact: Program for Appropriate Technology in Health, 4 Nickerson Street, Seattle, WA 98109; 206-285-3500; Fax: 206-285-6619; {www.path.org}.

> *"The Facts About Weight Loss Products and Programs"*
>
> *" Infertility Services"* - how to choose a good one
>
> *"The Skinny on Dieting"* - the facts about weight loss claims
>
> All free from Federal Trade Commission, Public Reference, Room 130, Washington, DC 20580; 202-326-2222; {www.ftc.gov}.

Legal Aid For Abused Women Who Are Not Eligible For Free Legal Services

If you have been turned down from state-offered services, and cannot afford a lawyer on your own, you can apply to *Legal Aid For Abused Women (LAAW),* a nonprofit organization that helps people when no other means are available.

You Can Get Free Medical Care and Food But Not Welfare

Welfare reform laws have caused local governments to actively try to discourage people from applying for welfare payments. But, by federal law, they cannot discourage anyone from immediately applying for free medical care (Medicaid) and food assistance (Food Stamps). They are completely separate programs, and officials in Washington, DC believe that many eligible people are not applying for these services because local officials don't tell them their rights. It's the law. You have the right to apply.

Source: New York Times, November 22, 1998, Section 4, page 4

LAAW can help you find a lawyer. LAAW provides a revolving fund for legal aid. Recipients reimburse up to 100% of the monetary assistance provided and/or volunteer their time to assist others affected by domestic violence.

Legal aid is provided regardless of race, nationality, gender, social status, orientation, or education level.

Contact: Legal Aid For Abused Women, 3524 S. Utah St., Arlington, VA 22206; 703 820-8393; Fax: 703 820-7968; {E-mail: 75700.655@ compuserve.com}; {http://ourworld. compuserve.com/homepages/laaw}.

30% of All Families Eligible For Free Health Services — Others Pay Sliding Scale

Many services provided by county governments are free and persons who don't qualify for free services are charged on a sliding scale based on income.

A typical fee chart is the one below from Denton, Texas. The data is based on 1996 Federal Poverty Rates from the Bureau of the Census. Denton also states that *NO ONE WILL BE REFUSED SERVICES FOR INABILITY TO PAY*, which is typical for most counties. **REMEMBER**, if you don't qualify for free services, everyone qualifies for services on a sliding scale.

Estimated Income Limits For Free Service			
Service	Single Person	Family of 2	Family of 4
Food Vouchers and Nutritional Info (185% of poverty)	$14,893	$20,073	$30,433
Prenatal Care During Pregnancy (200% of poverty)	$16,100	$21,700	$32,900
Child Medical Care (200% of poverty)	$16,100	$21,700	$32,900
Adult Health Care (150% of poverty)	$12,075	$16,275	$24,675
Dental Care (150% of poverty)	$12,075	$16,275	$24,675
HIV Counseling & Testing	No limits, $10.00 donation requested		
Sexually Transmitted Disease Clinic	No limits, $10.00 donation requested		
Tuberculosis	No limits, $4.00 for testing		
Overseas Vaccinations	No limits, $5.00 to $50.00		
Immunizations	No limits, up to $30 per family, no one refused		
Substance Abuse Screening & Referral	No limits, Free		

Estimate of Families Living At Poverty Levels

% Of Poverty Level	Number of Families	% of Total Families
100%	12,594,000	12.3%
150%	21,055,000	20.0%
185%	28,174,000	27.4%
200%	30,078,000	29.3%

(Poverty Data from Census Report P60-198 1996 ----One Person = $7,995,
Two Persons = $ 10,233, Four Persons = $16,063,
Household Income Data from Census Current Population Reports, P60-200)
(Poverty Data 7/1/98 USDA {www.usda.gov/fcs/cnp/ieg98-99.htm}
1=$8,050, 2=$10,850, 3=13,650, 4=16,450, 5=19,250, 6=22,050, 7=24,850, 8=27,650

Everything You Need To Know On Any Women's Health Topic: HOTLINE

This hotline sends out free publications and makes referrals to other organizations and groups on women related health topics. Contact National Women's Health Information Center, Office on Women's Health, U.S. Department of Health and Human Services, 200 Independence Ave., SW, Room 730B, Washington, DC 20201.

800-944-WOMEN; {www.4women.gov}.

Grants and Fundraising Help For Transplant Patients

Organizations like The National Foundation for Transplants and National Transplant Assistance Fund assist patients, their families, and friends in raising significant amounts of money for the patient's transplant care when there is no public or private insurance that will cover all the costs. They also provide grants to help pay for medications required after a transplant, or money for transplant-related emergencies, and one-time assistance grants of $1,000.

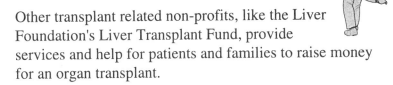

Other transplant related non-profits, like the Liver Foundation's Liver Transplant Fund, provide services and help for patients and families to raise money for an organ transplant.

- ☐ *National Foundation for Transplants*, 1102 Brookfield, Suite 200, Memphis, TN 38119; 800-489-3836; 901-684-1697; Fax: 910-684-1128; {www.transplants.org}.
- ☐ *National Transplant Assistance Fund*, 6 Bryn Mawr Avenue, P.O. Box 258, Bryn Mawr, PA 19010; 800-642-8399; Fax: 610-527-5210; {www.transplantfund.org}.
- ☐ *American Liver Foundation*, 75 Maiden Lane, Suite 603, New York, NY 10038; 800-GO LIVER; {www.liverfoundation.org}.

$5 For SEXually Transmitted Diseases Tests

If you are worried that you may have contracted a Sexually Transmitted Disease (STD) or even HIV, you can get tested and even treated for free or for very low cost at one of your local public health clinics, or other public and private clinics around the country. Contact your county office of health listed in your telephone book or your state Department of Health listed in the Appendix.

If you need more help in identifying local help or need further information about HIV or an STD, contact one of the following, run by the U.S. Department of Health and Human Service's Center For Disease Control:

Free Take Out Taxi For Seniors

People 60 and over who are homebound because of illness, incapacity, or disability, or who are otherwise isolated can receive hot meals delivered to their home. The program is funded in every state by the Older Americans Act.

Contact your local area agency on aging or your state Department on Aging listed in the Appendix. If that fails, contact the Eldercare Locator hotline at 1-800-677-1116. They are available to help anyone identify services for seniors.

- *STD Hotline* 1-800-227-8922; {www.cdcnpin.org/}

- *National AIDS Hotline* 1-800-342-AIDS; {www.cdcnpin.org/}.

- *National Herpes Hotline* 1-919-361-8488; {www.cdc.gov/nchstp/dstd/dstdp/html}

These hotlines can answer questions over the phone, send out educational literature about a wide variety of sexually transmitted diseases and prevention methods, and provide referrals to free and low cost clinics nationwide.

Low Cost Home Health Care

Montgomery County in Maryland provides home health care free or on a sliding scale, depending on income, through the local public health office. You don't have to be a senior to qualify.

A survey by the Center for Disease Control reports that about half of all local public health agencies provide similar services. To see what is available in your area, contact your county office of health listed in your telephone book or your state Department of Health listed in the Appendix. If you cannot get satisfaction from these offices, contact your local office of your state or federal elected official.

For similar services for seniors, contact your local area agency on aging or your state Department on Aging listed in the Appendix. If that fails, contact the Eldercare Locator hotline at 1-800-677-1116. They are available to help anyone identify services for seniors.

Do You Need A Break As A Caregiver?

If you're the only caregiver for a sick child or relative and get frustrated because you cannot leave the patient alone, you can get someone to take over for a few hours or a few days while you get rest or run errands.

The service is called Respite Care and depending on your income you can get this care for free or low cost through a number of different agencies:

★ *Your local public health services* : Contact your county office of health listed in your telephone book or your state Department of Health listed in the Appendix.

Free Video Describes What Medicare Covers For In-Home Health Care

Get a free VHS copy of *Home Health Care* from your local Medicare office or from 800-318-2596 or order on-line at {www.medicare.gov}.

★ *Your local office on aging*: Contact your local Area Agency on Aging or your state Department on Aging listed in the Appendix. If that fails, contact the Eldercare Locator hotline at 1-800-677-1116.

★ *Easter Seals office* or Easter Seals, 230 West Monroe Street, Suite 1800, Chicago, IL 60606; 800-221-6825; 312-726-6200; Fax: 312-726-1494; {www.seals.com}. This organization charges on ability to pay, but no person is refused service.

★ *Respite Locator Service*: National Resource Center or Respite & Crisis Care, 800 Eastowne Drive, Suite 105, Chapel Hill, NC 27514; 800-7 RELIEF; {www.chtop.com/locator.htm}.

INFERTILITY HELP LINE

Resolve is a non-profit organization that provides information, support and advocacy on the issues surrounding infertility. Their help line will help non-members with physician referrals, insurance questions, local support groups, and some free publications.

HELPLine hours are: Monday thru Friday 9:00 a.m to noon, and 1:00 p.m. to 4:00 p.m. Eastern Standard Time and Tuesday evenings 4:00 p.m. to 9:00 p.m.. Contact Resolve, Inc., 1310 Broadway, Somerville, MA 92144; 617-623-1156; Fax: 617-632-0252; HELPLine: 617-623-0744; {www.resolve.org}.

Choosing An Option

Deciding to have a child or children is an important step in anyone's life. Choosing a method of birth control is another big decision.

The Food and Drug Administration has several free publications dealing with specific types of birth control methods, along with a general overview of the different types of contraceptive methods. A good general overview publication is titled, *Protecting Against Unintended Pregnancy: A Guide to Contraceptive Choices.*

For your copies, contact Office of Communications, Food and Drug Administration, 5600 Fishers Lane, HFI-40, Rockville, MD 20857; 888-463-6332 (toll-free); {www.fda.gov}.

Join a Parkinson's Support Group - Or Start One!

The National Parkinson Foundation (NPF) has over 900 active support groups throughout the United States and Canada. If you are interested in starting a group or just want to find out about events in your area, contact: National Parkinson Foundation, Inc., 1501 NW 9th Ave., Miami, FL 33136; 305-547-6666; Fax 305-243-4403; 800-327-4545; 800-433-7022 (in FL); {E-mail: mailbox@npf.med.miami.edu}.

Hot Flash Hotline

Menopause doesn't have to be the hormonal hurricane women faced in the past. Taking estrogen and progesterone can help relieve the problems of menopause, although they may not be without problems of their own.

A free booklet entitled *Menopause* can answer many of your questions and outlines different forms of treatment. Contact: Information Center, National Institute on Aging, P.O. Box 8057, Gaithersburg, MD 20898; 800-222-2225; {www.nih.gov/nia}.

BLADDER PROBLEMS

Wetting the bed affects many young people, although it usually disappears over time. No matter when it happens or how often it happens, incontinence causes great distress. That's why it is important to understand that occasional incontinence is a normal part of growing up and that treatment is available for most children who have difficulty controlling their bladders.

Urinary Incontinence in Children is a free publication that looks at the causes of daytime and nighttime incontinence and describes treatments available and additional resources. For your copy, contact National Kidney and Urologic Diseases Information Clearinghouse, 3 Information Way, Bethesda, MD 20892; 301-654-4415; {www.niddk.nih.gov}.

DYSLEXIA

Has the school talked with you about some problems your child is having? Do they suspect a learning disability? *Facts About Dyslexia* is a free publication that describes what dyslexia is, how it is diagnosed, and what you can do to help your child.

For your free copy, contact National Institute for Child Health and Human Development, 31 Center Dr., Room 2A32, MSC 2425, Bethesda, MD 20892; 301-496-5133; {www.nih.gov/nichd}.

Plain Talk About Stress
Plain Talk About Adolescence
Plain Talk About Dealing with the Angry Child

For the above free publications, contact: Public Inquiries, National Institute of Mental Health, Room 7C-02, 5600 Fishers Lane, Rockville, MD 20857; 301-443-4513; {www.nimh.nih.gov}.

EAR INFECTIONS

There is not too much you can do at two in the morning when your child is crying because of an ear infection. You try to make the child as comfortable as possible and wait for the doctor's office to open.

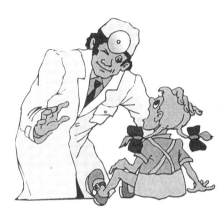

Ear infections are a common problem for children, but one they usually outgrow by the time they are six. The National Institute on Deafness and Other Communication Disorders has an *Ear Infection Packet* they can send to parents, explaining how these infections occur and current treatment options.

Average Home Has 3-10 Gallons of Hazardous Materials

And 92% of human poisonings reported to U.S. poison control centers took place in the home

Source: Children's Health Environmental Coalition Network, Malibu, CA {www.checnet.org/chec/index.html}.

For more information, contact National Institute on Deafness and Other Communication Disorders Clearinghouse, P.O. Box 37777, Washington, DC 20013; 800-241-1044; {www.nih.gov/nidcd/}.

ᕱᗗᗗᗗᗔᑎ ᗞᗗᑭᐸᐸᗞ

It seems as though there has been an increase in the diagnosis of Attention Deficit Disorder. Are we becoming more aware of this disorder or are we over-diagnosing it?

The National Institute of Mental Health funds research on a variety of learning disabilities and has published several helpful brochures and information packets on attention deficit disorder and learning disabilities in general.

Attention Deficit Hyperactivity Disorder describes symptoms, co-existing conditions, and possible causes, as well as treatment and education options. *Learning Disabilities* describes treatment options, strategies for coping, and sources of information and support.

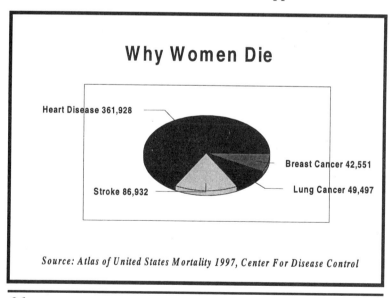

Why Women Die

Heart Disease 361,928

Breast Cancer 42,551

Stroke 86,932

Lung Cancer 49,497

Source: Atlas of United States Mortality 1997, Center For Disease Control

For more information, contact National Institute of Mental Health, 5600 Fishers Lane, Room 7C-02, Bethesda, MD 20892; 301-443-4513; {www.nimh.nih.gov}.

Service Organizations

Need help with child care, elderly services, substance abuse treatment? What about youth programs or disaster assistance? Many large service organizations have local offices that provide all this and more. Services vary depending upon the needs of the community, but before you fight your battles alone, contact these main offices to find out about local programs:

+ *Catholic Charities USA*, 1731 King St., #200, Alexandria, VA 23314; 703-549-1390; {www.catholiccharitiesusa.org}.
+ *Salvation Army*, 615 Slaters Lane, P.O. Box 2696, Alexandria, VA 22313; 703-684-5500; 800-SAL-

---

E-Mail A Friend Healthy Heart Greetings!

Create very special e-cards for those you love. Choose from lots of great images, heartwarming sayings and heart-healthy hints provided by the American Heart Association. And you can add your own personal message. You can send your free Heart to Heart e-card immediately, or schedule it to be sent any time during the ensuing twelve months. To create and send a free e-card, surf to: {www.americanheart.org/ecard/index.html}.

ARMY; {www.salvationarmyusa.org}.
+ *United Way of America*, 701 N. Fairfax St.,
  Alexandria, VA 22314; 800-411-UWAY;
  {www.unitedway.org}.

Hospice Care

Sometimes, there is nothing to be done for a terminally ill
patient other than to keep him or her comfortable. Hospice
can help your loved one live their remaining days fully and
comfortably.

To find a hospice provider near you, contact your doctor or
local hospital for a referral. The National Hospice
Organization is a non-profit organization dedicated to
hospice care and can connect you to over 2,400 hospices

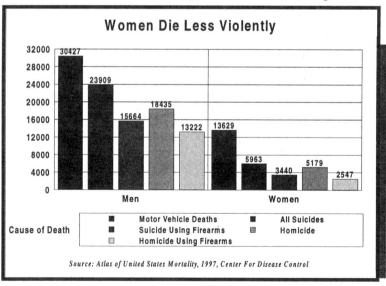

Women Die Less Violently

Cause of Death
- Motor Vehicle Deaths
- Suicide Using Firearms
- Homicide Using Firearms
- All Suicides
- Homicide

Source: Atlas of United States Mortality, 1997, Center For Disease Control

across the United States. You may contact the National Hospice Organization, 1901 North Moore St., Suite 901, Arlington, VA 22209; 703-243-5900; {www.nho.org}.

Get Money While You're Waiting For Government Money

General Public Assistance or just Public Assistance (it is known by many different names) is a welfare program offered in 42 states. This is a program of last resort for people either waiting to qualify for other government programs such as disability benefits, or who do not quality for any programs, yet need money to live.

The program eligibility and benefit levels vary within and across state lines. In some states, this benefit is only available in certain areas. There are strict income and asset levels that you must meet to qualify.

Do You Smoke?

You Can Quit Smoking Consumer Guide is a free publication that tells you how you can improve your chances of quitting and overcoming your addiction to nicotine. Contact: Agency for Health Care Policy and Research, P.O. Box 8547, Silver Spring, MD 20907; 800-358-9295; {www.ahcpr. gov}.

In Kansas, General Assistance pays families $278 per month while they are waiting for other government money. In California, the benefit is $225. Contact your local welfare office, your state Department of Social Service, or your state Temporary Assistance to Needy Families office listed in the Appendix to see what your state offers and the eligibility requirements.

On-Line Database of 650,000 Doctors

The American Medical Association's (AMA) Physician Select provides on-line information on virtually every licensed physician in the United States and its possessions, including more than 650,000 doctors of medicine (MD) and doctors of osteopathy or osteopathic medicine (DO). All physician credential data have been verified for accuracy and authenticated by accrediting agencies, medical schools, residency training programs, licensing

Report Bad Burgers

Or any other food, for that matter, that makes you, or someone you know, sick. Your local public health officials will take immediate action. They'll get you treated and make sure the problem does not spread. Contact your county office of public health listed in your telephone book, or your state Department of Health listed in the Appendix.

and certifying boards, and other data sources. You can search this database by name or medical specialty. You will also find health information on specific conditions from AMA Health Insight, a reference library.

Contact: American Medical Association, 515 North State Street, Chicago, IL 60610; 312-464-5000; {www.ama-assn.org/aps/amahg.htm} (Physician Select).

If Princess Diana Could Do It, You Can Do It. Get Control of Your Eating Disorder!

Do you suffer from anorexia nervosa, bulimia or binge eating disorder? Turn to the American Anorexia Bulimia Association (AABA) for help to get your lifeback on track!

AABA is a national, nonprofit organization of concerned members of the public and healthcare industry dedicated to the prevention and treatment of eating disorders. AABA's mission is carried out through many different free services, including help-lines, referral networks, public information, school outreach, support groups and prevention programs. AABA promotes social attitudes that enhance healthy body image and works to overcome the idealization of thinness that contributes to disordered eating.

Contact: AABA, 165 W. 46 Street #1108, New York, NY 10036; 212-575-6200; {E-mail: amanbu@aol.com}; {www.aabainc.org}.

Find Out, FOR FREE,
If You Have Diabetes

Sixteen million Americans have diabetes — one in three does not know it! Research proves that early detection and proper treatment for diabetes can lead to a longer, healthier life.

If you or the people you care about are at high risk for diabetes, you can call the American Diabetes Association's (ADA) "Diabetes Information and Action Line" (D.I.A.L.) where you can receive a free packet of information about

---

Find A Pediatrician!

If you need the services of a qualified pediatrician or pediatric subspecialist, contact the Pediatrician Referral Service of the American Academy of Pediatrics in writing, indicating the desired geographic area. Send a letter with a self-addressed, stamped envelope. At the time of publication, an online version of the referral service was still under construction, but it should be available now.

Contact: American Academy of Pediatrics, Attn: Pediatrician Referral Service, 141 Northwest Point Boulevard, Elk Grove Village, IL 60007-1098; {www.aap.org}.

---

diabetes and find out about free diabetes screenings and other diabetes alert activities in your area. D.I.A.L. is a national network of information and referral telephone lines for people with diabetes and their loved ones. This helpline can provide information on all aspects of diabetes management and refer callers to local diabetes programs and services, including diabetes education classes, year-round youth programs, counseling and support groups, and advocacy services.

Diabetes is more common in African Americans, Hispanics, Native Americans, Asian-Americans and Pacific Islanders. If you are a member of one of these ethnic groups, you need to pay special attention. Contact: American Diabetes Association, 1660 Duke Street, Alexandria, VA 22314; 800-DIABETES; 800-342-2383; {www.ada.org}.

New Benefits For Diabetes Patients

New Medicare benefits will make monitoring your blood glucose more affordable. The American Diabetes Association (ADA) with support from the makers of Accu-Chek has launched a web site to promote use of these new benefits. Patient and health care provider guides on the website explain how you can take advantage of these benefits. You also have the option of e-mailing your friends to help spread the word.

Contact: American Diabetes Association, 1660 Duke Street, Alexandria, VA 22314; 800-DIABETES; 800-342-2383; {www.ada.org}.

SURF & TURF FOR $3.00:
AQUATIC EXERCISE PROGRAM FOR PARKINSON'S PATIENTS

The National Parkinson's Foundation (NPF)/YMCA 's "Surf & Turf"Aquatic Exercise Programs provide:

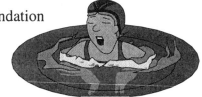

➥ An invigorating 90-minute program of chair and water exercise.
➥ Conducted by trained YMCA instructors.
➥ Muscle groups used for walking, activities of daily living, and speech are stimulated.
➥ A minimal fee of $3.00 per class will get and keep you moving.
➥ Program format may vary.

This program does not replace exercise prescribed by your doctor or therapist. Contact: National Parkinson Foundation, Inc., P.O. Box 010391, Miami, FL 33010-0391; 305-547-6666; Fax: 305-243-4403; 800-327-4545; 800-433-7022 (in FL); {E-mail: mailbox@npf.med. miami.edu}; {www.parkinson.org/services.htm}.

FAST CASH & FREE DRUGS FOR KIDNEY PATIENTS

The American Kidney Fund's (AKF) Individual Patient Grants pay for urgently needed transportation to treatment, over-the-counter medications, health insurance premiums and living kidney donor expenses. The AKF Pharmacy Program provides vital prescription medicines, nutritional supplements and medical equipment to qualified kidney patients.

> **Women Make 3/4ths of the Health Care Decisions In America and Spend 2 Out of Every 3 Health Care Dollars**
>
> *Source: Society for the Advancement of Women's Health Research; {www.womens-health.org}*

AKF establishes Patient Emergency Funds in dialysis and kidney transplant facilities. These funds enable facility staff to give immediate small cash grants to patients in emergency situations. AKF's Disaster Relief Program helps kidney patients get back on their feet when environmental crises strike their communities. AKF has helped victims of floods, hurricanes and earthquakes.

Contact: The American Kidney Fund, 6110 Executive Boulevard, Suite 1010, Rockville, MD 20852; 800-638-8299; 301-881-3052; Fax: 301-881-0898; {E-mail: helpline@akfinc.org}; {www.akfinc.org}.

Free Kidney Publications

The American Kidney Fund (AKF) has been educating the public about the prevention, causes, treatment, and psychosocial aspects of kidney disease for 25 years. The Fund will provide one copy of each title below free of charge. Additional copies may be obtained at a small charge. Titles include:

- *American Kidney Fund Helps* (English and Spanish)
- *Facts About Kidney Diseases and Their Treatment*
- *Kidney Disease: A Guide for Patients and Their Families*
- *Kidney Disease: A Guide for Patients...*(Spanish)
- *The Dialysis Patient: An Informative Guide for the Dentist*
- *Children and Kidney Disease*
- *Kidneys for Kids*
- *The Kid*
- *Understanding Nephrotic Syndrome*
- *Diabetes and the Kidneys*
- *Diabetes and the Kidneys* (Large Print)
- *Facts About Kidney Stones*
- *High Blood Pressure and Its Effects on the Kidneys*
- *Diet Guide for the CAPD Patient*
- *Diet Guide for the CAPD Patient* (Spanish)

- *Diet Guide for the Hemodialysis Patient*
- *Diet Guide for the Hemodialysis Patient* (Spanish)
- Bumper Stickers — Kidney Donors Save Lives
- *Give a Kidney — A Guide for Organ Donation*
- *Give a Kidney — A Guide for Organ Donation* (Spanish)
- *Kidney Disease Strikes African Americans*
- *Organ Donor Cards*

Contact: The American Kidney Fund, Attn: Publications Dept., 6110 Executive Boulevard, Suite 1010, Rockville, MD 20852; 800-638-8299; 301-881-3052; Fax: 301-881-0898; {E-mail: helpline@akfinc.org}; {www.akfinc.org}.

Life Line To Kidney Disease Treatment and Organ Donation

The American Kidney Fund (AKF) maintains a national, toll-free help line to answer questions from kidney patients, their families, and the general public. The help line provides information about kidney disease, its prevention and treatment, and organ donation. Referrals are made to other agencies as needed. The AKF help line provides general information only and cannot give medical advice.

Contact: American Kidney Fund, 6110 Executive Boulevard, Suite 1010, Rockville, MD 20852; 800-638-8299; 301-881-3052; {www.akfinc.org}.

Free Exercise Video, Publications and Professional Consultation for Renal Rehabilitation

The Life Options Rehabilitation Resource Center (RRC)

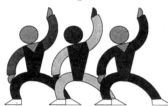

provides both professional and patient educational materials on renal rehabilitation, free of charge, courtesy of Amgen Inc. RRC staff can help answer your questions about which materials and resources will match your needs. Available materials include:

❏ *Renal Rehabilitation: Bridging the Barriers* (full report)
❏ *Renal Rehabilitation: Bridging the Barriers* (summary)
❏ *Bridging the Barriers: For Patients and Their Families*
❏ *Exercise: A Guide for People on Dialysis*
❏ *Feeling Better With Exercise: A Video Guide for People on Dialysis*
❏ *Employment: A Guide to Work, Insurance, and Finance for People on Dialysis*
❏ *New Life, New Hope: A Book for Families & Friends of Renal Patients* (limited copies available)
❏ Free Subscription to the *Renal Rehabilitation Report*

Contact: Rehabilitation Resource Center, Medical Media Associates, Inc., 603 Science Drive, Madison, WI 53711-

1074; 800-468-7777; Fax: 608-238-5046; {E-mail:
lifeoptions@medmed.com}; {www.lifeoptions.org/
contact.html}.

Free Clearinghouse For Kids Needing Critical Care

KidsPeace's National Referral Network is a free
referral service that helps callers locate behavioral health
treatment services for children, adolescents and families
right in their own community. Network specialists work
closely with callers to identify the most appropriate
resources from a database of 20,000 individual and group
practitioners.

Free Medical and Dental Services To Families in Southern California

Children's Network International (CNI) provides
free clinics to low-income children and their
families in Southern California and Central
America and wherever CNI is invited. CNI
recruits doctors, dentists and nurses for the clinics.
It also provides the medical and dental supplies
for the clinics. Contact: Children's Network
International, P.O. Box 1858, Los Angeles, CA
90078-1858; 323-980-9870; Fax: 323-980-9878;
{E-mail: info@cni2aid. org}; {www.geocities.com/
~cni2aid/}.

To contact KidsPeace Admissions and General Information, please call toll free at 800-8KID-123; {E-mail: admissions@kidspeace.org}; {www.kidspeace.org}. For emergency help, call the KidsPeace HelpLine at 800-334-4KID; {E-mail: helpline@kidspeace.org}; or 800-KID-SAVE; {E-mail: kidsave@kidspeace.org}.

Different Psychiatric Services

The *KidsPeace Child and Family Guidance Center* provides outpatient psychiatric services to low-income children, adolescents and families referred through the Lehigh County, Pennsylvania, Base Service Unit. Clients from the age of 2 through adult are accepted for a wide range of emotional, social, behavioral and learning-associated problems.

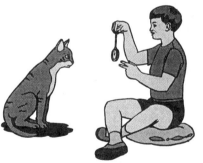

Childhood anxieties/ phobias, parent/child conflicts, adolescent depression, attention deficit disorders, separation/divorce issues, physical abuse/neglect, marital/couples conflict, parenting issues and special needs of foster care and adoptive children are examples of matters addressed by the outpatient program. Contact KidsPeace 800-8KID-123; {E-mail: admissions@kidspeace.org}; {www.kidspeace.org}.

Helping Kids Cope With Illness and Death

The Hospice of Lancaster County offers the following bereavement programs to children:

✳ *"Coping Kids"* is a non-clinical support group exclusively for kids dealing with the illness or death of a loved one.

✳ *"Camp Chimaqua"* is a three-day children's bereavement camp organized for children ages 6 and up who are grieving the loss of a loved one.

✳ The hospice's *SoulMates* pairs a teen affected by illness or loss with a teen of the same age. SoulMates partners basically "hang out" just like other teens: they talk on the phone, go to the movies or head for the mall. The aim of SoulMates is to provide reliable, unbiased friendship, compassion and support on a peer level to an adolescent in need.

✳ *"Good Grief Club"* materials provide elementary as well as middle to high school students with a background on grief and loss and an opportunity for personal reflection.

Contact: Hospice of Lancaster County, 685 Good Drive, P.O. Box 4125, Lancaster, PA 17604; 717-391-2412.

One-On-One Help For
Stroke Victims and Families

If you or someone you know has experienced stroke firsthand, call the American Heart Association's (AHA) Stroke Connection at 800-553-6321 or send an e-mail to {strokeconnection@heart.org}.

This is a network of over 1,600 stroke groups or clubs and more than 50,000 stroke survivors, caregivers and professionals throughout the country. You can receive

Free Risk Assessment for Women's Heart Disease

Heart disease and stroke kill more women than all forms of cancer, AIDS and accidents combined. The "Each One, Reach One" program at the American Heart Association offers free information and free risk assessment which can be used to help start modifying your lifestyle to reduce your risk of heart disease and stroke. They also tell you how to get a friend involved in the program.

Contact: Women's Health Information, American Heart Association, National Center, 7272 Greenville Avenue, Dallas, TX 75231; 888-MY-HEART; {http://women. americanheart.org/}.

information regarding stroke, how it affects the lives of stroke survivors and their families, how to find a support group near you, how to subscribe to the *Stroke Connection Magazine*, or to talk to someone who understands. The phone line is manned by stroke families who want to help. They are there for you to answer your questions and offer options.

Contact: Stroke Connection, American Heart Association, National Center, 7272 Greenville Avenue, Dallas, TX 75231; 800-553-6321; {E-mail: strokeconnection@ heart.org}; {www.americanheart.org}.

Video For Soccer Moms Who Fear Injuries

"Safety Guidelines For Youth Soccer" is a video produced by the American College of Sport Medicine's (ACSM) and the United States Youth Soccer Association (USYSA). It's designed for parents and coaches of young soccer players between 10 and 16. It covers pre-screening for competition, proper training, injury prevention, nutrition, first aid treatment, and rehabilitation.

The video, made possible by a grant from Snickers brand, is available for $4.00 from USYSA, 899 Presidential Drive,

Suite 117, Richardson, TX 75081; 800-4-SOCCER (476-2237); {http://usysa.org}.

ACSM also offers a public education brochure titled, *Nutrition, Training and Injury Prevention Guidelines: A Guide for Soccer Players.* A single copy of this information packed brochure is available free of charge by sending a self-addressed, stamped, business-size envelope to: ACSM, Attention: Soccer, P.O. Box 1440, Indianapolis, IN 46206-1440; {www.acsm.org}.

Heart Disease — The Leading Cause of Death In Women

This year alone, heart disease will kill over 500,000 women, and 39% of women who have heart attacks will die within a year. Nutrition intervention is effective in preventing and treating heart disease in women.

The major risk factors for this disease in women include elevated blood lipids and lipoproteins, excess body weight, hypertension, and cigarette smoking. Good nutrition can prevent and alleviate the most common risk factors associated with heart disease in women — high cholesterol, excess body weight and hypertension. Get the facts about coronary heart disease and nutrition!

To find out what is known and what is not known about the connection between nutrition and coronary heart disease, and to find out whether or not nutrition (low-fat/low saturated fat diet, vitamin E, and fish consumption) interventions affect coronary heart disease risk in women, read the fact sheet provided by the American Dietetic Association's (ADA) at its website.

Contact: American Dietetic Association, 216 West Jackson Boulevard, Chicago, IL 60606-6995; 312-899-0040; {www.eatright.org/womenshealth/osteoporosis.html}.

OVER $1 MILLION IN GRANTS/ LOANS FOR ABORTIONS

The National Network of Abortion Funds (NNAF), is a growing association of 57 grassroots abortion funds across the United States. NNAF provides direct financial aid in the form of loans and grants to low-income women/girls seeking to terminate an unwanted pregnancy. Also, some funds provide assistance for a variety of associated needs including: pregnancy testing, ultrasound, childcare, transportation and lodging.

To find your local organization, call the National Abortion Federation hotline at 800-772-9100. The National Network of Abortion Funds c/o CLPP, Hampshire College, Amherst, MA 01002-5001; 413-582-5645; Fax: 413-582-5620; {http://hamp. hampshire.edu/~clpp/nnaf}.

Free Medical Services and Legal Clinic For D.C. Residents

Bread for the City helps elderly disabled, parents with children and the homeless in Washington, DC. It also provides primary medical service, legal clinic, Jane Adams social work program (help people apply for food stamps, Medicaid, SSI), food program and clothing programs.

Free Burials For Jews

The Hebrew Free Burial Society Cemetery provides free services for financially needy Jews in hospitals, nursing homes, prisons and hospices. Contact: Hebrew Free Burial Society-Chesed Shel Emes,c/o Jewish Chaplaincy Service, 6101 Montrose Road, Rockville, MD 20852; 301-230-7294; 301-230-7260; TTY: 301-230-7272; {www.jirs.org/jirs/8f0lys4f.htm}.

Free medical care is provided to the uninsured and those who are not eligible for public benefits. Clinics include adult general medicine, pediatrics, OB/GYN care, and the city's only free job physicals.

Contact: Bread for the City, 1525 7th Street, NW, Washington, DC 20001; 202-265-2400; Fax: 202-745-1081; St. Thomas More Catholic Church, 4275 4th Street SE, Washington, DC 20032; 202-561-8587; {E-mail: breadz@mindspring.com}; {www.breadz.org}.

LEGAL RESOURCE KITS TO HELP WOMEN IN CRISIS

The National Organization for Women's Legal Defense Fund (LDEF) offers the following legal resource kits. Each kit contains a subject publications list, bibliographies, fact sheets, resource lists, statistical information and articles or pieces relevant to the topic. Topics include:

▲ A Guide to Court Watching in Domestic Violence and Sexual Assault Cases;

▲ Divorce and Separation;

▲ Domestic Violence and Child Custody;

▲ Employment Sexual Harassment & Discrimination (Spanish);

▲ Incest and Child Sexual Abuse;

▲ Pregnancy & Parental Leave; Sexual Harassment in Housing;

▲ Sexual Harassment in the Schools; Sexual Harassment in the Schools: A Blueprint for Action (Spanish);

▲ Stalking; Violence Against Women;

▲ How to Find a Lawyer (free).

To get a copy of the month's free legal resource kit, please print it directly from the web site. The kit is designed so that you can print it section by section. If you would like to order a hard copy of the kit, please send a letter requesting the kit you would like to receive along with a check or money order for $5.00 to cover the cost of reproduction and postage (made out to NOW LDEF) and your name and shipping address to: NOW LDEF, Attn: Publications Department, 395 Hudson Street, 5th Floor, New York, NY 10014; 212-925-6635; {www.nowldef.org/html/pub/kits.htm}.

SPECIAL DOGS FOR SPECIAL KIDS

Loving Paws Assistance Dogs is a non-profit organization which trains dogs to assist children under the age of 18 from around the United States who are physically disabled. These dogs can open and close doors, retrieve dropped items or things out of reach, turn lights on and off, push elevator buttons, pull wheelchairs, go get help, bark on command, pick up dropped coins.

To apply for a dog, an applicant need only write or e-mail Loving Paws for an application. The completed application will be evaluated and if appropriate, an interview will be scheduled. Trained assistance dogs are valued at over $12,000 each. The applicant pays only a small application fee. Loving Paws provides the dog free of charge, but at the time of writing there is a waiting list. When a dog is ready, the student attends a two- to three-week training class with one parent.

Contact: Loving Paws Assistance Dogs, P.O. Box 12005, Santa Rosa, CA 95406; 707-586-0798; Fax: 707-586-0799; {E-mail: lvgpaws@lovingpaws.com}; {www.lovingpaws. com}.

Free Medical Equipment Loaned To MS Patients

The Western Washington Chapter of the National Multiple Sclerosis Society provides medical equipment, such as wheelchairs and walkers, on loan to persons with MS who do not have insurance, or whose insurance will not cover needed equipment. They will help persons with MS purchase equipment. If you don't live in this area, contact the office below or your local Multiple Sclerosis Society to see if similar services are available near you.

Contact: Western Washington Chapter of the National Multiple Sclerosis Society, Central Washington Office, P.O. Box 1093, Yakima, WA 98907; 509-248-2350; 800-736-7312; Fax: 509-248-2352; {www.nmsswas.org/general/independence. html}.

Free Fitness Classes for People with MS

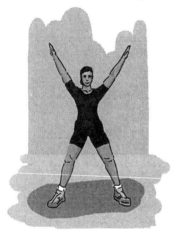

The Western Washington Chapter of the National Multiple Sclerosis Society offers financial assistance for specific populations of people (seniors, arthritis, etc.) with MS for fitness programs. Instructors must have special training in fitness programs for individuals who require low impact exercise, or have special needs.

Eligibility: individuals with MS with financial needs in the following counties in Washington state: King, Snohomish, Skagit, Whatcom, Clallam, Jefferson, Kitsap, San Juan, Island, Pierce, Thurston, Lewis, Skamania, Cowlitz, Wahkiakum, Pacific, Grays Harbor, and Mason counties. If you don't live in this area, contact the office below or your local Multiple Sclerosis Society to see if similar services are available near you.

Contact: Western Washington Chapter of the National Multiple Sclerosis Society, 192 Nickerson St. #100, Seattle, WA 98109; 206 284-4236; Fax: 206-284-4972; 800-800-7047; {E-mail: nmsswascw2@nwinfo.net}; {www.nmsswas.org/general/health.html}.

Financial Assistance To Pay For Counseling For People With MS

The Western Washington Chapter of the National Multiple Sclerosis Society offers financial assistance for counseling to people with Multiple Sclerosis and their families. This program is designed to assist individuals with MS and their families to cope with the disease by seeing a professional therapist for counseling. Financial assistance for counseling is limited to $300 per year for in-office counseling and $340 for in-home counseling.

Contact the Yakima office at: P.O. Box 1093, Yakima, WA 98907; 509-248-2350; 800-736-7312; Fax: 509-248-2352; {E-mail: nmsswascw2@nwinfo.net}; {www.nmsswas.org/living/counseling.html}.

FREE MONEY AND HELP FOR LUPUS PATIENTS

The S.L.E. (LUPUS) Foundation (a Chapter of the Lupus Foundation of America) offers individual entitlement counseling showing families how to obtain Medicaid, Medicare, social security income/social security disability, food stamps, housing assistance and legal aid. They also have a Grant-in-Aid Program that provides mini-grants to help people with Lupus survive emergency and crisis situations.

Contact: The S.L.E. Foundation Inc., 149 Madison Avenue, Suite 205, New York, NY 10016; 212-685-4118; Fax: 212-545-1843; {E-mail: Lupus@LupusNY.org}; {www.lupusny.org/programs.htm}.

Special Help For People in Hospitals, Nursing Homes or Jails

The League of Mercy (LOM) is a visitation program that connects volunteers and Salvation Army officers and soldiers to those with special needs in hospitals, nursing homes, and correctional facilities. They provide friendship, spiritual support, and comfort items, such as shampoo, stationery, postage stamps, combs, and lap robes. They also support special communities like in Aurora, Illinois where

A Private Army To Help With Your Disasters

The Salvation Army is an integral member of the community of disaster service organizations and is part of the Federal Relief Act of 1970 (PL 91-606) and the Disaster Relief Act of 1974 (PL93-288). For information on how it may be able to help you in disaster, contact: The Salvation Army National Headquarters Commissioner Robert A. Watson, National Commander, 615 Slaters Lane, P.O. Box 269, Alexandria, VA 22313; 703-684-5500; Fax: 703-684-3478; {www.salvationarmyusa.org}; {www.salvationarmyusa.org/disfol/disast2.htm}.

the 30-year-old Christmas gift distribution program benefits some 2,000 troubled teens in residential care. The teens receive candy and cards for both giving to others and for themselves—a gesture that equips them to reach out in a significant way as typical participants during holiday events.

Contact: The Salvation Army National Headquarters Commissioner Robert A. Watson, National Commander 615 Slaters Lane, P.O. Box 269, Alexandria, VA 22313; 703-684-5500; Fax: 703-684-3478; {www.salvationarmyusa.org}.

Christmas Dinners, Clothing, Toys, Financial Assistance To Families In Need

Each year, The Salvation Army provides Christmas dinners, clothing, and toys to families in need. Financial assistance helps families with basic necessities and seasonal aid. Families of prisoners are often included in these acts of charities. Additionally, volunteers distribute gifts to shut-ins in hospitals and nursing homes during Christmas. Many families receive additional aid over a period of months after the Christmas season. These people are usually struggling with family, emotional, or employment problems.

Contact: The Salvation Army National Headquarters Commissioner, Robert A. Watson, National Commander, 615 Slaters Lane, P.O. Box 269, Alexandria, VA 22313; 703-684-5500; Fax: 703-684-3478; {www.salvationarmyusa.org}.

Help For First-Time Offenders

For more than 20 years, the Florida Division of The Salvation Army has been involved in a program of service for first-time misdemeanants. In many counties throughout the state, The Salvation Army is responsible to the county judge for the supervision of these individuals' probation.

As part of the program, The Salvation Army provides counseling, supervision of any fines or restitution required by the court, and supervision of community service hours. In one year alone, more than 50,000 individuals on probation were supervised and assisted by The Salvation Army.

To find out about local programs like this one contact: The Salvation Army National Headquarters Commissioner Robert A. Watson, National Commander 615 Slaters Lane, P.O. Box 269, Alexandria, VA 22313; 703-684-5500; Fax: 703-684-3478; {www.salvationarmyusa.org}.

AFFORDABLE MENTAL HEALTH COUNSELING

The Community Institute for Psychotherapy is a non-profit agency whose mission is to provide mental health counseling services to low-income individuals in Marin County, CA so that they may re-establish mental and emotional well-being and live satisfying and productive lives. CIP offers outpatient psychotherapy on a sliding scale fee basis to adults, children, families, and couples who would otherwise be unable to afford such services.

To find out if similar programs like this exist in your area, contact your local Social Services Agency or look in "Local Free Health Clinics" section of this book. Contact: Community Institute for Psychotherapy, 1330 Lincoln Avenue, Suite 201, San Rafael, CA 94901; 415-459-5999; Fax: 415-459-5602; {E-mail: cip@wenet.net}.

Bus Passes, In-Home Counseling, Help With Pets, Etc. For People With HIV

The Monterey County AIDS Project (MCAP) provides the following practical support services to people infected with HIV and their family members and friends in Monterey County:

★ *Bus Passes* - *Up to 10 bus tickets per month*

★ *Ride Program Referrals* - Access volunteers and other community agencies.

★ *Home Visits* - All our counselors are happy to visit at home.

★ *Companions* - Special friends to provide support.

★ *Special Needs* - With volunteers, arrangements can be made for special projects, rides, and help with pets.

To find out if similar programs like this exist in your area, contact your local Social Services Agency or look in "Local Free Health Clinics" section of this book. Contact: The Monterey County AIDS Project, 12 E. Gabilan, Salinas, CA 93901; 831-772-8350; Fax: 831-424-9615; {E-mail: rhaase@mcap.org}; {www.mcap.org/practica.htm}.

Free Massage and Aromatherapy for HIV Patients

Reiki, deep massage, Swedish traditional full body massage, or aromatherapy is available for individuals infected with HIV from The Monterey County AIDS Project (MCAP). Massages are available on Tuesdays between 9:00 a.m.-5:00 p.m. Skilled volunteer practitioners have received their training from The Esalan Institute in Big Sur and The Monterey Institute of Touch. The Massage

Studio is located at: 780 Hamilton St. Seaside, CA 93955; 831-394-4747; {E-mail: LiteHands@aol.com}.

To find out if similar programs like this exist in your area, contact your local Social Services Agency or look in "Local Free Health Clinics" section in this book. Contact: The Monterey County AIDS Project, 12 E. Gabilan, Salinas, CA 93901; 831-772-8350; Fax: 831-424-9615; {E-mail: rhaase@mcap.org}; {www.mcap.org/massage.htm}.

FREE GROCERIES FOR HIV PATIENTS

The Monterey County AIDS Project (MCAP) offers its Food Pantry Clients one bag of groceries a week. The bags are meant to be supplemental, and are not intended to substitute for a proper diet and nutrition. Home deliveries are available to clients without transportation or resources.

To find out if similar programs like this exist in your area, contact your local Social Services Agency or look in "Local Free Health Clinics" section of this book. Contact: The Monterey County AIDS Project, 12 E. Gabilan, Salinas, CA 93901; 831-772-8350; Fax: 831-424-9615; {E-mail: rhaase@mcap.org}; {www.mcap.org/food.htm}.

Rehabilitation Centers for Those With Alcohol and Chemical Dependency

The Salvation Army maintains the largest resident substance abuse rehabilitation program in the United States. They provide housing, nourishing meals, medical care and engage in work therapy.

There are more than 125 Salvation Army Adult Rehabilitation centers throughout the U.S. In the follow-up period (six months after graduation from a center), results show:

➡ 57 percent drink less.

➡ 50 percent have good jobs (with almost double their previous earnings).

➡ 25 percent show total sobriety.

➡ Good social adjustment and steady employment.

Contact: The Salvation Army, 615 Slaters Lane, P.O. Box 269, Alexandria, VA 22313; 703-684-5500; Fax: 703-684-3478; {www.salvationarmyusa.org}.

NATIONAL INSTITUTE's of HEALTH TOLL-FREE INFORMATION LINES

AIDS Clinical Trials	800-TRIALSA
AIDS Treatment Information Service	800-HIV-0440
National Institute on Aging Information Center	800-222-2225
Alzheimer's Disease Education and Referral Center	800-438-4380
Cancer Information Service	800-4-CANCER
Patient Recruitment and Public Liaison Office	800-411-1222
National Institute of Child Health and Human Development	800-370-2943
National Diabetes Outreach Program	800-438-5383
National Institute on Deafness and Other Communication Disorders	800-241-1044
National Clearinghouse for Alcohol and Drug Information	800-729-6686
EnviroHealth: Information Service of the National Institute of Environmental Health Sciences	800-643-4794
National Heart, Lung, and Blood Institute Information Line	800-575-WELL
National Institute of Diabetes and Digestive and Kidney Diseases Bladder Control for Women Campaign	800-891-5388
National Institute of Mental Health Anxiety	888-8-ANXIETY

National Institute of Mental Health Depression	800-421-4211
National Institute of Mental Health Panic	800-64-PANIC
National Network of Libraries of Medicine	800-338-7657
National Institute of Neurological Disorders and Stroke Information	800-352-9424
National Center for Complementary and Alternative Medicine	888-NIH-6226
NIH Ovulation Research	888-644-8891
Osteoporosis and Related Bone Diseases	800-624-BONE
Weight-Control Information Network	800-WIN-8098

Discounts On Bicycle Helmets

The Department of Health in Mesa County Colorado offers discounts on bicycle helmets for children in the county. Check with your local office of health to see if there are any programs like this in your area.

If not, you can start one with a free *Toolkit for Organizers of Bicycle Helmet Programs* from Bicycle Helmet Safety Institute, 4611 Seventh Street South, Arlington, VA 22204; 703-486-0100; Fax: 703-486-0576; {www.helmets.org}. This organization will also send you a free copy of *A Consumer's Guide to Bicycle Helmets.*

Free Prescription Drugs

Make $40,000 and Get Free Prescription Drugs — Everything But Viagra

Valium, Prozac, Dilantin, Insulin, the smoking patch and almost anything but Viagra you can get FREE directly from the drug companies themselves.

That's right: drug companies don't want everybody to know this, but they will give their drugs free of charge to certain people who can't afford their medications. I guess they don't want to tarnish their greedy bad guys image by publishing these benevolent programs.

So, what's the catch? It sounds too easy. All that many of these companies require is that your doctor write them a note stating that you will have difficulty paying for the drugs you need. Some companies have income requirements, but the income levels go up to $40,000.

You can also be your own advocate and make the process work for yourself.

First: Check the list of drugs below and identify the manufacturer.

Second: From the listing of pharmaceutical firms that follows the drug listing, contact the company directly and request information about their program.

Third: More than likely, you will have to bring in forms to your doctor for a signature. If your doctor won't sign the form, consider getting another doctor.

Fourth: Once the forms are filled out, the company will send the drugs either directly to you, or to your doctor or to a local pharmacy for you to pick up.

Fifth: If you can't find your drug in the list, contact the following to obtain the latest edition of this information:

Pharmaceutical Manufacturers Association
1100 15th St., NW
Washington, DC 20005
800-PMA-INFO
www.pharma.org

Sixth: Be sure you also look on page 99 to see if your state provides help with prescription drugs.

Alphabetical Listing by Drug

This section identifies the name of medications frequently prescribed for older Americans and the manufacturers of the drugs that are covered under an indigent patient program listed in this directory. If a drug that you take is NOT listed here, it still may be provided under a medication assistance program; it is suggested that your physician call the company to determine if it is covered by an assistance program.

If the manufacturer of a particular drug is not listed in this directory, it is suggested that the patient or physician call the company directly to determine if the company has an indigent patient program. Drug Manufacturer telephone numbers can be found in the *Physician's Desk Reference.*

Drug/Manufacturer

A
A/T/S/Hoechst Marion
Abelcet/Liposome Company
Accolate/Zeneca
Accutane/Roche Laboratories
Aclovate/Glaxo Wellcome
Actigall/Novartis
Acupril/Parke Davis
Adalat/Bayer Corporation
Adriamycin/Pharmacia and
    Upjohn
Albuterol/Bristol-Myers
    Squibb
Aldactazide/Searle
Aldomet/Merck
Alkeran/Glaxo Wellcome
Allegra/Hoechst Marion

Almaryl/Hoechst Marion
Alphagan/Allergan
Altace/Hoechst Marion
Alu-Tab/3M
Alu-Cap/3M
Alupent/Boehringer Ingleheim
Amantadine/Bristol-Myers Squibb
Amicar/Immunex
Amin-Aid/R&D Laboratories
Aminohuppurate/Merck
Amoxil/Smithkline Beecham
Amoxicillin/Bristol-Myers Squibb
Ampicillin/Bristol-Myers Squibb
ANA/Bayer Corporation
Anafranil/Novartis
Anaprox/Roche Laboratories
Ancobon/Roche Laboratories

Antivenin/Merck
Antivert/Pfizer Inc
Anturane/Novartis
Apresazide/Novartis
Apresoline/Novartis
AquaMephyton/Merck
Aralen/Sanofi Winthrop
Aramine/Merck
Aredia/Novartis
Arimidex/Zeneca
Asacol/Procter and Gambel
Atarax/Pfizer Inc
Atenolol/Bristol-Myers Squibb
Atrovent/Boehringer Ingleheim
Attenuvax/Merck
AVC/Hoechst Marion
Azactam/Bristol-Myers Squibb
Azmacort/Rhone-Poulenc Inc

B

Bactrim/Roche Laboratories
Bactroban/Smithkline Beecham
Barotras/Rhone-Poulenc Inc
Beclovent/Glaxo Wellcome
Beconase/Glaxo Wellcome
Bentyl/Hoechst Marion
Benztropine/Bristol-Myers
  Squibb
Berocca/Roche Laboratories
Betagan/Allergan
Betapace/Berlex
Betaseron/Berlex
Biavax/Merck
BiCNU/Bristol-Myers Squibb
Biltricide/Bayer Corporation
Blenoxane/Bristol-Myers Squibb
Breonesin/Sanofi Winthrop
Brethaire/Novartis
Brethine/Novartis
Bricanyl/Hoechst Marion
Bronkometer/Sanofi Winthrop
Bumex/Roche Laboratories
BuSpar/Bristol-Myers Squibb

C

Calan/Searle
Calci-Chew/R&D Laboratories
Calci-Mix/R&D Laboratories
Calcimar/Rhone-Poulenc Inc
Calcium Disodium Versenate/3m
Calel-D/Rhone-Poulenc Inc
Cantil/Hoechst Marion
Capoten/Bristol-Myers Squibb
Capozide/Bristol-Myers Squibb
Captopril/Bristol-Myers
Carafate/Hoechst Marion
Cardene/Roche Laboratories
Cardizem/Hoechst Marion
Cardura/Pfizer Inc
Casodex/Zeneca
Cataflam/Novartis
Catapres/Boehringer Ingleheim
Caverjject/Pharmacia and Upjohn
Ceclor/Eli Lilly
CeeNU/Bristol-Myers Squibb
Cefaclor/Bristol-Myers Squibb
Cefadroxil/Bristol-Myers Squibb
Cefadyl/Bristol-Myers Squibb
Cefazolln/Bristol-Myers Squibb
Ceftin/Glaxo Wellcome
Cefzil/Bristol-Myers Squibb
CellCept/Roche Laboratories
Cephalexin/Bristol-Myers
Cephulac/Hoechst Marion
Chibroxin/Merck
Chlo-Amine/Bayer Corporation
Cholestyramino/Bristol-Myers
  Squibb
Chronulac/Hoechst Marion
Cimetidine/Bristol-Myers Squibb
Cipro I.V/Bayer Corporation
Claforan/Hoechst Marion
Cleocin/Pharmacia and Upjohn
Clinoril/Merck
Clomid/Hoechst Marion
Cloxacillin/Bristol-Myers Squibb
Clozaril/Novartisd

Cogentin/Merck
Cortosporin/Glaxo Wellcome
Cognex/Parke Davis
Colestid/Pharmacia and Upjohn
Collagenase Santyl/Knoll
Compazine/Smithkline Beecham
Cordarone/Wyeth-Ayherst
  Laboratories
Cort dome Suppositories/Bayer
  Corporation
Cortenama/Solvay
Cortone/Merck
Corvert/Pharmacia and Upjohn
Cosmegen/Merck
Coumadin/DuPont Merck
Cozaar/Merck
Creon/Solvay
Crixivan/Merck
Crystodigin Tablets/Eli Lilly
Cuprimine/Merck
Curretab/Solvay
Cutivate/Glaxo Wellcome
Cyyclobenzebprine/Bristol-Myers
  Squibb
Cyclospasmol/Wyeth-Ayherst
  Laboratories
Cyclospotrin/Novatis
Cytadren/Novartis
Cytotec/Searle
Cytoxan/Bristol-Myers Squibb
Cytovene/Roche Laboratories

D
d-Biotin/R&D Laboratories
Dalmane/Roche Laboratories
Danocrine/Sanofi Winthrop
Dantrium Capsules/Procter and
  Gambel
Daranide/Merck
Daraprim/Glaxo Wellcome
Darvocet/Eli Lilly
Darvon/Eli Lilly
DDAVP/Rhone-Poulenc Inc
Decadron/Merck

Demser/Merck
Depo-Provera/Pharmacia and
  Upjohn
Dermacort/Solvay
Dermatop/Hoechst Marion
Desferal/Novartis
Desyrel/Bristol-Myers Squibb
Dexedrine/Smithkline Beecham
Dexone/Solvay
Diabe Vite/R&D Laboratories
Diabinese/Pfizer Inc
Dialume/Rhone-Poulenc Inc
DiBeta/Hoechst Marion
Dibezyline/Smithkline Beecham
Dicioxacillin/Bristol-Myers
  Squibb
Didronel/Procter and Gambel
Diflucan/Pfizer Inc
Dilacor/Rhone-Poulenc Inc
Dilantin/Parke Davis
Dipentum/Pharmacia and Upjohn
Diprolen/Schering
  Laboratories/Key
Diprosone/Schering
  Laboratories/Key
Disalcid/3M
Ditropan/Hoechst Marion
Dlltiazem/Bristol-Myers Squibb
Dobutrex/Eli Lilly
Domepaste Bandages/Bayer
  Corporation
Doxyeyellne/Bristol-Myers
  Squibb
Drisdol/Sanofi Winthrop
DTIC Dome/Bayer Corporation
Duricef/Bristol-Myers Squibb
Duiril/Merck
Duphalac/Solvay
DURAGEXIC/Janssen
Duricef/Bristol-Myers Squibb
Dyazide/Smithkline Beecham
Dycill/Smithkline Beecham
Dynapen/Bristol-Myers Squibb

E

EC-Naprosyn/Roche Laboratories
Edecrin Sodium/Merck
Edecrin/Merck
Efudex/Roche Laboratories
Emete-con/Pfizer Inc
Emgel/Glaxo Wellcome
Epifrin/Allergan
Epivir/Glaxo Wellcome
Epogen/Amgen, Inc
Ergamisol/Janssen
Esdrix/Novartis
Esophotrast/Rhone-Poulenc Inc
Estrace/Bristol-Myers Squibb
Estraderm/Novartis
Estradiol/Bristol-Myers Squibb
Estratab/Solvay
Etopophos/Bristol-Myers Squibb

F

Famvir/Smithkline Beecham
Feldene/Pfizer Inc
Fertinex/Serono Laboratories Inc
Flexeril/Merck
Flonase/Glaxo Wellcome
Flovin I.V./McNeil
Floxin Tablets/McNeil
Fludara/Berlex
Fluorouracil/Roche Laboratories
Fosamax/Merck
Foscavir Injection/Astra
Fungizone/Bristol-Myers Squibb
Fulvicin/Schering
   Laboratories/Key

G

Gantanol/Roche Laboratories
Gemfibrozil/Bristol-Myers Squibb
Geocillin/Pfizer Inc
Glipizide/Bristol-Myers Squibb
Glucagon/Eli Lilly
Glucophage/Bristol-Myers Squibb
Glucotrol/Pfizer Inc
Grifulvin V/Ortho

H

Habitrol/Novartis
Halcion/Pharmacia and Upjohn
Haldol Decanoate/McNeil
Halotestin/Pharmacia and Upjohn
Heparin Sodium/Eli Lilly
Hiprex/Hoechst Marion
Hismanal/Janssen
Hivid/Roche Laboratories
HP Achta/Rhone-Poulenc Inc
Humalog/Eli Lilly
Humatrope/Eli Lilly
Humorsol/Merck
Humulin/Eli Lilly
Hycamtin/Smithkline Beecham
Hydrea/Bristol-Myers Squibb
Hydrocortone/Merck
Hydroxychlorquine/Bristol-Myers
   Squibb
Hygroton/Rhone-Poulenc Inc
Hytakerol/Sanofi Winthrop
Hyzaar/Merck

I

Idamycin/Pharmacia and Upjohn
Ifex/Bristol-Myers Squibb
Iletin/Eli Lilly
Imitrex/Glaxo Wellcome
Imodium/Janssen
Imogam/Pasteur Merieux
   Connaught
Imovax/Pasteur Merieux
   Connaught
Imuran/Glaxo Wellcome
Indapamide/Bristol-Myers Squibb
Indocin/Merck
Inversine/Merck
Invirase/Roche Laboratories
Ismelin/Novartis
Isoptin SR/Knoll
Isordil/Wyeth-Ayherst
   Laboratories
Isuprel/Sanofi Winthrop

K
K-Lyte/Bristol-Myers Squibb
Kadian/Zeneca
Kefurox/Eli Lilly
Kefzol/Eli Lilly
Kemadrin/Glaxo Wellcome
Kantrex/Bristol-Myers Squibb
Kenalog/Bristol-Myers Squibb
Klatrix/Bristol-Myers Squibb
Klonopin/Roche Laboratories
Kytril/Smithkline Beecham

L
L-Carnitine/R&D Laboratories
Lacrisert/Merck
Lamictal/Glaxo Wellcome
Lamprene/Novartis
Lanoxicaps/Glaxo Wellcome
Lanoxin/Glaxo Wellcome
Larodopa/Roche Laboratories
Lasix/Hoechst Marion
Leucovorin/Immunex
Leukeran/Glaxo Wellcome
Leukine/Immunex
Leustatin/Ortho Biotech Inc
Levo-Dromoran/Roche
  Laboratories
Levoprome/Immunex
Librax/Roche Laboratories
Limbritol/Roche Laboratories
Lioresal/Novartis
Lithobid/Solvay
Lithonate/Solvay
Lithotabs/Solvay
Lodosy/DuPont
Loestrin/Parke Davis
Lopressor/Novartis
Loprox/Hoechst Marion
Lorabid/Eli Lilly
Lotensin/Novartis
Lotensin HCT/Novartis
Lotrel/Novartis
Lotrimin/Schering
  Laboratories/Key

Lotrisone/Schering
  Laboratories/Key
Lovenox/Rhone-Poulenc Inc
Lozol/Rhone-Poulenc Inc
LPF/Immunex
Ludiomil/Novartis
Luvox/Solvay
Lysodren/Bristol-Myers Squibb

M
M-R-Vax/Merck
M-M-R/Merck
Macrobid/Procter and Gambel
Macrodantin/Procter and Gambel
Mag-Carb/R&D Laboratories
Mandol/Eli Lilly
Marax/Pfizer Inc
Marinol/Roxane
Matulane/Roche
Maxair/3M
Maxaquin/Searle
Maxlplme/Bristol-Myers Squibb
Medihaler/3M
Mefoxin/Merck
Megace/Bristol-Myers Squibb
Menest/Smithkline Beecham
Mephyton/Merck
Mepron/Glaxo Wellcome
Meruvax/Merck
Mesnex/Bristol-Myers Squibb
Methotrexate/Immunex Novatrone
Metipirone/Novartis
Metoclopramide/Bristol-Myers
  Squibb
Metoprolol Tartrate/Bristol-Myers
  Squibb
Metrodin/Serono Laboratories Inc
Mevacor/Merck
Mexitil/Boehringer Ingleheim
Mezlin/Bayer Corporation
Microbuten/Pharmacia and
  Upjohn
Micronase/Pharmacia and Upjohn

Midamor/Merck
Minipress/Pfizer Inc
Minizide/Pfizer Inc
Mintezol/Merck
Mithracin/Bayer Corporation
Monistat-Derm/Ortho
  Pharmaceutical
Monocid/Smithkline Beecham
Monopril/Bristol-Myers Squibb
MRV/Bayer Corporation
Mucomyst/Bristol-Myers Squibb
MumpsVax/Merck
Mustargen/Merck
Mutamycin/Bristol-Myers Squibb
Mycelex/Bayer Corporation
Mycostatin/Bristol-Myers Squibb
Myleran/Glaxo Wellcome
Mytelease/Sanofi Winthrop

N
Nadolol/Bristol-Myers Squibb
Nafcillin/Bristol-Myers Squibb
Nalcecon/Bristol-Myers Squibb
Naprosyn/Roche Laboratories
Naproxin/Bristol-Myers Squibb
Nasacort/Rhone-Poulenc Inc
Nasalide/Roche Laboratories
Nasarel/Roche Laboratories
Natalins/Bristol-Myers Squibb
Navane/Pfizer Inc
Navelbine/Glaxo Wellcome
Nebcin/Eli Lilly
NebuPent/Fujisawa
NegGram/Sanofi Winthrop
Neoatigmine/Bristol-Myers
  Squibb
Neodecadron/Merck
Neoral/Novartis
Neosporin Opthalmic/Glaxo
  Wellcome
NephrAmine/R&D Laboratories
Nephro-Fer/R&D Laboratories
Nephro-Calci/R&D Laboratories

Nephro-Vite/R&D Laboratories
Nephro-Derm/R&D Laboratories
Neupogen/Amgen, Inc.
Neurotin/Parke Davis
Niacin/Bristol-Myers Squibb
Nicobid/Rhone-Poulenc Inc
Nicolar/Rhone-Poulenc Inc
Nimotop/Bayer Corporation
Nitrazine/Bristol-Myers Squibb
Nitro-Bid/Hoechst Marion
Nitrolingual/Rhone-Poulenc Inc
Nizoral/Janssen
Nolvades/Zeneca
Norflex/3M
Norgesic/3M
Normodyne/Schering
  Laboratories/Key
Noroxin/Merck
Norpace/Searle
Norplant/Wyeth-Ayherst
  Laboratories
Norpramin/Hoechst Marion
Norvasc/Pfizer Inc
Nydrazid/Bristol-Myers Squibb

O
Ocusert/Alza
Ogen/Pharmacia and Upjohn
Omni/Smithkline Beecham
Oncaspar/Rhone-Poulenc Inc
Oncovin/Eli Lilly
Ophithaine/Bristol-Myers Squibb
Optimine/Schering
  Laboratories/Key
Oramorph/Roxane
Orasone/Solvay
Oratrast/Rhone-Poulenc Inc
Ornade/Smithkline Beecham
Orudis/Wyeth-Ayherst
  Laboratories
Ovcon/Bristol-Myers Squibb
Oxacillin/Bristol-Myers Squibb
Oxistat/Glaxo Wellcome

P
Pancrease Capsules/McNeil
Parafon Forte DSC/McNeil
Paraplayten/Bristol-Myers Squibb
Parlodel/Novartis
Pavabid/Hoechst Marion
Paxil/Smithkline Beecham
PBZ/Novartis
Pediotic Suspension/Glaxo
 Wellcome
PedvaxHib/Merck
Penetrex/Rhone-Poulenc Inc
Penicillin/Bristol-Myers Squibb
Pentasa/Hoechst Marion
Pepcid/Merck
Periactin/Merck
Permax/Athena Neurosciences
Phenergan/Wyeth-Ayherst
 Laboratories
pHisoHex/Sanofi Winthrop
Photophrin/Sanofi Winthrop
Pilagan/Allergan
Plaquenil/Sanofi Winthrop
Platinol/Bristol-Myers Squibb
Plendil/Astra Merck
Pneumovax/Merck
Pollen Extract/Bayer Corporation
Polycillin/Bristol-Myers Squibb
Polysporin Opthalmic/Glaxo
 Wellcome
Potassium CI/Bristol-Myers
 Squibb
Pravachol/Bristol-Myers Squibb
Precose/Bayer Corporation
Premarin/Wyeth-Ayherst
 Laboratories
Prilosec/Astra Merck
Primaquine/Sanofi Winthrop
Primaxin/Merck
Principen/Bristol-Myers Squibb
Prinivil/Merck
Prinizide/Merck
Procardia/Pfizer Inc

Prochlorperazine/Bristol-Myers
 Squibb
Procrit/Ortho Biotech Inc
Progestasert/Alza
Prograf/Fujisawa
Proloprim/Glaxo Wellcome
Prollxin/Bristol-Myers Squibb
Pronestyl/Bristol-Myers Squibb
Propine/Allergan
Propulsid/Janssen
Prolixin/Bristol-Myers Squibb
Pronestyl/Bristol-Myers Squibb
Proscar/Merck
Protamine Sulfate/Eli Lilly
Proventil/Schering
 Laboratories/Key
Provera/Pharmacia and Upjohn
Purinethol/Glaxo Wellcome
Q
Questran/Bristol-Myers Squibb

R
Rauzide/Bristol-Myers Squibb
Recombivax/Merck
Regroton/Rhone-Poulenc Inc
Relafen/Smithkline Beecham
Renova/Ortho
ReoPro/Eli Lilly
Retin-A/Ortho
Retrovir/Glaxo Wellcome
Ridaura/Smithkline Beecham
Rifadin/Hoechst Marion
Rifamate/Hoechst Marion
Rifater/Hoechst Marion
Riultek/Rhone-Polenc Inc
Rimactane/Novartis
Risperdal/Janssen
Rocaltrol/Roche Laboratories
Rocephrin/Roche Laboratories
Roferon-A/Roche Laboratories
Romazicon/Roche Laboratories
Rowasa/Solvay
Roxanol/Roxane

Roxicodone/Roxane
Rubex/Bristol-Myers Squibb
Rythmol/Knoll

S

Sandimmune/Novartis
Sandoglubulin/Novartis
Sandostatin/Novartis
Seconal/Eli Lilly
Sectral/Wyeth-Ayherst
  Laboratories
Seldane/Hoechst Marion
Semprex-D/Glaxo Wellcome
Septra/Glaxo Wellcome
Ser-Ap-Es/Novartis
Serentil/Boehringer Ingleheim
Serevent/Glaxo Wellcome
Serostim/Serono Laboratories Inc
Silvadene/Hoechst Marion
Sinemet CR/DuPont Merck 1
Sinemet/DuPont Merck
Sinequan/Pfizer Inc
Slo-Phylllin/Rhone-Poulenc Inc
Slo-bid/Rhone-Poulenc Inc
Slow-K/Novartis
SMZ-TMP/Bristol-Myers Squibb
Sorbitrate/Zeneca
Sorzone/Bristol-Myers Squibb
Spectazole/Ortho
Spec-T Sore/Bristol-Myers Squibb
Sporanox/Janssen
Stadol/Bristol-Myers Squibb
Stelazine/Smithkline Beecham
Stilphostrol/Bayer Corporation
Sumycin/Bristol-Myers Squibb
Symmetrel/DuPont Merck
Synalar/Roche Laboratories
Synthroid Tablets/Knoll
Syprine/Merck

T

Tace/Hoechst Marion
Tagamet/Smithkline Beecham
Tambocor/3M

Taxol/Bristol-Myers Squibb
Taxotere/Rhone-Poulenc Inc
Tazidime/Eli Lilly
Tegison/Roche Laboratories
Tegretol/Novartis
Tegretol-XR/Novartis
Temovate/Glaxo Wellcome
Tenuate/Hoechst Marion
Teslac/Bristol-Myers Squibb
Testoderm/Alza
Theolair/3M
TheraCys/Pasteur Merieux
  Connaught
Theragran/Bristol-Myers Squibb
Thioguanne/Glaxo Wellcome
Thioplex/Immunex
Ticlid/Roche Laboratories
Tilade/Rhone-Poulenc Inc
Timentin/Smithkline Beecham
Timolide/Merck
Timoptic/Merck
Tobramycin/Bristol-Myers Squibb
Tofranil/Novartis
Tolectin/McNeil
Tonocard/Astra Merck
Topicort/Hoechst Marion
Trancopal/Sanofi Winthrop
Trandate/Glaxo Wellcome
Transdermal Nitro and
  Voltaren/Novartis
Trental/Hoechst Marion
Trexan and Vaseretic/DuPont
Tridesilon/Bayer Corporation
Trimox/Bristol-Myers Squibb
Trimpex/Roche Laboratories
Trinalin/Schering
  Laboratories/Key
Trusopt/Merck
Tubocurarine/Bristol-Myers
  Squibb
Tussar/Rhone-Poulenc Inc
Tylenol with Codeine/McNeil
Tylox Capsules/McNeil

U
Ultram/McNeil
Urecholine/Merck
Urex/3M

V
Vagistat-1/Bristol-Myers Squibb
Valium/Roche Laboratories
Valtrex/Glaxo Wellcome
Vancenase/Schering
  Laboratories/Key
Vancocin HCI/Eli Lilly
Vantin/Pharmacia and Upjohn
Vaqta/Merck
Varivax/Merck
Vascor/McNeil
Vaseretic/Merck
Vasodilan/Bristol-Myers Squibb
Vasotec/Merck
Velban/Eli Lilly
Veetids/Bristol-Myers Squibb
Velosef/Bristol-Myers Squibb
Venomil Maintenance/Bayer
  Corporation
Venomil Individual/Bayer
  Corporation
Ventolin/Glaxo Wellcome
VePesid/Bristol-Myers Squibb
Vermox/Janssen
Vesanoid/Roche Laboratories
Vesprin/Bristol-Myers Squibb
Vibra-Tabs/Pfizer Inc
Vibramycin/Pfizer Inc
Videx/Bristol-Myers Squibb

Viramune/Roxane
Viroptic/Glaxo Wellcome
Vistaril/Pfizer Inc
Vistide/Gilead
Vivactil/Merck
Vivelle/Novartis
Voltaren-XR/Novartis
Vumon/Bristol-Myers Squibb

W
Wellbutrin/Glaxo Wellcome
Wellcovorin/Glaxo Wellcome
Wytensin/Wyeth Ayherst
  Laboratories

X
Xanax/Pharmacia and Upjohn

Z
Zantac/Glaxo Wellcome
Zarotin/Parke Davis

Zerit/Bristol-Myers Squibb
Zestoretic/Zeneca
Zestril/Zeneca
Zinecard/Pharmacia and Upjohn
Zithromax/Pfizer Inc
Zocor/Merck
Zyrtec/Pfizer Inc
Zofran/Glaxo Wellcome
Zoladex/Zeneca
Zoloft/Pfizer Inc
Zovirax/Glaxo Wellcome
Zyloprim/Glaxo Wellcome

Directory of Pharmaceutical Manufacturers Programs

ALZA Pharmaceuticals
Contact: Indigent Patient Assistance Program, c/o Comprehensive Reimbursement Consultants (CRC), 8990 Springbrook Drive, Suite

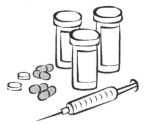

200, Minneapolis, MN 55433; 800-577-3788. Products covered are: Bicitra, Ditropan, Elmiron, Mycelex, Neutra-Phos, Neutra-Phos-K, Ocusert, PolyCitra, PolyCitra-K, Progestasert, Testoderm. Eligibility is determined by ALZA Pharmaceuticals and is based on patient's insurance status and income level. Patients must be ineligible for any other third-party reimbursement or support.

Amgen, Inc.
Contact: Safety Net Program for Epogen (Epoetin alfa); 800-272-9376. For patients on dialysis only. Eligibility is based on patient's insurance status and income level; patients may be uninsured or underinsured. Any dialysis center, physician, hospital or home dialysis supplier may sponsor a patient by applying to the program on his or her behalf.

Safety Net Program for Infergen (Interferon alfacon-1); 888-508-8088. For patients with chronic hepatitis C only. Eligibility is based on patient's insurance status and income level; patients may be uninsured or underinsured. Providers may enroll a patient or the patient may enroll him or herself.

Safety Net Program for Neupogen (Filgrastim); 800-272-9376.

Astra Merck, Inc.
Contact: Patient Assistance Program; 800-355-6044. Products covered are: Lexxel (enalapril maleate-felodipine), Plendil (felodipine), Prilosec (omeprozole), Tonocard (tocainide HCI). Health care provider must apply on behalf of a patient who has a medical need and a financial

hardship that would prevent the patient from filling a prescription. Astra Merck's Patient Assistance Program is available to patients who do not have insurance, are not eligible for governmental assistance programs (e.g., Medicaid), or who do not have other means to pay for their medication.

Astra USA, Inc.
Contact: F.A.I.R. (Foscavir Assistance and Information on Reimbursement) Program, State and Federal Associates, 1101 King St., Alexandria, VA 22314; 800-488-3247, 703-683-2239 (fax). Products covered are: Foscavir (foscarnet sodium). If patient is not covered for outpatient prescription drugs under private insurance or a public program, patient's income must fall below level selected by the company. Patient may or may not be poor, but retail drug purchase would cause hardship. If patient is covered for outpatient prescription drugs, he or she may be eligible for assistance with deductibles or maximum benefit limits. Eligibility is determined by the company based on income information provided by the physician.

Athena Neurosciences, Inc.
Contact: Athena Indigent Patient Program, Athena Neurosciences, Inc., 800 Gateway Blvd., South San Francisco, CA 94080. Products covered are: Permax (pergolide mesylate), Zanaflex (tizanadine hydrochloride), Diastat (diazepam rectal gel). The patient must be a resident of the United States, have a net worth of less than $30,000 and no third-party prescription drug coverage.

Bayer Corporation, Inc
Contact: Bayer Indigent Program, P.O. Box 29209, Phoenix, AZ 85038-9209, 800-998-9180. Most Bayer prescription medications used as recommended in prescribing information. An application form must be completed. Physician must certify patient is not eligible for, or covered by, government-funded reimbursement or insurance program for medication; patient is not covered by private insurance; and patient's income is below federal poverty-level guidelines. Physician must indicate condition for which drug is to be prescribed and certify that drug will be used for indicated use only. Physician must agree to follow patient through therapy. All applications are subject to a case-by-case evaluation by Bayer Corporation.

Biogen, Inc.
Contact: Avonex Access program, Avonex Support Line; 800-456-2255. Product covered is: Avonex (interferon beta-la). Eligibility is based on patient's insurance status and income level.

Boehringer Ingleheim Pharmaceuticals, Inc.
Contact: Partners in Health, Beohringer Ingelheim Pharmaceuticals, P.O. Box 368, Ridgefield, CT 06877-0368, 800-556-8317 (for information and form). Products covered are: Atrovent, Alupent MDI, Combivent, Flomax, Catapres-TTS, Mexitil, Serentil for FDA-approved incidations only. Patient must be a U.S. citizen ineligible for Medicaid prescription coverage. Patient must meet established financial criteria.

Bristol-Myers Squibb
Contact: Bristol-Myers Squibb, Patient Assistance Program, P.O. Box 4500, Princeton, NJ 08543-4500, Mailcode P25-31; 800-332-2056. Call for current information on specific pharmaceutical products. This program is designed to provide temporary assistance to patients with a financial hardship who are not eligible for prescription drug coverage through Medicaid or any other public or private health programs.

Ciba Pharmaceuticals
See Novartis Pharmaceuticals.

DuPont Merck Pharmaceutical Company
Contact: DuPont Merck Pharmaceutical Company Patient Assistance Program, c/o Michelle Paoli, P.O. Box 80723, Wilmington, DE 19880-0723, 800-474-2762. All marketed non-controlled prescription products are covered. Eligibility is based on the patient• s insurance status and income level/assets. Patients should have exhausted all third-party insurance, Medicaid, Medicare, and all other available programs. Patients must be residents of the United States.

Eisai Inc.
Contact: The Aricept Patient Assistance Program; 800-226-2072. Product covered is: Aricept (donepezil HCI). Eligible patients are U.S. residents without prescription drug coverage through either public or

private insurance. Patients must be diagnosed by a physician as having mild to moderate dementia of the Alzheimer's type.

Fujisawa USA, Inc.
Contact: Susan Lindsey, NebuPent Product Manager, Fujisawa USA, Inc., 3 Parkway North Center, Deerfield, IL 60015-2548; 847-317-8874. Product covered is: NebuPent (pentamidine isethionate). This program is designed to provide NebuPent to AIDS patients who would not otherwise be able to afford this treatment. All requests for consideration must be written by a physician and should include the patient's medical, financial, and insurance information.

Contact: Prograf Patient Assistance Program, c/o Medical Technology Hotlines, P.O. Box 7710, Washington, DC 20044-7710; 800-4-PROGAF, 800-477-6472, or 202-393-5563 in the Washington, DC area. Products covered are: Prograf capsules (tacrolimus, FK506). Fujisawa USA, Inc., developed the Prograf Patient Assistance Program to help improve access to oral Prograf for patients who have no health insurance for Prograf and limited financial resources. To be eligible for this program, patients must meet income and insurance requirements set by Fujisawa USA. Please call the Prograf Reimbursement Hotline (800-4-PROGRAF) for an application or for information about eligibility. If you describe a patient's insurance and financial situation, Hotline staff can determine whether the patient is likely to qualify for the Program Patient Assistance Program.

Genentech, Inc.
Contact: Uninsured Patient Assistance Program, Genentech, Inc., P.O. Box 2586, Mail Stop #13, S. San Francisco, CA 94083-2586; 800-879-4747, 415-225-1366 (fax). Products covered are: Actimmune (interferon gamma-lb), Activase (alteplase recombinant), Protropin (somatrem for injection), Nutropin (somatropin for injection), Nutropin AQ (somatropin for injection), Rituxan (rituximab). A completed application form must be submitted for all products and must contain required medical, financial, and insurance information. The required information for Actimmune, Nutropin, Protropin, and Rituxan applications is provided by the physician and patient. Required

information for Activase is provided by the hospital. For consideration for any of the programs, the patient must not be eligible for public or private insurance reimbursement. Specifically for Activase, the patient must have an annual gross income of $25,000 or less. Once patient eligibility has been verified for Actimmune, Nutropin, Nutropin AQ, and Protropin, future shipments will be directed to the physician's office on behalf of the patient. Once patient eligibility has been verified for Activase and Rituxan, Genentech will provide replacement of the amount of product used to treat the patient. These programs may be subject to change.

Genetics Institute, Inc.
Contact: The Benefix Reimbursement and Information Program; 888-999-2349. Product covered is: Benefix Coagulation Factor IX (recombinant). Eligible patients must be without prescription drug coverage from a third-party payer.

Contact: The Neumega Access Program; 888-638-6342. Product covered is: Neumega (oprelvekin). This program is for uninsured or underinsured patients who have limited financial resources.

Genzyme Corporation
Contact: Ceredase/Cerezyme Access Program (CAP), Wytske Kingma, M.D., Medical Affairs, Genzyme Corp., One Kendall Square, Cambridge, MA 01239-1562; 800-745-4447, ext. 7808. Products covered are: Ceredase (alglucerase injection) and Cerezyme (imiglucerase for injection). Eligibility is based on financial and medical need. Patient must be uninsured and lack the financial means to purchase the drug. This program is considered to be a temporary funding program.

Gilead Sciences, Inc.
Contact: Gilead Sciences Support Services, 800-445-3235. Product covered is: Vistide (cidofovir injection) for the treatment of cytomegalovirus (CVM) retinitis in patients with AIDS. Gilead Sciences Support Services assists both insured and uninsured patients. To determine eligibility, physicians or patients should request a Patient Assistance Program application from the Gilead Sciences Support Services office listed above.

Glaxo Wellcome Inc.
Contact: Glaxo Wellcome Inc., Patient Assistance Program, P.O. Box
52185, Phoenix, AZ 85072-2185; 800-722-9294 or {www.Helix.com}.
All marketed Glaxo Wellcome prescription products are covered.
Glaxo Wellcome is dedicated to assuring that no one is denied access to
our marketed prescription products as a result of their inability to pay.
The Patient Assistance Program is intended to serve patients who do
not have or qualify for private insurance or government-funded
programs, and is not intended to supplant or replace government
sponsored programs. The Patient Assistance Program is designed as an
interim solution to assist financially disadvantaged individuals until
alternative funding can be found. Income eligibility is based upon
multiples of the U.S. poverty level adjusted for household size. The
Patient Assistance Program is committed to an equitable distribution of
available resources among both patient populations and geographies,
and is dedicated to providing patients and their providers with
information or guidance in finding alternative reimbursement venues
for needed medicines. The provision of free medication is a
philanthropic activity of Glaxo Wellcome, and therefore, the Patient
Assistance Program is considered the payer of last resort.

Hoechst Marion Roussel, Inc.
Contact: Indigent Patient Program, Hoechst Marion Roussel, Inc., P.O.
Box 9950, Kansas City, MO 64134-0950, 800-221-4025. All
prescription products, except Rifadin, Rifamate, Rifater, and Tenuate
are covered by this program. Eligibility is determined by the physician
based on patient's income level and lack of insurance. Physicians are
encouraged to participate in the spirit of this partnership by also
providing their services free of charge. The intent of the program is to
provide access to products for patients who fall below the federal
poverty level and have no other means of health care coverage. The
program is restricted to indigent patients.

Janssen Pharmaceutical
Contact: Janssen Patient Assistance Program. 1800 Robert Fulton
Drive, Reston, VA 22091-4346; 800-544-2987. Products covered are:
Duragesic (fentanyl transdermal), Ergamisol (levamisole), Hismanal
(astemizole), Imodium (loperamide), Nizoral Cream (ketaconazole
cream), Nizoral Shampoo (ketaconazole shampoo), Nizoral Tablet

(ketaconazole tablet), Propulsid (cisapride), Sporanox (itraconazole), Vermox (mebendazole). These products will be offered free of charge to any persons who meet specific medical criteria and lack financial resources and third-party insurance.

Contact: The Risperdal Assistance Program, c/o Janssen Cares, 4828 Parkway Plaza Blvd., Suite 120, Charlotte, NC 28217-1969, 800-652-6227. Product covered is: Risperdal (risperidone).Risperdal will be free of charge to any persons who meet specific medical criteria and lack financial resources and third-party insurance.

Knoll Pharmaceutical Company
Contact: Knoll Indigent Patient Program, Knoll Pharmaceutical Company, Telemarketing, 3000 Continental Drive North, Mount Olive, NJ 07828-1234, Attn: Telemarketing. Products covered are: Isoptin SR (verapamil HCI), Rythmol (propafenone HCI), Collagenase Santyl, Synthroid Tablets (levothyroxine sodium, USP), Mavik (trandolapril), Tarka (trandolapril and verapamil). Physician must submit appropriate documentation proving patient indigence to company.

Lederle Laboratories
See Wyeth-Ayerst Laboratories Indigent Patient program.

Eli Lilly and Company
Contact: Lilly Cares Program Administrator, Eli Lilly and Company, P.O. Box 25768, Alexandria, VA 22313; 800-545-6962. Most Lilly prescription products and insulins (except controlled substances) are covered. Gemzar is covered under a separate program. Eligibility is determined on a case-by-case basis in consultation with the prescribing physician. Eligibility is based on the patient's inability to pay and lack of third-party drug payment assistance, including insurance, Medicaid, government subsidized clinics, and other government, community, or private programs. Inpatients and those who can obtain drug reimbursement from any source are not eligible. Requests for replacement drugs cannot be honored. Medications are provided directly to the physician for dispensing to the patient. Quantity of supply is dependent upon type of product being prescribed. All Lilly medications must be used as recommended in product labeling.

Contact: Gemzar Patient Assistance Program, 888-443-6927. Product covered is: Gemzar (gemcitabine hydrochloride). Applicants determined to be eligible based on program income criteria will be approved on the basis of these additional criteria: no medical insurance, and ineligibility for any programs with a drug benefit provision, including Medicaid, third-party insurance, Medicare, and all other programs have denied coverage for Gemzar in writing and all appeals have been exhausted.

The Liposome Company, Inc.
Contact: Financial Assistance Program for Abelcet, The Liposome Company, Inc., One Research Way, Princeton, NJ 08540-6619; 800-335-5476. Product covered is: Abelcet (amphotericin B lipid complex injection). Patients must be uninsured (not eligible to receive reimbursement through any other third-party drug reimbursement program) and be unable to pay for the product out-of-pocket.

Merck & Co., Inc.
Contact: Merck Patient Assistance Program, 800-994-2111. Most Merck products are covered. Requests for vaccines and injectibles are not accepted, with the exception of anti-cancer injectable products. Crixivan is covered under a separate program (listed below). This program provides temporary assistance to patients who have no access to insurance coverage for prescription medications and are truly unable to afford prescription medications. The patient must have exhausted all options for prescription benefits and coverage.

Contact: SUPPORT, Reimbursement Support and Patient Assistance Services for Crixivan (indinavir sulfate); 800-850-3430. The SUPPORT program assists patients who are prescribed Crixivan and are uncertain of their insurance coverage in locating payment sources for Crixivan. Free product is provided to those uninsured patients who qualify and for whom no alternative source of coverage can be identified.

Novartis Pharmaceuticals
Contact: Patient Assistance Program, P.O. Box 52052, Phoenix, AZ 85072-9170; 800-257-3273. Products covered include certain single-

source and/or life-sustaining products. Controlled substances are not included. Physicians should call for more information.

Ortho Biotech, Inc.
Contact: The Ortho Biotech FAP (Financial Assistance Program) Program, 1800 Robert Fulton Drive, Suite 300, Reston, VA 20191-4346; 800-553-3851. Products covered are Procrit (Epoetin alfa), for non-dialysis use, Leustatin (cladribine) Injection. Program will ensure that Procrit and/or Leustatin are made available free of charge to any persons who meet specific medical criteria and lack financial resources or third-party insurance necessary to obtain treatment. A reimbursement specialist determines eligibility for a patient. Ortho Biotech requests that physicians not charge FAP patients for professional services.

Ortho Dermatological and Ortho-McNeil Pharmaceutical, Inc.
Contact: Ortho Dermatological Patient Assistance Program or Ortho-McNeil Patient Assistance Program, 1800 Robert Fulton Drive, Suite 300, Reston, VA 20191-4346; 800-797-7737. Products covered include prescription products. Patient sshould not have insurance coverage for prescription medications. Patients should not be eligible for other sources of drug coverage; they need to have applied to public sector programs and been denied. Patients' income must fall below the federal poverty level and retail purchase would cause hardship.

Parke Davis
Contact: Parke Davis Patient Assistance Program, P.O. Box 9945, McLean, VA 22102; 800-755-0120. Products covered are: Acupril, Cognex, Dilantin, Neurontin, Zarontin, and Rezulin. Lipitor is covered under a separate program (see below). Patients must not be eligible for other sources of drug coverage and must be deemed financially eligible based on company guidelines.

Contact: Lipitor Patient Assistance Program, P.O. Box 1058, Somerville, NJ 08876; 908-218-0120. Product covered is: Lipitor (atorvastin calcium) Patients must not be eligible for other sources of drug coverage and must be deemed financially eligible based on company guidelines and physician certification.

Pasteur Merieux Connaught
Contact: Customer Account Management, Pasteur Merieux Connaught, Route 611, P.O. Box 187, Swiftwater, PA 18370-0187, 800-822-2463. Products covered are: Imovax Rabies, ravies vaccine; Imogam Rabies-HT, rabies immune globulin (human); TheraCys BCG live intravesical. (Imovax and Imogam Rabies-HT are provided on a post-exposure basis.) Eligibility is determined on a case by case basis and limited to those individuals who have been identified as indigent, uninsured and ineligible for Medicare and Medicaid.

Pfizer Inc.
Contact: Pfizer Prescription Assistance, P.O. Box 25457, Alexandria, VA 22313-5457; 800-646-4455. Most Pfizer outpatient products with chronic indications, except Diflucan and Zithromax, are covered by this program. Difucan and Zithromax are covered by a separate program. Any patient that a physician is treating as indigent is eligible. Patients must have incomes below $12,000 (single) or $15,000 (family). Patients must not be receiving or be eligible for third-party or Medicaid reimbursements for their medications. No copayment or cost-sharing is required by the patient.

Contact: Diflucan and Zithromax Patient Assistance Program; 800-869-9979. Products covered are: Diflucan (fluconazole), Zithromax (azithromycin). Patient must not have insurance or other third party coverage, including Medicaid, and must not be eligible for a state AIDS drug assistance program. Patient must have an income of less than $25,000 a year without dependents, or less than $40,000 a year with dependents.

Contact: Aricept Patient Assistance program (See Eisai, Inc.)

Contact: Lipitor Patient Assistance Program (See Parke-Davis)

Contact: Sharing the Care, Pfizer Inc., 235 E. 42nd St., New York, NY 10017-5755; 800-984-1500. Pfizer single-source products are covered. The program is a joint effort of Pfizer, the National Governors' Association, and the National Association of Community Health Centers. It works solely through community, migrant, and homeless health centers that are certified by the federal government as meeting criteria for Section 330 of the Public Health Service Act. A center must have an in-house pharmacy to participate. To be eligible, the patient must be a patient of a participating health center and must be uninsured, not eligible for government entitlement programs that cover pharmaceuticals, and at or below the federal poverty level.

State Health Care Access Programs. All Pfizer products are covered. Must be a state resident to qualify. Patients must be below the federal poverty guidelines who do not have health insurance benefits and do not qualify for any government entitlement programs. No copayment or cost-sharing is required from the patient. Physician must waive his or her fee for the initial visit. This program does not apply to individuals during hospital inpatient stays.

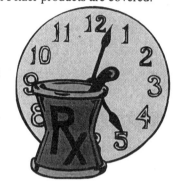

Arkansas: Ms. Pat Keller, Program Director, Arkansas Health Care Access Foundation, P.O. Box 56248, Little Rock, AK 72215; 800-950-8233, 501-221-3033. Eligible individuals are certified by the Arkansas Local County Department of Human Services.

Kentucky: Mr. Keith Knapp, Executive Vice President, Kentucky Health Care Access Foundation, 12700 Shelbyville Rd., Suite 1000, Louisville, KY 40243; 800-633-8100, 502-244-4214, 402-244-4209 (fax). Eligible individuals are certified by the Kentucky Cabinet for Human Resources.

South Carolina: Ms. Parker Sparrow, Director, Commun-I-Care, P.O. Box 12054, Columbia, SC 29211; 800-763-0059, 803-779-4875, 803-254-0320 (fax). Individuals are certified by Commun-I-Care.

Pharmacia and Upjohn, Inc.
Contact: RxMAP Prescription Medication Assistance Program, P.O. Box 29043, Phoenix, AZ 85038, 800-242-7014. Numerous products are covered. Eligibility is based on federal poverty level and no prescription drug coverage.

Proctor & Gamble Pharmaceuticals Inc.
Contact: Procter & Gamble Pharmaceuticals, Inc., P.O. Box 231, Norwich, NY 13815, Attn: Customer Service Department; 800-448-4878. Products covered are: Alora, Asacol, Dantrium Capsules, Didronel, Helidac, Macrodantin, Macrobid. Procter & Gamble Pharmaceuticals has always tried to ensure that all patients have full access to its products. To qualify, patients should not have insurance coverage for prescription mediciness or be eligible for Medicaid reimbursements. The intent of the program is to ensure access to products for patients who fall below the federal poverty level and have no other means of health coverage. Each patient's case is handled strictly on an individual basis. The company relies on the physician's assessment of need to determine eligibility. Application forms are provided by the company for the physician to complete. An original prescription duly signed by the attending physician for one of the company's products is required.

Rhone-Poulenc Rorer Inc.
Contact: Medical Affairs/Patient Assistance Program, Rhone-Poulenc Rorer Inc., Mailstop #4C29, P.O. Box 5094, 500 Arcola Rd., Collegeville, PA 19426; 610-454-8110, 610-454-2102 (fax). All products are included, with some limitations. Rhone-Poulenc Rorer's Patient Assistance Program is administered on a case-by-case basis. A patient is eligible to apply to the program if there is a medical and financial need for assistance as identified by a physician, social agent or agency, and if the effort to obtain assistance from all third-party payers, Medicaid, Medicare, and all other local, state or federal government support has been exhausted. The physician is requested to fill out a form provided by RPR and to send the completed form along with a valid prescription to the above address. Determination of eligibility is made by the company based on the information in the completed form. Once eligibility has been determined, the prescribed medication is sent to the physician for dispensing to the patient.

Roche Laboratories
Contact: Roche Medical Needs Program, Roche Laboratories, Inc., 340 Kingsland St., Nutley, NJ 07110, 800-285-4484. Most Roche products are covered. Drugs used in transplants and the treatment of cancer and AIDS have separate programs, which are listed below. The Roche

Medical Needs Program is designed as an interim solution for patients who lack third-party outpatient prescription drug coverage under private insurance, government-funded programs (Medicaid, Medicare, Veterans Affairs, etc.), or private/community sources and are unable to afford to purchase Roche products on their own. This program is for outpatients who meet the program criteria and is offered through licensed practitioners. The program is not intended for clinics, hospitals, and/or other institutions.

Contact: Roche Transplant Reimbursement Hotline; 800-772-5790. Products covered are: CellCept (mycophenolate mofetil), Cytovene (ganciclovir capsules), and Cytovene-IV (ganciclovir sodium for injection), and Cytovene products for use with transplant patients.

Contact: Roche HIV Therapy Assistance Program; 800-282-7780. Products covered are: Fortovase (saquinavir), Invirase (saquinavir mesylate), Cytovene (ganciclovir capsules), Cytovene-IV (ganciclovir sodium for injection) and HIVID (zalcitabine), Cytovene products for use with HIV/AIDS patients.

Contact: Oncoline/Hepline Reimbursement Hotline; 800-443-6676 (press 2 or 3). Products covered are: Roferon-A (Interferon alpha-2a, recombinant), Vesanoid (tretinoin) and Fluorouracil injection.

Roxane Laboratories, Inc.
Contact: Nexus Healthcare, 4161 Arlingate Plaza, Columbus, OH 43228; 800-274-8651. Products covered are: Duraclon, Marinol (dronabinol) Capsules 2.5 mg, Oramorph SR (morphine sulfate sustained release) Tablets 15 mg, 30 mg, 60 mg, and 100 mg, Roxanol (morphine sulfate concentrated oral solution) 20 mg/mL and 120 mL bottles, Roxanol 100 (morphine sulfate concentrated oral solution) 100 mg/5 mL and 240 mL bottles, Roxicodone (oxycodone) Tablets 5 mg, Oral solution 5 mg/mL, Roxicodone Intensol 20 mg/mL, Viramune (nevirapine). Product will be provided free of charge to patients through their pharmacist, provided the patient is uninsured and meets annual income requirements.

Sandoz Pharmaceuticals Corporation
See Novartis Pharmaceuticals.

Sanofi Pharmaceuticals
Contact: Sanofi Pharmaceuticals, Needy Patient Program, c/o Product Information Department, 90 Park Avenue, New York, NY 10016; 800-446-6267. Products covered are: Aralen, Breonesin, Danocrine, Drisdol, Hytakerol, Mytelase, NegGram, pHisoHex, Plaquenil, Primaquine, Photofrin, PrimaCor, Skelid. Eligibility is determined on a financial case by case basis.

Schering Laboratories/Key Pharmaceuticals
Contact: For Intron/Eulexin Products: 800-521-7157. For other products: Schering Laboratories/Key Pharmaceuticals, Patient Assistance Program, P.O. Box 52122, Phoenix, AZ, 85072, 800-656-9485. Most products are covered. The program is designed to assist those patients who are truly in need — indigent — who are not eligible for private or public insurance reimbursement and cannot afford treatment. Patient eligibility is determined on a case-by-case basis based on economic and insurance criteria. Eligibility criteria are currently being evaluated and may be subject to change.

Searle
Contact: Administrator, Searle Patients in Need Foundation, 5200 Old Orchard Rd., Skokie, IL 60077; 800-542-2526 or Local Searle Sales Representative. Products covered are: Antihypertensives: Aldactazide (spironolactone with hydrochlorothiazide), Aldactone (spironolactone), Calan SR (verapamil HCI) sustained-release, Kerlone (betaxolol HCI). Antihypertensive/Anti-Anginal/Antiarrhythmic: Calan (verapamil HCI). Antiarrhythmics: Norpace (disopyramide phosphate), Norpace CR (disopyramide phosphate) extended-release. Prevention of NSAID-induced gastric ulcers: Cytotec (misoprostol). The physician is the sole determinant of a patient's eligibility for the program based on medical and economic need. Searle provides guidelines for physicians to consider, but they are not requirements. Searle does not review documentation for eligibility. The guidelines suggest that: patient suffers from conditions for which a Searle product in the Patients in Need program may be appropriate; patient does not qualify for outpatient prescription drugs under private insurance, a public program, or other assistance that pays in whole or in part for prescription drugs; patient's income falls below a level suggested by Searle.

Serono Laboratories, Inc.
Contact: Gina Cella, Executive Director, Corporate Communications, Serono Laboratories, Inc., 100 Longwater Circle, Norwell, MA 02061; 617-982-9000, 617-982-1369 (fax). Products covered are: Saizen (somatropin [rDNA origin} for injection) for treatment of pediatric growth hormone deficiency; Fertinex (urofollitropin for injection, purified), Gonal-F (follitropin alfa for injection) for treatment of infertility, Serostim (human growth hormone {rDNA origin} for treatment of AIDS wasting.

Sigma-Tau Pharmaceuticals, Inc.
Contact: Carnitor Drug Assistance Program, c/o NORD, P.O. Box 8923, New Fairfield, CT 06812; 800-999-NORD. Product covered is: Carnitor (levocarnitine). Eligibility is determined by medical and financial criteria and applied to a cost-share formula.

SmithKline Beecham Pharmaceuticals
Contact: SB Access to Care Program, SmithKline Beecham Pharmaceuticals, One Franklin Plaza-FP1320, Philadelphia, PA 19101; 800-546-0420. SmithKline Beecham outpatient prescription products are covered. Controlled substances are not covered. Eligibility is based on patient's insurance status and financial need. The patient must have exhausted all third-party insurance, Medicaid, Medicare, and all other available programs.

Contact: Access to Care Paxil Certificate Hotline. Physicians may enroll in a certificate program by calling 800-729-4544.

Contact: Oncology Access to Care Program Hotline, 800-699-3806. Products covered are: Kytril (granisetron HCI), Hycamtin (topotecan HCI). Eligibility is based on patient's insurance status and financial need. The patient must have exhausted all third-party insurance, Medicaid, Medicare, and all other available programs. Patients must meet the program's income requirements.

Solvay Pharmaceuticals, Inc.
Contact: Patient Assistance Program, Solvay Pharmaceuticals, Inc., c/o Phoenix Marketing Group, One Phoenix Drive, Lincoln Park, NJ 07035, 800-788-9277. Products covered are: Creon Minimicrospheres

Delayed-Release Capsules, Dexone (dexamethasone tablets, USP), Estratab (esterified estrogens tablets, USP), Estratest (esterified estrogens and methyltestosterone), Estratest HS (esterified estrogens and methyltestosterone), Lithobid (lithium carbonate, USP) Slow-Release Tablets, Lithonate (lithium carbonate) capsules, Lithotabs (lithium carbonate) tablets, Luvox (fluvoxamine maleate) tablets, Orasone (prednisone tablets, USP), Amantadine HCl Capsules, Advanced Formula Zenate Prenatal Multivitamin/Mineral Supplement Tablets. The patient's eligibility is determined on a case-by-case basis in consultation with each prescribing physician and is based on a patient's inability to pay, lack of insurance, and ineligibility for Medicaid. The patient must be a resident of the United States. The physician is encouraged to waive his or her fee. The free product must be provided to the patient for whom it is requested.

3M Pharmaceuticals
Contact: Indigent Patient Pharmaceutical Program, Medical Services Department, 275-3E-3M Center, P.O. Box 33275, St. Paul, MN 55133-3275; 800-328-0255, 612-733-6068 (fax). Most drug products sold by 3M Pharmaceuticals in the United States are covered. Patients whose financial and insurance circumstances prevent them from obtaining 3M Pharmaceuticals drug products considered to be necessary by their physician are eligible. Consideration is on a case-by-case basis.

The Upjohn Company
See Pharmacia & Upjohn, Inc.

Wyeth-Ayerst Laboratories
Contact: The Norplant Foundation, P.O. Box 25223, Alexandria, VA 22314; 703-706-5933. Product covered is: the Norplant (levonorgestrel implants) five-year contraceptive system. Eligibility is determined on a case-by-case basis and limited to individuals who cannot afford the product and who are ineligible for coverage under private and public sector programs.

Contact: Wyeth-Ayerst Laboratories Indigent Patient Program, John E. James, Professional Services, IPP, 555 E. Lancaster Ave., St. Davids, PA 19087. Various products (not including schedule II, III, or IV products) are covered. Eligibility is limited to individuals, on a case-by-case basis, who have been identified by their physicians as "indigent," meaning: a. Low or no income; b. Not covered by any third-party agency.

Zeneca Pharmaceuticals
Contact: Zeneca Pharmaceuticals Foundation Patient Assistance Program, Zeneca Pharmaceuticals Foundation, P.O. Box 15197, Wilmington, DC 19850-5197; 800-424-3727. Products covered are: Accolate (zafirlukast), Arimidex (anastrozole), Casodex (bicalutamide), Kadian (morphine sulfate, sustained release), Nolvadex (tamoxifen citrate), Seroquel (quetiapine fumarate), Sorbitrate (isosorbide dinitrate), Sular (nisoldipine), Tenoretic (atenolol/chlorthiazide), Tenormin (atenolol), Zestril (lisinopril), Zestoreticlisinopril/ hydrochlorthiazide), Zoladex (goserelin acetate implant), Zomig (zomitriptan). Determination is made by the Foundation based on income level/assets and absence of outpatient private insurance or participation in a public program.

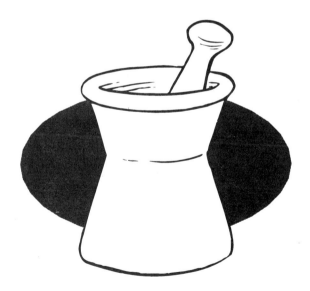

STATES WITH DISCOUNT DRUG PROGRAMS

Help can be just a phone call away. Eleven states have special drug programs that give huge discounts to qualifying state residents. Although many of these programs are geared toward senior citizens, Maine and Maryland provide support for all qualifying low-income residents. Participation in these programs usually depends upon your having exhausted other sources of support such as Medicaid or private insurance.

Often all it takes is a phone call and filling out a simple form. You will have to meet income eligibility, but you can make upwards of $24,400 a year and still qualify in New York, for example. If your state is not listed below, contact your state Department of Aging in the back of this book, but also check out other free drug programs sponsored by non-profit groups and the drug manufacturers themselves. You will find a detailed description of these programs following the listing of the state-by-state drug programs.

Connecticut
Conn PACE
P.O. Box 5011
Hartford, CT 06102
800-423-5026 (in CT)
860-832-9265

Eligibility Requirements:
♦ You must be 65 years old or older, or receive Social Security disability.

♦ You must have lived in Connecticut for six months.
♦ Your income cannot exceed $14,500 if you are single, and $17,500 if you are married.
♦ You may not have an insurance plan that pays for all or a portion of each prescription, a deductible insurance plan that includes prescriptions, or Medicaid.

Cost:
♦ You pay a $25 yearly registration fee.
♦ Your co-pay is $12 for each prescription.
♦ You must get generic drugs whenever possible, unless the doctor writes on the prescription, brand drug only.

Delaware
Nemours Health Clinic Program
1801 Rockland Rd.
Wilmington, DE 19803
302-651-4400
800-763-9326

Eligibility Requirements:
♦ You must be a Delaware resident.
♦ You must be a U.S. citizen.
♦ You must be 65 or older.
♦ Your income must be less than $12,500 if you are single, or $17,125 if you are married.

Cost:
♦ You must pay 25% of the prescription drug cost.

Illinois
Pharmaceutical Assistance Program
Illinois Department of Revenue
P.O. Box 19021
Springfield, IL 62794
800-624-2459
217-524-0435

Eligibility Requirements:
◆ You must be 65 years of age or older, or over 16 and totally disabled, or a widow or widower who turned 63 before spouse's death.
◆ You must be a resident of Illinois.
◆ Your income must be less than $16,000.
◆ You must file a Circuit Breaker claim form.

Cost:
◆ Pharmaceutical Assistance card will cost either $40 or $80, depending upon your income.
◆ Your monthly deductible will be $15 if the cost of your card is $40, and $25 if the cost of your card is $80.
◆ You must choose the generic brand when available, unless you are willing to pay the difference in price.

Maine

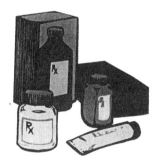

Maine Residents Low-Cost Drug Program
Maine Revenue Services
State Office Building
State House Station 24
Augusta, ME 04333-0024
207-626-8475
TDD: 207-287-4477 (8:00am-4:30pm, Monday-Friday)

Call the Maine Revenue Services at the number above to find out if you are eligible to receive a Maine Residents Low-Cost Drug Card. The Bureau of Medical Services, which administers the program, can provide you with current information on what drugs are covered. You can contact them at:

Department of Human Services
Bureau of Medical Services
State House Station 11
Augusta, ME 04333-0011
800-321-5557, ext. 1818

Maryland

Maryland Pharmacy Assistance Program
P.O. Box 386
Baltimore, MD 21203-0386
410-767-5397
800-492-1974

Eligibility Requirements:
- ◆ For anyone in the state who cannot afford medications and is not on medical assistance. Income requirements vary, so it is best to call.
- ◆ Permanent resident of Maryland.

Michigan

MEPPS (Michigan Emergency Pharmaceutical Program for Seniors)
Office of Services to the Aging
611 West Ottowa
P.O. Box 30676
Lansing, MI 48909
517-373-8230

Eligibility Requirements:
Seniors (65 or older) currently residing in Michigan who have no other current prescription drug coverage and do not qualify for Medicaid.

Cost:
There is a voluntary co-pay of 25 cents for each prescription.

New Jersey

Pharmaceutical Assistance to the Aged and Disabled (PAAD)
Special Benefit Programs
P.O. Box 715
Trenton, NJ 08625
800-792-9745
609-588-7049

Eligibility Requirements:
♦ You must be a New Jersey resident.
♦ Your income must be less than $18,151 if you are single, or less than $22,256 if you are married.
♦ You must be at least 65 years of age.
♦ Drugs purchased outside the state of New Jersey are not covered, nor any pharmaceutical product whose manufacturer has not agreed to provide rebates to the state of New Jersey.

Cost:
♦ You pay $5 for each covered prescription. PAAD collects payments made on your behalf from any other assistance program, insurance, or retirement benefits which may cover prescription drugs.

New York
Elderly Pharmaceutical Insurance Coverage (EPIC)
P.O. Box 15018
Albany, NY 12212
800-332-3742
518-452-6828
www.health.state.ny.us/nysdoh/epic/faq.htm

Eligibility Requirements:
♦ You must be 65 or older.
♦ You must reside in New York State.
♦ Your income must not exceed $18,500 if you are single; or $24,400 if you are married.
♦ You are not eligible if you receive Medicaid benefits or have other prescription coverage that is better than EPIC.

Cost:
♦ Seniors may join EPIC by enrolling in one of two plans; the right one for you depends upon your income. The Fee Plan entitles you to a substantial cost reduction on prescription drugs after you have paid an annual fee that ranges, depending upon your financial circumstances, from $10 to $220 per person. The Deductible Plan,

which is only available to those with moderate incomes, requires you to pay full price for prescriptions until you meet an annual deductible. After the deductible is met, these enrollees save more than half of their prescription costs per year. Deductibles start at $468 per person annually, depending upon income level. At the drugstore, you pay between $3 and $23 per prescription depending upon the prescription cost (Deductible Plan enrollees must have first met their annual deductions).

Pennsylvania

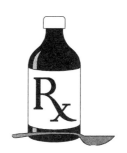

PACE Card and PACENET
(Pennsylvania Pharmaceutical Assistance
    Contract For The Elderly)
Pennsylvania Department of Aging
P.O. Box 8806
400 Market St., 6th Floor
Harrisburg, PA 17101-2301
717-787-7313
800-225-7223
www.state.pa.us/PA_Exec/Aging/srhe-pac.html

Eligibility Requirements:
♦ You must be 65 or older.
♦ Your income must be less than $14,000 if you are single, or have a combined income of less than $17,200 if you are a couple. PACENET, a modified program for seniors with slightly higher incomes, raises income ceilings by $2,000.
♦ You must be a Pennsylvania resident for at least 90 days prior to the date you apply.

Cost:
♦ PACE participants have a $6 co-payment for each prescription. PACENET enrollees must meet a $500-per-person annual deductible before qualifying for co-pays ranging from $8 for generics to $15 for brand names per prescription.
♦ PACE limits drug amounts to no more than a 30-day supply or 100 pills.

Rhode Island

Rhode Island Pharmaceutical Assistance to the Elderly (RIPAE)
Rhode Island Department of Elderly Affairs
160 Pine St.
Providence, RI 02903
401-222-3330
800-322-2880

Eligibility Requirements:
♦ You must be a Rhode Island resident.
♦ You must be 65 years old.
♦ Your income must not exceed $15,558 if you are single; $19,449 if you are married.
♦ Any other prescription drug coverage benefits must be exhausted before you would be eligible for RIPAE.

Cost:
♦ Members pay 40% of the cost of prescription drugs used to treat certain illnesses.

Vermont

VScript Program
Office of Vermont Health Access (OVA)
103 South Main St.
Waterbury, VT 05671
802-241-2880
Eligibility Requirements:
♦ You must be at least 65 or disabled.
♦ You may not have income in excess of 175% of the federal poverty guidelines.
♦ You may not be in a health insurance plan that pays for all or a portion of the applicant's prescription drugs.

Cost:
♦ Co-payments are $1 to $2 per prescription, depending upon the drug.

Free Medical Care for Rich and Poor By the Best Doctors in the World

Each year close to 75,000 patients receive free medical care by some of the best doctors in the world. Medical research professionals receive millions of dollars each year to study the latest causes, cures and treatments to various diseases or illnesses. If your health condition is being studied somewhere, you may qualify for what is called a "clinical trial" and get treatment for free. These clinical trials can also be used when your doctor recommends an experimental new treatment.

There are several ways to find out about ongoing clinical trials across the nation. Your first call should be to the National Institutes of Health (NIH) Clinical Center. NIH is the federal government's focal point for health research and is one of the world's foremost biomedical research centers. The Clinical Center is a 325-bed hospital that has facilities and services to support research at NIH. They also have an

and services to support research at NIH. They also have an adjacent 13-story Ambulatory Care Research Facility that provides additional space and facilities for outpatient research. Your doctor should contact

The Patient Referral Line
800-411-1222

to find out if your diagnosis is being studied, and to be put in contact with the primary investigator who can then tell if you meet the requirements for the study. An information brochure is available describing the Clinical Center programs.

Contact:
Clinical Center
National Institutes of Health
Building 61
10 Cloister Center
Bethesda, MD 20892
800-411-1222
301-496-2563
www.cc.nih.gov

If your doctor diagnoses you for a disease, but you can't afford treatment, you should check to see whether the National Institutes of Health is studying the disease and looking for patients to be treated at no cost.

In 1998, the Clinical Center at NIH in Bethesda, MD, treated 75,000 patients—so it's not as if only the lucky or the rich get to take part in the clinical studies. Keep in mind, though, that most doctors aren't even aware of what is being studied at NIH and probably won't think of a clinical study as an option for you—so *you* may very well have to tell your doctor that NIH is looking for patients with your diagnosis. The list of diseases studied at NIH includes almost everything from writers' cramp and lupus, to AIDS and PMS.

Referring doctors and dentists are welcome to visit their patients at the Clinical Center. When a patient is discharged, the referring doctor or dentist receives a full report on the results of studies and the treatment given. Cooperation of doctors, dentists and patients is appreciated for follow-up observation of patients after they have been discharged.

Patient Referrals

Again, patients are admitted to the Clinical Center *only* on referral by a doctor or dentist and only for research purposes. A complete diagnosis and medical history is necessary for admission.

Your doctor should make preliminary inquiries by telephone to determine if your diagnosis may be of interest to investigators. If your disease is under active investigation, your doctor may be asked to submit the diagnosis and medical history in writing to the principal investigator.

Financial Assistance

If necessary, the Clinical Center Social Work Department
will help prospective patients with personal problems
concerning their admission. This department *cannot*
provide financial assistance to individuals and their families
except in certain emergency situations. For more information, contact the Social Work Department at 301-496-2381.

Patients are not financially responsible for medical, surgical
or other hospital services performed at the Clinical Center;
however, the patient's transportation costs *usually* cannot be
paid.

Eligibility Requirements

1. You must be referred by a physician or dentist in
    private practice, hospital, clinic or other medical
    organization.

2. Your specific disease or condition must be under active
    investigation by NIH physicians at the time of
    admission.

3. Each Institute considers your age, weight, sex, general
    health and the length of their waiting list to qualify you
    as a patient for admission. Possibilities for long-term
    inpatient status and extended follow-up observations
    may also be considered. Apart from the medical

considerations listed above, there are no other restrictions based on race, creed, age, sex or color.

4. You must have a reasonable understanding of your role in a research study.

Length of Stay

You will be returned to the care of your referring doctors or institutions, or to your family, when your participation in a study has been completed and your medical condition permits. The clinical director of the Institute in which you are under study is responsible for making these determinations.

Accuracy of Information

The information in this section is the most up-to-date possible at the time of publication of this book. However, each year the Clinical Center publishes a new directory of clinical studies that includes the most recently funded studies, along with those that continue to be funded. So to ensure that the following studies are still underway and looking for patients, you'll have to contact the Center. Also, an up-to-date index of the current clinical studies is carried on the AMA/GTE Telenet Medical Information Network. Quarterly index updates are available on the information network to Telenet subscribers.

Clinical Studies

The Clinical Center has a searchable database where you can search using diagnosis, sign, symptom, or other key words or phrases. You will find a summary of study, eligibility criteria, and more. Search {www.cc.nih.gov}.

Doctors Who Get Grants To Study Your Illness

In addition to the free clinical studies at NIH described in the preceding section, there are thousands of other doctors who get research money and may be able to treat your condition for free. You can locate these doctors through the Division of Research Grants at NIH. This office can conduct a CRISP (Computer Retrieval for Information on Scientific Projects) search for you at no charge. The search can provide you with information on grants awarded to the National Institutes of Health, Food and Drug Administration, and other government research institutions, universities, or hospitals that deal with the topic in which you are interested. They have a free brochure available that describes their services.

Contact:
Division of Research Grants
Rockledge 2, MSC 7772
6701 Rockledge Dr.
Bethesda, MD 20892
301-435-0656
http://grants.nih.gov/grants/oer.htm

You can search online using search terms and a variety of parameters.

A second place to look is at the National Library of Medicine where you can conduct a search on their MEDLINE database (part of their MEDLARS databases). This search can provide you with citations and abstracts on your diagnosis and clinical trials from 6.6 million articles from approximately 4,300 biomedical journals published in the United States and abroad. You can access this system online at {www.nlm.nih.gov}.

Contact:
MEDLARS Management Section
National Library of Medicine
Bldg. 38A, Room 4N421
8600 Rockville Pike
Bethesda, MD 20894
800-638-8480

Free Health Care At Your Hospital

Do you need an operation? Has an unexpected health crisis occurred? Are you worried about paying your hospital bills?

Many hospitals, nursing homes, and clinics offer free or low-cost health care under the Hill-Burton free care program. You are eligible if your income falls within the Poverty Income Guidelines.

You must request and apply for Hill-Burton assistance (you can even apply after you have been discharged). Each Hill-Burton facility can choose which types of services to provide at no charge or reduced charge, and must give you a written individual notice that will tell you what types of services are covered. They also must provide a specific amount of free care each year, but can stop once they have given that amount.

A special hotline has been established that distributes information on applying for Hill-Burton assistance, and can answer questions regarding eligibility guidelines, facilities obligated to provide services, and help with filing a complaint. If you do not qualify for Hill-Burton assistance, don't worry: many hospitals have special funds to provide care for the poor. The hospital business offices can help you apply for various forms of government assistance, as well as set up payment plans you can afford. They can't help you if they don't know you have a problem. For more information on Hill-Burton:

Contact:
Office of Health Facilities
Health Resources and Services Administration
Department of Health and Human Services
5600 Fishers Lane, Room 11-03
Rockville, MD 20857
800-638-0742
800-492-0359 (in MD).
www.hrsa.dhhs.gov/OSP/dfcr/index.htm

Local Free Health Services

Your local health department (found in the blue pages of your phone book) often operates free or sliding-fee scale clinics and screening centers to handle non-emergency health problems. Many operate prenatal and well-baby clinics as well. The services and fees vary from place to place, so contact the health department to find out about eligibility, hours of service, and services provided.

According to the National Association of Community Health Centers, federally sponsored community health centers serve six million people, and four to six million people are served at other-sponsored health centers. However, some problems exist. Because of the increase demand for low-cost health care, many centers are closing off registration and are carrying waiting lists of 15 to 20 percent of their current case load. The demand and availability of local health centers do vary, so don't overlook this resource. To find out about local clinics:

Your State Department of Public Health
(See listing below)

Public Health Hotlines

Alabama
Alabama Department of Public
Health
RSA Tower
201 Monroe Street
Montgomery, AL 36104
Mailing Address:
  RSA Tower
  P.O. Box 303017
  Montgomery, AL 36130-
  3017
334-206-5300
www.alapubhealth.org
E-mail: webmaster@
alapubhealth.org

Alaska
Alaska Department of Health
& Social Services
350 Main Street
Room 503
Juneau, AK 99801
Mailing Address:
  P.O. Box 110610
  Juneau, AK 99811-0610
907-465-3090
Fax: 907-586-1877
http://health.hss.state.ak.us
E-mail: petern@
health.state.ak.us

Arizona
Arizona Department of Health
Services
Office of Women's &
Children's Health

411 North 24th Street
Phoenix, AZ 85008
602-220-6550
Fax: 602-220-6551
TDD: 602-256-7577
www.hs.state.az.us

Arkansas
Arkansas Department of
Health
4815 West Markham
Little Rock, AR 72201
501-661-2000
800-482-5400
http://health.state.ar.us
E-mail: wbankson@
mail.doh.state. ar.us

California
California Department of
Health Services
Office of Women's Health
714 P Street, Room 792
Sacramento, CA 95814
906-653-3330
Fax: 916-653-3535
www.dhs.ca.gov

Colorado
Colorado Department of Public
Health & Environment
4300 Cherry Creek Dr. South
Denver, CO 80246-1530
303-692-1000
www.state.co.us/gov_dir/
cdphe_dir/

Connecticut
Connecticut Department of
Public Health
410 Capitol Avenue
P.O. Box 340308
Hartford, CT 06134-0308
860-509-8000
TDD: 860-509-7191
www.state.ct.us/dph/
E-mail: donna.winiarski@
po.state.ct.us

Delaware
Delaware Division of Public
Health
P.O. Box 637
Federal & Water Streets
Dover, DE 19903
302-739-4701
Fax: 302-739-6657
www.state.de.us/govern/
agencies/dhss/irm/dph/
dphhome.htm

District of Columbia
District of Columbia
Department of Health
800 9th Street, SW, 3rd Floor
Washington, DC 20024
202-645-5556

Florida
Florida Department of Health
2020 Capital Circle SE
Tallahassee, FL 32399-1700
850-487-2945
www.doh.state.fl.us
E-mail: Dorothy_Bruce@
doh.state.fl.us

E-mail: JoAnn_Steele@doh.
state.fl.us

Georgia
Georgia Division of Public
Health
Two Peachtree Street, NW
Atlanta, GA 30303-3186
404-657-2700
www.ph.dhr.state.ga.us/
E-mail: gdphinfo@
dhr.state.ga.us

Hawaii
Hawaii Department of Health
1250 Punchbowl Street
Honolulu, HI 96813
808-586-4400
Fax: 808-586-4444
www.state.hi.us/health/
E-mail: pijohnst@ health.
state.hi.us

Idaho
Idaho Department of Health &
Welfare
450 W. State St., 10th Floor
P.O. Box 83720
Boise, ID 83720-0036
208-334-5500
Fax: 208-334-6558
TDD: 208-334-4921
www.state.id.us/dhw/
hwgd_www/home.html

Illinois
Illinois Dept. of Public Health
535 West Jefferson Street
Springfield, IL 62761

217-782-4977
Fax: 217-782-3987
TTY: 800-547-0466
www.idph.state.il.us

Indiana
Indiana State Department of
Health
2 North Meridian Street
Indianapolis, IN 46204
317-233-1325
www.ai.org/doh/index.html
E-mail: OPA@isdh.state.in.us

Iowa
Iowa Department of Public
Health
Lucas Building
321 East 12th Street
Des Moines, IA 50319
517-281-5787
www.idph.state.ia.us

Kansas
Kansas Division of Health &
Environment
Capitol Tower
400 Eighth Avenue, Suite 200
Topeka, KS 66603-3930
785-296-1500
Fax: 785-368-6368
www.kdhe.state.ks.us

Kentucky
Kentucky Cabinet for Health
Services
275 East Main Street
Frankfort, KY 40621
502-564-3970

Fax: 502-564-6533
http://cfc-chs.chr.state.ky.us

Louisiana
Louisiana Department of
Health and Hospitals
1201 Capitol Access Road
P.O. Box 629
Baton Rouge, LA 70821-0629
225-342-9500
Fax: 225-342-5568
www.dhh.state.la.us
E-mail: Webmaster@
dhhmail.dhh.state.la.us

Maine
Maine Department of Human
Services
221 State Street
Augusta, ME 04333
207-287-3707
Fax: 207-626-5555
TTY: 207-287-4479
www.state.me.us/dhs/main/
welcome.htm

Maryland
Maryland Department of
Health & Mental Hygiene
State Office Building Complex
201 West Preston Street
Baltimore, MD 21201-2399
410-767-6860
TDD: 800-735-2258
www.dhmh.state.md.us/index.
html

Massachusetts
Massachusetts Department of
Public Health

250 Washington Street
Boston, MA 02108-4619
617-624-5700
Fax: 617-624-5206
www.magnet.state.ma.us/dph/
dphhome.htm

Michigan
Michigan Department of
Community Health
Lewis Cass Building
Sixth Floor
320 South Walnut Street
Lansing, MI 48913
517-373-3500
www.mdch.state.mi.us/
E-mail: arias@state.mi.us

Minnesota
Minnesota Department of
Health
717 Delaware Street Southeast
Minneapolis, MN 55440-9441
612-676-5000
www.health.state.mn.us
E-mail: webmaster@
health.state.mn.us

Mississippi
Mississippi State Department
of Health
2423 North State Street
P.O. Box 1700
Jackson, MS 39215-1700
601-576-7400
Fax: 601-576-7364
www.msdh.state.ms.us/
msdhhome.htm
E-mail: info@msdh.state.ms.us

Missouri
Missouri Department of Health
930 Wildwood
P.O. Box 570
Jefferson, MO 65102-0570
573-751-6001
Fax: 573-751-6041
www.health.state.mo.us
E-mail: info@mail.health.
state.mo.us

Montana
Montana Department of Public
Health & Human Services
111 North Sanders
Helena, MT 59620
Mailing Address:
P.O. Box 4210
Helena, MT 59604-4210
406-444-2596
Fax: 406-444-1970
www.dphhs.mt.gov
E-mail: kpekoc@mt.gov

Nebraska
Nebraska Health & Human
Services System
Department of Services
P.O. Box 95044
Lincoln, NE 68509-5044
402-471-2306
www.hhs.state.ne.us/index.htm
E-mail: hhsinfo@ www.hhs.
state.ne.us

Nevada
Nevada State Health Division
505 E. King St., Room 201
Carson City, NV 89710

775-687-3786
Fax: 775-687-3859
www.state.nv.us/health/

New Hampshire
New Hampshire Department of
Health & Human Services
6 Hazen Drive
Concord, NH 03301-6505
603-271-4939
www.dhs.state.nh.us/index.htm

New Jersey
New Jersey Department of
Health & Senior Services
P.O. Box 360
John Fitch Plaza
Trenton, NJ 08625-0360
609-292-7836
Fax: 609-633-9601
www.state.nj.us/health/

New Mexico
New Mexico Department of
Health
1190 St. Francis Drive
Harold Runnels Building
Sante Fe, NM 87504
505-827-2619
Fax: 505-827-2530
www.state.nm.us/state/
doh.html

New York
New York Department of
Health
Corning Tower Building
Empire State Plaza
Albany, NY 12237

518-486-9002
www.health.state.ny.us
E-mail: ljr06@health.
state.ny.us

North Carolina
North Carolina State Center
for Health Statistics
Cotton Classing Building
222 North Dawson Street
Raleigh, NC 27603-1392
Mailing Address:
  P.O. Box 29538
  Raleigh, NC 27626-0538
919-733-4728
Fax: 919-733-8485
http://hermes.sches.chnr.state.
nc.us/SCHS/main.html

North Dakota
North Dakota Department of
Health
600 East Boulevard Avenue
Bismarck, ND 58505-0200
701-328-2372
Fax: 701-328-4727
www.ehs.health.state.nd.
us/ndhd/
E-mail: rfrank@state.nd.us

Ohio
Ohio Department of Health
246 North High Street
P.O. Box 118
Columbus, OH 43266-0118
614-466-3543
www.odh.state.oh.us
E-mail: questions@
gw.odh.state.oh.us

Oklahoma
Oklahoma State Department of
Health
1000 NE 10th Street
Oklahoma City, OK 73117
405-271-5600
800-522-0203
www.health.state.ok.us
E-mail: webmaster@
health.state.ok.us

Oregon
Oregon Health Division
800 NE Oregon Street
Portland, OR 97232
503-731-4000
www.ohd.hr.state.or.us˜
E-mail: ohd.info@state.or.us

Pennsylvania
Pennsylvania Department of
Health
P.O. Box 90
Health & Welfare Building
Harrisburg, PA 17108
800-692-7254
www.health.state.pa.us
E-mail: webmaster@
heath.state.pa.us

Rhode Island
Rhode Island Department of
Health
3 Capitol Hill
Providence, RI 02908
401-222-2231
Fax: 401-222-6548
TTY: 800-745-5555
www.health.state.ri.us/

E-mail: library@health.
state.ri.us

South Carolina
South Carolina Department of
Health & Environmental
Control
2600 Bull Street
Columbia, SC 29201
803-898-3432
www.state.sc.us/dhec/
E-mail: menchima@
columb29.dhec.state.sc.us

South Dakota
South Dakota Department of
Health
Health Building
600 East Capitol
Pierre, SD 57501-2563
800-738-2301
Fax: 605-773-5683
www.state.sd.us/state/executiv
e/ doh/doh.html
E-mail: Info@doh.state.sd.us

Tennessee
Tennessee Department of
Health
425 5th Avenue North
Nashville, TN 37247
615-741-3111
www.state.tn.us/health
E-mail: DDenton@mail.
state.tn.us

Texas
Texas Department of Health
1100 West 49th Street

Austin, TX 78756-3199
512-458-7111
www.tdh.texas.gov/

Utah
Utah Department of Health
P.O. Box 1010
Salt Lake City, UT 84114-
1010
801-538-5101
http://hlunix.ex.state.ut.us/
E-mail: pwightma@doh.
state.ut.us

Vermont
Vermont Department of Health
108 Cherry Street
Burlington, VT 05402-0070
800-464-4343
Fax: 802-863-7475
www.state.vt.us/health

Virginia
Virginia Department of Health
Main Street Station
Richmond, VA 23219
804-786-5916
Fax: 804-371-4110
www.vdh.state.va.us/
E-mail: rnash@vdh.state.va.us

Washington
Washington State Department
of Health
1112 SE Quince Street
P.O. Box 47890
Olympia, WA 98504-7890

360-236-4010
www.doh.wa.gov/
E-mail: gkm0303@
doh.wa.gov

West Virginia
West Virginia Bureau for
Public Health
Building 3, Room 518
State Capitol Complex
Charelston, WV 25305
304-228-2971
Fax: 304-558-1035
http://wvbph.marshall.edu

Wisconsin
Wisconsin Department of
Health & Family Services
1 West Wilson Street
Madison, WI 53702-0007
608-266-1865
TTY: 608-267-7371
www.dhfs.state.wi.us

Wyoming
Wyoming Department of
Health
2300 Capitol Avenue
Mailing Address:
    117 Hathaway Building
    Cheyenne, WY 82002
307-777-7657
Fax: 307-777-7439
TTY: 307-777-5648
http://wdhfs.state.wy.us/wdh/
E-mail: wdh@missc.
state.wy.us

It's The Law: Care At Hospital Emergency Rooms

If you walk into an emergency room, do they have to treat you? Emergency rooms are now required by federal law to provide an initial screening to assess a patient's condition, which is designed to stop the automatic transfer of people unable to pay. Emergency rooms must also treat emergency situations until they are stabilized, then they can refer you to other hospitals or clinics for further treatment.

Emergency medicine encompasses the immediate decision making and action necessary to prevent death or any further disability for patients in health crises. It also includes interventions necessary to stabilize the patient, as well as short-term assessment of the patient's condition beyond the immediate life, limb, and disability threats.

If you feel you have been denied service, or received insufficient care, you should complain to your regional Health Care Financing Administration, who then will investigate your complaint. Because of the increase in the number of people who cannot afford or do not qualify for health insurance, many people wait to seek treatment until the situation becomes so terrible they end up in the emergency room. People are also using the emergency room as their primary care physician. By using some of your other options to receive health care, you can receive needed treatments sooner and from more appropriate sources.

Regional Health Care Financing Administration Offices

Region 1
JF Kennedy Federal Building
Government Center
Boston, MA 02203
617-565-1188

Region 2
26 Federal Plaza
JK Javits Federal Building
New York, NY 10278
212-264-4488

Region 3
The Public Ledger Building
150 S. Independence Mall
Suite 216
Philadelphia, PA 19106
215-861-4154

Region 4
61 Forsyth St., SW
Suite 4T20

Atlanta, GA 30303
404-562-7150

Region 5
105 W. Adams St.
Chicago, IL 60603
312-886-6432

Region 6
1301 Young St.
Dallas, TX 75202
214-767-6427

Region 7
601 E 12th St.
Federal Building
Kansas City, MO 64106
816-426-5233

Region 8
1961 Stout St.
Federal Office Building

Denver, CO 80294
303-844-2111

Region 9
75 Hawthorne St.
San Francisco, CA 94105
415-744-3502

Region 10
2201 Sixth Ave.
Blanchard Plaza
Mail Stop RX-40
Seattle, WA 98121
206-615-2306

Finding Doctors Who Work For Free! That's Right

Where are the free clinics in your area?
Do you have volunteer physician groups
near you? Your local medical society
can be a great resource to answer these
questions.

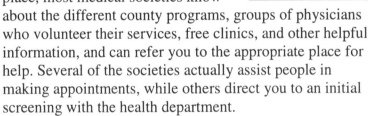

Although service varies from place to
place, most medical societies know
about the different county programs, groups of physicians
who volunteer their services, free clinics, and other helpful
information, and can refer you to the appropriate place for
help. Several of the societies actually assist people in
making appointments, while others direct you to an initial
screening with the health department.

According to a recent American Medical Association
survey, physicians average 6.6 hours per week of free or
reduced fee care. This amounts to $6.8 billion annually. To
find out if there are local opportunities available for you:

Contact:
Your State Medical Association for assistance in locating
your local medical society
(See listing below)

Medical Association Hotlines

Alabama
Medical Association of the
State of Alabama
19 S. Jackson St.
Montgomery, AL 36102
334-263-6441
www.masalink.org

Alaska
Alaska State Medical
Association
4107 Laurel St.
Anchorage, AK 99508
907-562-2662

Arizona
Arizona Medical Association
810 W. Bethany Home Rd.
Phoenix, AZ 85103
602-246-8901
www.armadoc.com

Arkansas
Arkansas Medical Society
P.O. Box 5776
Little Rock, AR 72205
501-224-8967
www.arkmed.org

California
California Medical Association
P.O. Box 7690
San Francisco, CA 94120
415-541-0900
www.cmanet.org

Colorado
Colorado Medical Society
P.O. Box 17550
Denver, CO 80217
303-779-5455

Connecticut
Connecticut State Medical
Society
160 St. Ronan St.
New Haven, CT 06511
203-865-0587

Delaware
Medical Society of Delaware
1925 Lovering Ave.
Wilmington, DE 19806
302-652-6512
www.medsocdel.org

District of Columbia
D.C. Medical Society
2215 M St., NW
Washington, DC 20037
202-466-1800

Florida
Florida Medical Association
760 Riverside Ave.
P.O. Box 2411
Jacksonville, FL 32204
800-762-0233
904-356-1571
http://flmed.net

Georgia
Georgia Medical Association
938 Peachtree St., NE
Atlanta, GA 30309
404-876-7535
www.mag.org

Hawaii
Hawaii Medical Association
1360 S. Bevetania
Honolulu, HI 96814
808-536-7702

Idaho
Idaho Medical Association
P.O. Box 2668
Boise, ID 83701
208-344-7888
www.idmed.org

Illinois
Illinois Medical Society
20 N. Michigan Ave.
Suite 700
Chicago, IL 60602
800-782-ISMS
312-782-1654
www.isms.org

Indiana
Indiana State Medical
Association
322 Canal Walk
Indianapolis, IN 46202
317-261-2060
www.ismanet.org

Iowa
Iowa Medical Society
1001 Grand Ave.
W. Des Moines, IA 50265
515-223-1401
www.iowamedicalsociety.org

Kansas
Kansas Medical Society
623 SW 10th Ave.
Topeka, KS 66612
913-235-2383
www.inlandnet.net/~ksmedsoc
/kms.html

Kentucky
Kentucky Medical Association
4965 US Hwy. 42, Suite 2000
Louisville, KY 40222
502-426-6200
www.kyma.org

Louisiana
Louisiana State Medical
Society
6767 Perkins
Baton Rouge, LA 70808
504-763-8500
www.lsms.org

Maine
Maine Medical Association
P.O. Box 190
Manchester, ME 04351
207-622-3374
www.mainemed.com

Maryland
Maryland Medical Society
1211 Cathedral St.
Baltimore, MD 21201
410-539-0872
www.medchi.org

Massachusetts
Massachusetts Medical Society
860 Winter St.
Waltham, MA 02451
800-322-2303
781-893-4610
www.massmed.org

Michigan
Michigan Medical Society
120 W. Saginaw St.
E. Lansing, MI 48823
517-337-1351
www.msms.org

Minnesota
Minnesota Medical
Association
Suite 300
3433 Broadway St. NW
Minneapolis, MN 55413
612-378-1875
www.mnmed.org

Mississippi
Mississippi Medical
Association
P.O. Box 5229
Jackson, MS 39296
601-354-5433
www.msmed.org

Missouri
Missouri Medical Association
113 Madison St.
P.O. Box 1028
Jefferson, MO 65102
573-636-5151
www.msma.org

Montana
Montana Medical Association
2021 11th Ave.
Suite #1
Helena, MT 59601
406-443-4000
www.montanamedical.org

Nebraska
Nebraska Medical Association
233 S. 13th St.
Suite #1512
Lincoln, NE 68508
402-474-4472
www.nebmed.org

Nevada
Nevada Medical Association
3660 Baker West #3101
Reno, NV 89509
775-825-6788
www.nsmadocs.org

New Hampshire
New Hampshire Medical
Society
7 North State St.
Concord, NH 03301
603-224-1909

New Jersey
New Jersey Medical Society
2 Princess Rd.
Lawrenceville, NJ 08648
609-896-1766
http://msnj.org

New Mexico
New Mexico Medical Society
7770 Jefferson NE
Suite #400
Albuquerque, NM 87109
505-828-0237
www.nmms.org/nmms

New York
New York Medical Society
420 Lakeville Rd.
Lakesuccess, NY 11042
516-488-6100

North Carolina
North Carolina Medical
Society Alliance
P.O. Box 27167
Raleigh, NC 27611
919-833-3836
www.ncmsalliance.org

North Dakota
North Dakota Medical
Association
P.O. Box 1198
Bismarck, ND 58502
701-223-9475
www.ndmed.com

Ohio
Ohio State Medical
Association
1500 Lake Shore Dr.
Columbus, OH 43017
614-486-2401

Oklahoma
Oklahoma State Medical
Association
601 NW Expressway
Oklahoma City, OK 73118
405-843-9571
www.osmaonline.org

Oregon
Oregon State Medical
Association
5210 South Corbett
Portland, OR 97201
503-226-1555
www.ormedassoc.org

Pennsylvania
Pennsylvania State Medical
Society
777 E. Park Dr.
P.O. Box 8820
Harrisburg, PA 17105
717-558-7750
www.pamedsoc.org

Rhode Island
Rhode Island State Medical
Society
106 Francis St.

Providence, RI 02903
401-331-3207

South Carolina
South Carolina State Medical
Association
P.O. Box 11188
Columbia, SC 29211
800-327-1021
803-798-6207
www.scmanet.org

South Dakota
South Dakota State Medical
Association
1323 S. Minnesota Ave.
Sioux Falls, SD 57105
605-336-1965

Tennessee
Tennessee State Medical
Association
P.O. Box 120909
Nashville, TN 37212
615-385-2100
www.medwire.org

Texas
Texas State Medical
Association
401 W. 15th St.
Austin, TX 78701
512-370-1300
www.texmed.org

Utah
Utah State Medical
Association
540 East 500 South

Salt Lake City, UT 84102
801-355-7477
www.xmission.com/~utahmed/
index.html

Vermont
Vermont State Medical
Association
Box 1457
Montpelier, VT 05601
802-223-7898

Virginia
Medical Society of Virginia
4205 Dover Rd.
Richmond, VA 23221
804-353-2721
www.msv.org

Washington
Washington State Medical
Association
2033 6th Ave., Suite 900
Seattle, WA 98121
800-552-0612
206-441-9762
www.wsma.org

West Virginia
West Virginia State Medical
Association
4307 MacCorkle Ave., SE
Charleston, WV 25304
304-925-0342
www.wvsma.com

Wisconsin
Wisconsin State Medical
Association

P.O. Box 1109
Madison, WI 53701
800-362-9080
608-257-6781
www.wismed.com

Wyoming
Wyoming State Medical
Association
P.O. Drawer 4009
Cheyenne, WY 82003
307-635-2424

Free and Low Cost Dental and Vision Care

Discounts On Dental And Vision Care

If you live near a university that has a dental or optometry school, then you may be in luck. Many of these schools offer reduced fee services for dental care or vision screening. You will receive treatment from students, but they will be supervised by some of the best people in the field.

These schools also often conduct research studies, so you if you qualify, you may be able to receive treatment for free. My 11-year-old daughter gets glasses, contacts, plus free contact solution for three years, because she is part of a study on nearsightedness in children. Not a bad deal! To locate schools near you, you can contact American Association of Dental Schools, 1625 Massachusetts Ave., NW, Suite 60, Washington, DC 20036; 202-667-9433; {www.aads.jhu.edu}. You can also contact American Optometric Association, 243 N. Lindbergh Blvd., St. Louis, MO 63141; 314-991-4100; {www.aoanet.org}.

Free Guide Dogs and Training to Help the Blind

Since 1946, the Guide Dog Foundation for the Blind, Inc. has provided guide dogs free of charge to blind people who seek enhanced mobility and independence.

To qualify for admission to this program, you must be: legally blind, in good physical and mental health, at least high school age, able to provide adequate housing and care for the dog, in need of the dog for mobility purposes.

FREE GUIDE DOGS FOR VISUALLY IMPAIRED

The Eye Dog Foundation is a non profit organization, whose mission is to provide trained guide dogs to visually impaired individuals, free of charge. The Foundation trains German Shepherds exclusively. Instruction, room and board, as well as the dog and related equipment are given free of charge. You can fill out the application form on the web site, or contact: The Eye Dog Foundation, Headquarters: 211 S. Montclair St., Bakersfield, CA 93309-3165; 661-831-1333; 800-393-3641; Fax: 661-831-0681; {E-mail: eyedog@lightspeed.net}; {www.eyedogfoundation.org/application.html}.

Contact: The Guide Dog Foundation For The Blind, Inc., 371 East Jericho Tpke, Smithtown, NY 11787-2976; 516-265-2121; Fax: 516-361-5192; 800-548-4337; {www.guidedog.org/getdox.htm}.

SIGHTLESS GET FREE SEEING EYE DOGS, TRAINING, TRAVEL AND AIR FARE

Pilot Dogs gives its trained animals to the blind at absolutely no charge. They also include four weeks of training in using the dog and will pay for room and board, all equipment, and round trip transportation. For more information, contact:

✻ *Pilot Dogs, Inc.*, 625 West Town Street, Columbus, OH 43215; 614-221-6367; fax: 614-221-1577; {www.pilotdogs.org/index.shtml}.

✻ *Southeastern Guide Dogs, Inc.*, 4210 77th St., East, Palmetto, FL 34221; 941-729-5665; Fax: 941-729-6646; {www.guidedogs.org}, {E-mail: SEGD@ bhip.infi.net}.

Free Eye Care

If you or someone you love needs eye care, but cannot afford it, the following organizations can help:

♥ For those 65 and older: *National Eye Care Project*, American Academy of Ophthalmology (AAO), P.O Box 429098, San Francisco, CA 94142; 415-561-8500; 800-222-3937; {www.eyenet.org}.

♥ For low-income families and children, applications are accepted on a first come-first serve basis in January with treatment following later in the year: *VISION USA*, American Optometric Association, 243 North Linbergh Blvd., St. Louis, MO 63141; 314-991-4100; 800-766-4466; {www.aoanet.org}.

♥ *Lions Clubs International*, 300 22nd St., Oak Brook, IL 60523; 630-571-5466; {www.lionsclubs.org}.

♥ *Glaucoma 2001*, American Academy of Ophthalmology (AAO), P.O Box 429098, San Francisco, CA 94142; 415-561-8500; 800-391-EYES; {www.eyenet.org}.

Free Eyeglasses, Cornea Transplants, and Glaucoma Screenings

Each year Lions Clubs around the country provide 600,000 free professional glaucoma screenings, perform 25,000 cornea transplants, collect over 3 million pairs of glasses, and provide thousands with free quality eye care. Services are provided based on need, and programs and services can be developed according to specific community needs. Lions Clubs conduct Hometown Day that brings people to Lenscrafters for eye exams and eyeglasses free of charge.

Consult your telephone directory for a Lions Club in your area or contact: Lions Club International, 300 22nd St., Oak Brook, IL 60523; 630-571-5466; Fax: 630-571-5735; {www.lionsclubs.org}.

Free Dental Care for People With Severe Disabilities

The United Cerebral Palsy Association of King-Snohomish Counties Therapeutic Services Northwest (TSN) has a Dental Clinic that provides specialized, hard-to-find dental care services to people with severe disabilities. The Dental Clinic is staffed by 16 volunteer dentists and four dental hygienists. If you don't live in this area, contact the office below or your local Multiple Sclerosis Society to see if similar services are available near you. Contact: Therapeutic Services Northwest, 4200 Stone Way Avenue North, Seattle, WA 98103; 206-633-6725; {E-mail: mikeh@ucpks.org}; {www.ucpks.org/tsn/tsn.html}.

$1,300 Worth Of Dental Care For Seniors and Disabled

The National Foundation of Dentistry for the Handicapped started the Donated Dental Services program to help disabled and elderly persons who are low-income by matching them with volunteer dentists. Homeless and mentally ill people are also helped.

Volunteer dentists agree to treat one or two people each year with dental problems, and dental laboratories that make dentures, crowns, and bridges also donate services. The program now serves over 500 people each year with each patient receiving an average of $1,300 worth of services. In some areas of the country, Dental House Call projects have been started where dentists will come to homes or centers to provide dental care.

To learn where services are located in your area, contact National Foundation of Dentistry for the Handicapped,

1800 15th St., Unit 100, Denver, CO 80202; 303-534-5360, Fax: 303-534-5290.

Free Dental Services For Children

The SmileMobile is a program of free or low-cost dental services for children from low-income families in Washington State. The SmileMobile is a modern dental office on wheels that brings dental services — at little or no charge — directly to children from low-income families who otherwise may not have access to dental care. It features three dental chairs and an X-ray machine.

To see the SmileMobile's schedule for the year, go to the Web site and click on: SmileMobile Schedule. If you don't live in this area, contact your local state department of health listed in your state capital for similar facilities in your area. Contact: The SmileMobile Project Manager: Jo Marrapodi, 206-517-6303; 800-367-4104; {E-mail: jmarrapodi@ddpwa.com}; or the Washington Dental Foundation, P.O. Box 75688, Seattle, WA 98125; 206-528-2331; 800-367-4104; {E-mail: foundation@ddpwa.com}; {www.ddpwa.com/comserv.htm#Foundation}.

Free and Low-Cost Dental Care

Don't let your teeth fall out just because you can't afford to go to a dentist. There are hundreds of programs across the country that offer free and low-cost dental care for seniors and practically anyone else who needs it, *often regardless of your income level.* If you know where and when to look, you may be able to get:

- free or low-cost dentures and repairs,
- automatic senior discounts of 15% to 80%,
- free at-home dental care if you can't get out,
- free dental implants by the best doctors in the world.

Most health insurance plans don't include dental coverage, and this means people often go without regular dental care simply because they think they can't afford it. But you may not be aware of the hundreds of programs that are designed for people like you — programs that actually require that you *don't* have dental insurance so that you can qualify to receive free or largely discounted dental care.

Here are some general examples of the kinds of programs funded all across the country:

Dental Care for the Elderly

You'll find that most states have special programs just for the elderly, especially those who have trouble finding money to pay for dental care on a limited income. Often dentists donate their time and services to make sure the elderly are taken care of. See the state-by-state listing on page 146.

Dental Schools for Everyone

The best-kept secrets about low-cost dental care are the 53 dental schools across the country. They offer quality dental care at a fraction of the cost of private dentists. Many will even set up a repayment plan for you if you can't afford to pay the bill.

Also, researchers at many dental schools receive big money from the federal government to do cutting edge dental research, and these researchers often need patients to work on for free. Be sure to ask about any clinical research underway at the dental school nearest you. See state-by-state listing on page 146.

Free and Low Cost Dental Clinics

Many state and local health departments support dental clinics that offer their services for free or on a sliding fee scale basis. Services are usually limited to those with limited income or those with special needs. See state-by-state listing on page 146.

Free Dental Care For Children

Almost every state runs some kind of dental care program to make sure that kids keep their teeth in good shape. Many of these programs offer their services for free or at huge discounts based upon your 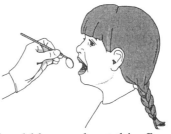 ability to pay. Your grandkids should know about this. See state-by-state listing on page 146.

Dental Care for Disabled and Handicapped

There are special programs just for those with mental or physical disabilities, including those with mental retardation, cerebral palsy, multiple sclerosis, and much more.

Many states also have special programs that offer free care for children born with cleft palates. See the state-by-state listing on page 146.

Free Tooth Implants and Impacted Molar Removal

These are just two of the many subjects that top dental researchers are studying at the National Institute of Dental Research which is part of the National Institutes of Health in Bethesda, Maryland. Also underway are studies on facial pain, taste disorders, herpes simplex, and dry mouth conditions.

Patients who participate in these clinical trials receive their dental care during that period free of charge. For information about the clinical studies program at the National Institutes of Health, you or your doctor can contact: Clinical Center, National Institutes of Health, Bldg. 10, 10 Center Dr., Bethesda, MD 20892, 301-496-2563, or the Patient Recruitment and Referral Center, Bldg. 61, 10 Cloister Ct., Bethesda, MD 20892; 301-402-6481; 800-411-1222; {www.cc.nih.gov}.

Dentists Who Get Government Grants to do Work for Free

Washington is not the only place where doctors receive government grants to conduct dental research and treat patients for free. Each year hundreds of dental schools and other dental research facilities around the country receive money to work on everything from gum disease to denture satisfaction.

You can contact the following office to receive information about on-going or up-coming dental research in your area.

National Institute of Dental Research
Research Data and Management
Information Section
45 Center Dr., Room 4AF-19, MSC 2190
Bethesda, MD 20892-2290
301-496-4261
www.nidr.nih.gov

Another method of finding these doctors is by contacting the "Dental Schools" in the state-by-state listing on page 146. Dental schools normally receive a good portion of available research.

Dental Societies — Dentists Who Volunteer

Each state's Dental Society keeps track of free and low-cost dental programs in their state, so it's a good idea to call them if you have any questions or if you're interested in learning about any new dental programs that start up.

Some Dental Societies also act as a clearinghouse for identifying dentists who volunteer their services to those facing emergencies or those who have other special problems. See the state-by-state listing on page 146.

Free Dentures for Seniors

Don't sit around with false teeth that keep falling out when you eat or hurt so badly that you can't keep them in your mouth. Many states have discount denture programs where you can receive big savings on false teeth, no matter what your age. See the state-by-state listing on page 146.

Dentists on Wheels

If you have trouble getting around because of a handicap or other infirmity, some states, like Illinois, Arizona, Missouri, New Jersey, and Colorado have mobile dental vans that will actually come to your home or nursing home and provide you with dental care right there on the spot. See the state-by-state listing on page 146.

State-by-State Listing

Alabama
Dental Programs
Department of Public Health
Dental Health Division
P.O. Box 303017
Montgomery, AL 36130
334-206-5673
www.alatubhealth.org
Call your nearest Community Health Center or Clinic for information on reduced fees for dental care. Usually clinics offer a sliding fee scale- qualifications vary. For example, some clinics will treat only children and senior citizens. They can help you find a doctor through Donated Dental Services.

Dental School
School of Dentistry
University of Alabama
1919 Seventh Ave., South
Birmingham, AL 35394
205-934-3000
205-934-4546 (children)
Annual patient visits: 49,617.

Dental Society
Alabama Dental Association
836 Washington Ave.
Montgomery, AL 36104-3893
334-265-1684
The Dental Society can help you find a dentist through Donated Dental
Services.

Donated Dental Services
P.O. Box 231403
Montgomery, AL 36123-1403
334-834-1114
They help qualified seniors locate dentists who will offer dental care at
no cost.

Poarch Creek Indian Health Dept.
5811 Jack Springs Rd.
Atmore, AL 36502
334-368-8630/Indians only
They provide free dental services to members of federally recognized
tribes.

Mostellar Dental Center
525 North Wintzell Ave.
Bayou La Batre, AL 36509
334-824-2347

Jefferson County Health Dept.
1400 6th Ave. South
Birmingham, AL 35202
205-933-9110
The Health Department offers discounts for adults over 62, based on
your social security income.

The Children's Hospital
1600 7th Ave. South
Birmingham, AL 35233-1785
205-934-3000
Emer. pts. at hosp.

UAB School Dentistry Dental Cl.
University Station
1919 7th Ave. South
Birmingham, AL 35294
205-934-4011

Houston County Health Dept.
301 West Lafayette St.
Dothan, AL 36301
334-712-1542

West AL Health Service
E.A. Maddos Center
607 Wilson Ave.
P.O. Box 599
Eutaw, AL 35462
205-372-9225

West AL Health Care Center
2209 W. Main St.
P.O. Box 47
Greensboro, AL 36744
334-624-0159
They use a sliding fee scale to determine cost. Bring proof of income.

Franklin Memorial Primary Care Center
1303 Dr. Martin Luther King Ave.
Mobile, AL 36603
334-432-4117

Mobile County Health Dept.
251 N. Bayou
Mobile, AL 36652
334-690-8140
They treat children under 21. Low rates are available.

Lister Hill Health Center
1000 Adams Ave.
Montgomery, AL 36104

334-263-2301
They use a sliding fee scale, based on the size of your family and your income. $24.50 first visit; $15.50 second visit; discounts on every service afterward.

Montgomery Primary Health Care
3060 Mobile Hwy.
Montgomery, AL 36108
334-293-6670
They use a sliding fee scale, based on your income.

Henderson (Charles) Child Health Center
P.O. Box 928
Troy, AL 36081
334-566-7600/Pts. 13 & under

West AL Dist. Health Dept.
1101 Jackson Ave.
P.O. Box 2789
Tuscaloosa, AL 35403
205-391-5415/children only

Whatley (Maud) Health Center
2731 M.L. King, Jr. Blvd.
P.O. Box 2400
Tuscaloosa, AL 35403
205-758-6647

Health Departments

Central AL/Complete Health/Midway Clinic
203 W. Lee St.
Tuskegee Inst., AL 36087
334-727-7488

Uniontown Health Services
330 Old Hamburg Rd.
Uniontown, AL 36786
334-628-2661
Discounts are based on your income.

Alaska
Dental Programs
Social Services
Department of Public Health
P.O. Box 110612
Juneau, AL 99811-0612
907-465-8628
Limited dental care is available. Call your Community Health Center to
get information about whether they offer dental. There are several
Indian dental health clinics. Many of these clinics operate on a sliding
fee scale.

Anchorage Neighborhood Health Center
1217 East 10th Ave.
Anchorage, AK 99501
907-257-4600
Call or write Anchorage Neighborhood Health Center to get
information on reduced-fee dental services for adults and children. A
sliding fee scale based on income is available.

Senior Citizen Discounts
Anchorage Dental Society
3400 Spenard Rd., Suite 10
Anchorage, AK 99503
907-279-9144
There are no special programs through the Dental Society; however,
they do keep a list of referrals of dentists who will give discounts to
senior citizens and are available for emergency dental help.

Dental Society
Alaska Dental Society
3305 Arctic Blvd. #102
Anchorage, AK 99503
907-563-3003

Arizona
Dental Programs
Department of Health Services
Office of Oral Health
1740 West Adams St., Room 10

Phoenix, AZ 85007
602-542-1866
www.hs.state.az.us\cfhs\ooh\
Low cost dental services are available through various Dental Clinics. Individuals must contact the Office of Dental Health to get eligibility requirements. They provide referrals to specific dentists.

Fluoride Mouth Rinse and Sealant Programs are also available through the public schools. Some Indian Health Centers offer dental for tribal members.

McDowell Dental Clinic
125 W. McDowell St.
Phoenix, AZ 85003
602-224-0030
The McDowell Clinic provides basic dental work for individuals with HIV. The Area on Aging has contracted with the Office of Dental Health to provide dental services using portable equipment set up at local Senior Centers.

Dental Society
Arizona State Dental Association
4131 N. 36th St.
Phoenix, AZ 85018-4761
602-957-4777
www.azda.org

Arkansas
Dental Programs
Department of Health
Dental Division
5800 West 10th St.
Little Rock, AR 72204
501-661-2279
Limited dental care is available. Three clinics offer dental care at a reduced fee. Low-income is a major factor in determining eligibility. They will also see anyone who is in severe pain due to an emergency. All hospitals keep a listing of dentists who volunteer to treat emergencies. No special programs are available for handicapped or elderly.

Dental Society
Arkansas State Dental Association
2501 Crestwood Dr., Suite 205
N. Little Rock, AR 72216
501-771-7650
http://www.dental.asda.org

California
Dental Programs
Health Services Department
Oral Health
714 P St., Room 550
Sacramento, CA 95814
916-654-0348
www.dhs.cahwnet.org/org.pcfh\pcrh\index.htm
Very limited dental care is available through some local Health Centers
or Clinics on a sliding fee scale based on income. You'll have to call
each individually to see if dental is available.

Senior-Dent
California Dental Association
1201 K Street Mall
P.O. Box 13749
Sacramento, CA 95853
916-443-0505
800-736-7071 (CA only)
www.cda.org
The *Senior-Dent Program* offers dental care at reduced fees to all
qualified senior citizens. To qualify you must meet three eligibility
requirements: 1) be 60 or older; 2) have an annual income of $20,000
or less; 3) not be receiving dental benefits from Denti-Cal or a dental
insurance plan. Participating dentists offer at least a 15% discount. Call
for additional information and a participating dentist.

Dental Schools
School of Dentistry
University of California, San Francisco
707 Parnassus Ave.
San Francisco, CA 94143

415-476-1891
www.edu.ucsf
Annual patient visits: 52,017.

School of Dentistry
University of California, Los Angeles
School of Dentistry
Box 951668
10833 LeConte Ave.
Los Angeles, CA 90095-1668
310-206-3904, to become a new patient, or
310-825-2337
Annual patient visits: 75,000.

School of Dentistry
University of Southern California
925 W. 34th St.
Los Angeles, CA 90089-0641
213-740-2800
www.usc.edu
Annual patient visits: 31,000.

Dental Society
California Dental Association
P.O. Box 13749
Sacramento, CA 95853-4749
916-443-0505
http://www.cda.org

Colorado
Dental Programs
Department of Health
Family and Community Health Services
Dentistry
4300 Cherry Creek Dr., South, A4
Denver, CO 80222
303-692-2360
www.cdthe.state.co.us

Call your local Health Department or Clinic to get information about reduced fee dental care. When dental care is offered, it is usually on a sliding fee scale based on income. Some will treat both children and adults. The Old Age Pension Dental Program is a special program for seniors.

Dental Care for the Handicapped
Donated Dental Services
1800 15th St., Suite 100
Denver, CO 80202
303-534-5360
Certain handicapped individuals who meet the following guidelines may be eligible to receive free or low-cost dental care. Patients must meet the following guidelines: 1) mentally or physically disabled including mental retardation, cerebral palsy, MS, or other disabilities; 2) advanced age; 3) Colorado resident; 4) each patient is screened to find those in most need; limited income due to handicap is a major factor. Call for additional information.

Old Age Pension Dental Program
Colorado Dept. of Public Health and Oral Health Program
4300 Cherry Creek Dr. South
Denver, CO 80246-1530
303-692-2360
The *Old Age Pension Dental Program* is a cooperative effort to provide dental services to a segment of elderly that have an urgent need. Most services offered are denture-related. Individuals must be low income and at least 60 years old. Call to get additional information. You must be receiving a Colorado old age pension first.

Community Health Center
Dental Program
722 S. Wahsatch
Colorado Springs, CO 80903
719-475-0783
The Community Health Center, Dental Program provides dental care on a sliding fee scale. Call for more information. They are also a medical aid clinic for seniors and adults.

Kids In Need of Dentistry
2465 S. Downing, Suite 207
Denver, CO 80210
303-733-3710
Call KIND at this number for a
referral to one of their five locations
nearest you. This program is for
children from the ages of newborn to 18
years of age only. They do not take
Medicaid.

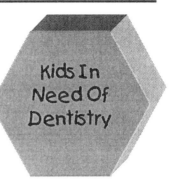

Salud Clinic
6075 Parkway Dr., Suite 160
Commerce City, CO 80022
303-286-8900
The Salud Clinic accepts both children and adult patients, and fees are
based on a sliding scale. They offer a discount for seniors based on a
sliding fee scale.

Dental Society
Colorado Dental Association
3690 S. Yosemite Ave., Suite 100
Denver, CO 80237-1808
303-740-6900

Connecticut
Dental Programs
Department of Public Health
Dental Health Division
150 Washington St.
Hartford, CT 06106
860-509-7561, Dental Licensing Dept.
www.state.ct.us\dph\
Call your nearest Local Health Department or Clinic to find out
information about reduced fees for dental care. Most clinics offer a
sliding fee schedule and will accept Medicaid and insurance, though
low-income is usually a requirement. Handicap access is also available.
Preventive programs are run through the various public school systems
and nursing homes. Area dentists volunteer their services to provide

low-income elderly with reduced-fee dental care. The Department of Public Health does not provide referrals or dental care.

Dental School
School of Dental Medicine
University of Connecticut
263 Farmington Ave.
Farmington, CT 06032
860-679-3437
http://www.uchc.edu
Annual patient visits: 19,496

Dental Society
Connecticut Dental Association
62 Russ St.
Hartford, CT 06106-1589
860-278-5550
http://www.ctdental.org

Delaware
Dental Programs
Division of Public Health
William Center Dental Clinic
805 River Rd.
Dover, DE 19901
302-739-4755
Children in pain, as well as children on Medicaid, are treated. There is very limited reduced fee dental care available in Delaware; however, there are two clinics that treat children and adults on a sliding fee scale. Call 302-428-4850 to get additional information and qualifications.

Nemours Health Clinic
1801 Rockland Rd.
Wilmington, DE 19803
800-292-9538
302-651-4400
The Nemours Health Clinic offers a Dental Program for senior citizens over 65. There are no income requirements, so be sure to call for additional information. Reduced cost for dentures and visits.

Dental Society
Delaware Dental Society
1925 Lovering Ave.
Wilmington, DE 19806
302-654-4335

District of Columbia
Dental Programs
Department of Public Health
Dental Health Division
4130 Hunt Place, NE
Washington, DC 20019
202-727-0530
Low income is a major factor in determining eligibility for free and low-cost dental care through the DC government health division. They provide care, not referrals. They have OB/GYN and pediatrics. For more elderly care service, call the Benning Health Center, 202-645-4161. They provide cleaning, filling and more on a sliding scale based on your ability to pay.

Dental School
College of Dentistry
Howard University
600 W St., NW
Washington, DC 20059
202-806-0007
Annual patient visits:
128,886.

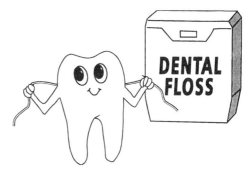

Dental Society
District of Columbia Dental
Society
502 C St., NE
Washington, DC 20002-5810
202-547-7613
www.dcdental.org
The Society will give referrals to clinics that offer low-cost dental care. There are no programs for the elderly.

Florida
Dental Programs
Department of Health and Rehabilitative Services
Public Health Dental Program
2020 Capital Circle
Tallahassee, FL 32399-1724
850-487-1911
Call your local County Health Department or Clinic for information on
low cost dental care. Clinics usually offer a sliding fee scale.
Qualifications vary and emphasis is on children. Guidelines are 200%
of poverty standards but offer sliding fee scale based on ability to pay.
They have a listing of health centers and dentists, and will refer you to
a dentist.

Dental School
College of Dentistry
University of Florida
1600 Archer Rd.
Gainesville, FL 32610
352-392-4261
www.dental.ufl.edu
Annual patient visits: 47,441.

Dental Society
Florida Dental Association
1111 E. Tennessee St.
Suite 102
Tallahassee, FL 32308
800-877-9922
http://www.floridadental.org

Georgia
Dental Programs
Department of Human Resources
Oral Health Section
Two Peachtree St., 6th Floor
Atlanta, GA 30303
404-657-2574
www.ph.dhr.state.ga.us/org/oralhealth.htm

Call your local Health Department or Clinic to get information on low-cost dental care. The oral health section will treat children, but will refer adults to low-cost dental programs. Low-income is a major factor in determining your eligibility. Fluoride and Sealant Programs are available through various public school systems. The Georgia Board of Dentistry has a list of voluntary dental services and can provide referrals.

Dental School
School of Dentistry
Medical College of Georgia
1459 Laney Walker Blvd.
Augusta, GA 30912
706-721-2696
www.mcg.edu
Annual patient visits: 3,444.

Dental Society
Georgia Dental Association
7000 Peachtree 3200, Bldg. 17
Atlanta, GA 30328
404-636-7553
http://www.godental.org
They can refer you to a dentist for reduced cost services.

Hawaii
Dental Programs
Department of Health
Dental Health Division
1700 Lanakila Ave., Room 202
Honolulu, HI 96817
808-832-5710
www.hawaii.gov/health
Dental care is available for very low-income individuals who are in the GAP Group, which includes children and adults. A sliding fee scale is used to determine what you pay based on your income. Dental care is also available for the mentally or physically handicapped, as well as homeless individuals. To be treated, you must meet certain criteria, which you can get by calling your local clinic.

Dental Society
Hawaii Dental Association
1000 Bishop St., Suite 805
Honolulu, HI 96813-4281
808-593-7956

Idaho
Dental Programs
Department of Health and Welfare
Dental Program
P.O. Box 83720
450 West State St., 1st Floor
Boise, ID 83720-0036
208-334-5966
www.idhw.state.id.us
Idaho has a limited dental care program for low-income individuals, but it is very limited for adults. Some restorative dental work is performed. Emergency service for women or children under the age of 21 is available. Call for eligibility requirements. Also, contact your nearest Community Health Center or Clinic to see if they offer dental assistance. Their fee scales are usually a sliding fee schedule, based on your ability to pay. *Preventive Programs* are offered through district health departments. Also, Senior Access for Boise residents offers low cost dental assistance. These programs are designed to help educate people on the importance of preventing dental problems before they occur.

Senior Care Program
Boise City/Ada County
3010 W. State St., Suite 120
Boise, ID 83703-5949
208-345-7783
The *Dental Access Program* helps low-income people receive assistance with the cost of dentures, denture repair, and extractions. Those eligible include: 1) Age 60 or older; 2) Residents of southwest Idaho; 3) Have limited or fixed income and no available resources to pay for dental work; 4) Must have a dental need that is denture related, 5) No Medicaid.

Dental Society
Idaho Dental Association
1220 W. Hays St.
Boise, ID 83702-5315
208-343-7543

Illinois
Dental Programs
Total Dent Program
Illinois Dental Society
P.O. Box 376
Springfield, IL 62705
800-252-2930 (IL only)
217-525-1406
www.idph.state.il.us
Call your local clinics or health centers to get information about
reduced-fee dental services. Income is a major factor used to determine
your eligibility, and sliding fee schedules are used based on your ability
to pay. Preventive programs, which will be expanding, are available for
children through the various school systems.

Total Dent Program
Illinois Dental Society
P.O. Box 376
Springfield, IL 62705
217-525-1406
http://www.isds.org
The *Total Dent Program* is designed to help low- or fixed-income
individuals receive needed dental care at a discount rate. To qualify,
you must meet ALL of the following requirements: 1) You cannot be
eligible for the Public Aide Dental Program or other dental insurance
coverage; 2) You must meet Title 20 income requirements; 3) You
must be willing to sign a form certifying the above. Dentists who
participate in this program offer a fee reduction of at least 20% to
participating Illinois residents. Call for additional information.

Denture Referral Service
Illinois Dental Society
P.O. Box 376

Springfield, IL 62705
217-523-8495
800-323-1743
The Illinois Retired Teachers Foundation sponsors the *Denture Referral Service* program, which provides dentures to eligible participants through volunteer dentists. Although you do NOT have to be a retired teacher to participate, you do need to fulfill the following requirements: 1) Resident of Illinois; 2) 65 years or older; 3) Have no public assistance or private dental insurance; 4) You must qualify for the Illinois *Circuit Breaker Program* which requires earnings of less than $14,000 per year.

Portable Dental Equipment
Illinois Dental Society
P.O. Box 376
Springfield, IL 62705-0376
217-525-1406
www.isds.org
In order to provide needed dental care for the homebound, elderly and physically and mentally handicapped, the Illinois State Dental Society maintains ten portable dental equipment units located throughout the state. Any licensed dentist in the state of Illinois may use the equipment to provide on-site dental care to these special individuals who meet the specified income and physical requirements.

Dental Schools
Dental School
Northwestern University
240 E. Huron, 1st Floor
Chicago, IL 60611
312-503-6837
www.nudc.nwu.edu
Annual patient visits: 96,044
This school has a geriatric clinic.

School of Dental Medicine
Southern Illinois University
2800 College Ave.
Building 263

Alton, IL 62002
618-474-7000
www.siue.edu
Annual patient visits: 33,258

College of Dentistry
University of Illinois
801 S. Paulina St.
Chicago, IL 60612
312-996-7558
http:\\dentistry.usc.edu\isdent
Annual patient visits: 70,510
This school also has a program for geriatrics. A doctor with an assistant
will visit nursing homes and retirement homes.

Dental Society
Illinois Dental Society
P.O. Box 376
Springfield, IL 62705-0376
217-525-1406
http://www.isds.org

Indiana
Dental Programs
Department of Public Health
Dental Health Division
2 N. Meridan St.
Indianapolis, IN 46204-3003
317-233-7417
www.isdh.state.in.us/
Call your local health center for more information. They can refer you
to local clinics that offer reduced rates for adults. They also organize
several preventive programs in schools.

Senior Smile Program
Dental Care for Senior Citizens
Indiana Dental Association
401 West Michigan St.
P.O. Box 2467

Indianapolis, IN 46206
317-634-2610
www.indental.org
Dental care at reduced fees is available at participating dentists to those
who meet the following guidelines: 1) 65 or older; 2) have no private
dental insurance nor federal, state or other dental health insurance; 3)
income no more than $10,000/single or $14,000 for married couples.
Call the Indiana Counsel on Aging at 317-254-5465 for more
information.

Donated Dental Services
Dental Care for Handicapped
P.O. Box 872
Indianapolis, IN 46206
317-631-6022
Participating dentists provide free
and low-cost dental care to
handicapped individuals who meet
the following guidelines: 1)
mentally or physically disabled
including mental retardation, cerebral

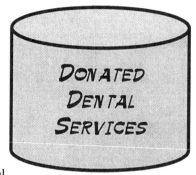

palsy, MS, or other disabilities; 2) live in Indiana; 3) each patient
screened to find those in most need. Limited income due to handicap is
a major factor in determining eligibility. Hours are Monday, Tuesday,
and Thursday, 9 a.m. to 4 p.m.

Dental School
School of Dentistry
Indiana University
1121 West Michigan St.
Indianapolis, IN 46202
317-274-7957
Annual patient visits: 58,495.
Clinic: 317-274-8111 (children)
            317-274-3547 (adults)

Dental Society
Indiana Dental Association
401 West Michigan St.

Suite 1000
P.O. Box 2467
Indianapolis, IN 46206-2467
317-634-2610
http://www.indental.org

Iowa
Dental Programs
Department of Public Health
Dental Division
321 East 12th St.
Lucas State Office Building
Des Moines, IA 50319-0075
515-281-5787
www.idph.state.ia.us
Call local Clinics or Health Centers to get information about reduced-fee dental services. A sliding fee schedule based on income is most often used, and most services are for children. Very limited adult care is available with low-income levels used to determine eligibility. Please call the clinics listed below for information.

Broadlawns Medical Center
Dental Clinic
1801 Hickham Rd.
Des Moines, IA 50314
515-282-2421

Des Moines Health Center
1111 Ninth St., Suite 190
Des Moines, IA 50314
515-244-9136

Siouxland Community Health Center
P.O. Box 2118
Sioux City, IA 51104-0118
712-252-2477

Community Health Care, Inc.
428 Western Ave.

Davenport, IA 52801
712-319-3222

Dental Health Center of East Central Iowa
855 A Ave., NE, Suite LL 1
Cedar Rapids, IA 52402
319-369-7730

Iowa Dental Elderly Access Program (IDEA)
Iowa Dental Association
505 Fifth Ave., Suite 333
Des Moines, IA 50309-2379
515-282-7250
This program makes dental services available to Iowa Senior Citizens
with limited financial means. Those eligible: 1) 65 or older; 2)
Residents of Iowa; 3) Income is 225% or less of the Federal income
poverty level; 4) Have no medical or dental insurance coverage for the
dental procedures being requested. Discounts off the dentists regular
fee will be made available and are determined on an individual basis in
consultation with a participating dentist. Call to get more information
and an application.

Dental School
College of Dentistry
University of Iowa
322 Dental Science Bldg.
Elliot Ave.
Iowa City, IA 52242-1001
319-335-7499
http://dentistry.vh.org/
Annual patient visits: 56,817.
Special care clinic for Geriatrics and Handicapped: (319) 335-7373

Dental Society
Iowa Dental Association
505 Fifth Ave., Suite 333
Des Moines, IA 50309-2379
515-282-7250

Kansas
Dental Programs
Department of Health and Environment
Dental Program
Attn: Dr. Corinne Miller
Landon State Office Bldg.
900 SW Jackson, Room 1051 South
Topeka, KS 66612
785-926-6215
www.kdhe.state.ks.us
A Health Clinic in Wichita offers reduced-fee dental services for
individuals with low income. A sliding fee scale is used. There is also a
Fluoride Rinse Program available in the public school systems where
needed. Dental care for children on Medicaid is available.

Senior Care Program
Kansas Dental Association
5200 SW Huntoon St.
Topeka, KS 66604-2398
800-432-3583
913-272-7360
Dental care at reduced fees is available by participating dentists to
those who meet the following guidelines: 1) 60 years or older; 2) have
no private, federal or state dental insurance; 3) income no more than
$10,000/single or $15,000 for married couples. Fees vary but are
reduced. Call for additional information.

Dental Society
Kansas Dental Association
5200 SW Huntoon St.
Topeka, KS 66604-2398
913-272-7360

Kentucky
Dental Programs
Department of Health
Dental Health Division
275 East Main St.
Frankfort, KY 40621

502-564-3246
www.csc.chs.chr.state.ky.us
Call your nearest Health Clinic for information on who offers free and
low-cost dental care. Income is a major factor used in determining
eligibility. There are three such programs now running in Kentucky.
All ages are treated using a sliding fee scale to determine ability to pay.

Jefferson County Dental
Park Duval Health Facility
1817 South 34th St.
Louisville, KY 40211
502-774-4401
Those eligible to participate in the dental care program at this facility
must meet the following guidelines: 1) Must be a resident of Jefferson
County; 2) Must meet low-income guidelines; 3) Must pay on a sliding
fee scale based on income level. Services include cleaning, dentures
and other services at reduced cost.

Kentucky Physicians Program
Kentucky Health Care Access Foundation
275 East Main St.
Frankfort, KY 40621
502-564-3246
www.csc.chs.chr.state.ky.us
Under the Kentucky Physicians Program, all dental work is done by
volunteer dentists. Those eligible to receive treatment include: 1)
Individuals with no insurance, no Medicaid and be within the Federal
Poverty Guidelines; 2) Must be registered as a program participant. The
first visit is free. Pharmacies donate medication based on need. Call to
get additional information

Denture Access Program
Kentucky Dental Association
1940 Princeton Dr.
Louisville, KY 40205-1873
502-459-5373
The Denture Access Program offers full dentures at a reduced rate.
There are no age requirements to participate. Call for additional
information and a referral to a participating dentist.

Dental Schools
College of Dentistry
University of Kentucky
800 Rose St.
Lexington, KY 40536
For appointments to the college clinic: 606-323-6525
www.mc.uky.edu/dentistry
Annual patient visits: 38,723.
The university has some programs for the elderly, and a few satellite
programs where they go to nursing homes.

University of Louisville
School of Dentistry
Louisville, KY 40292
502-852-5096 (adult)
502-852-5642 (children)
www.dental.louisville.edu
Annual patient visits: 65,914.

Dental Society
Kentucky Dental Association
1940 Princeton Dr.
Louisville, KY 40205-1873
502-459-5373

Louisiana
Dental Programs
Department of Public Health
Dental Health Division
200 Henry Clay Ave.
New Orleans, LA 70118
504-896-1337
The Dental Program offers reduced-rate dental care through your
nearest clinic. Louisiana State University offers dentures for those in
need, and also restorative work for those under 18 years of age that
receive Medicaid. This office also provides referrals for patients with
AIDS. For the 24-hour Emergency Dental Service, call 504-897-8250
for more information.

Donated Dental Services
Dental Care for Handicapped
NFDH-Louisiana
LSDU Dept. Pediatric Dentistry
1100 Florida Ave., Box 139
New Orleans, LA 70119-2799
504-948-6141
Certain handicapped individuals who meet the following guidelines can receive reduced-rate and free dental care through this programs: 1) mentally or physically disabled including mental retardation, cerebral palsy, MS, or other disabilities; 2) live in Louisiana; 3) each patient must be screened to find those in most need • limited income due to handicap is a major factor in determining eligibility.

Dental School
School of Dentistry
Louisiana State University
1100 Florida Ave.
New Orleans, LA 70119
504-619-8700
www.isusd.isumc.edu
Annual patient visits: 47,247.

Dental Society
Louisiana Dental Association
7833 Office Park Blvd.
Baton Rouge, LA 70809
225-926-1986
www.ladental.org

Maine
Dental Programs
Department of Human Services
Oral Health Program
Bureau of Health
11 State House Station #11
151 Capitol St.
Augusta, Maine 04333
207-287-3121

Call your nearest Community Health Center or Clinic for information on reduced fees for dental care. Usually fees are based on a sliding scale. Insurance is accepted. Both children and adults are eligible. *American Indian/Alaska Native Tribal Programs* offer direct and/or referral medical/dental services for registered members of federally recognized American Indian/Alaska Native Tribes. These are tribally-directed programs and may differ significantly in eligibility requirements and services.

Senior Dent Program
Maine Dental Association
P.O. Box 215
Association Dr.
Manchester, ME 04351
207-622-7900
The Senior Dent program offers comprehensive dental care to low-income elderly at reduced fees. Those eligible must: 1) be residents of Maine; 2) be 62 or older; 3) Have no

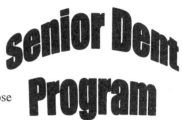

dental benefits under a private insurance plan or the Medicaid program; 4) Have an annual income that qualifies them for *Maine's Low Cost Drug Program*. Those eligible will receive at least a 15% discount from the usual and customary fees. Contact your local agency on aging.

Dental Society
Maine Dental Association
P.O. Box 215
Association Dr.
Manchester, ME 04351-0215
207-622-7900

Maryland
Dental Programs
Maryland State Health Department
Dental Health Division - Baltimore
201 West Preston St.
Baltimore, MD 21201-3046
410-767-5688

www.mdpublichealth.org
Under the Maryland Access to Care program, low-income individuals under 21 or over 65 years of age. The program offers reduced fee dental care. Fee schedule for care is based on ability to pay. Medicaid recipients also can receive free dental care when necessary through the health department. The Donated Dental Services program is also helpful, 410-964-1944.

Dental Care for Handicapped
Donated Dental Services
6450 Dobbin Rd.
Columbia, MD 21045-4744
410-964-1944
Certain handicapped individuals who meet the following guidelines may be eligible to receive free dental care: 1) mentally or physically disabled including mental retardation, cerebral palsy, MS, or other disabilities; 2) Maryland resident; 3)doctors volunteer to help people of all ages with a handicap, who are in need of dental care and cannot afford it. Limited income due to handicap is a major factor. Call Joey Holley, Unis Jaeger or Jessica Young for more information.

Dental School
Baltimore College of Dental Surgery
University of Maryland
666 W. Baltimore St.
Baltimore, MD 21201
410-706-5603
www.dental.umaryland.edu
Annual patient visits: 5,892.

Dental Society
Maryland Dental Association
6450 Dobbin Rd., Suite F
Columbia, MD 21045-5824
410-964-2880
http://www.msda.com
Referral service for physically or mentally handicapped people of any age to receive free dental care.

Massachusetts
Dental Programs
Department of Health and Hospitals
Community Dental Programs
1010 Massachusetts Ave.
Boston, MA 02118
617-534-4717
www.state.ma.us/dph
Eighteen Health Center Programs throughout Boston offer low-cost
dental care to Boston residents, usually on a sliding fee scale based on
your income. Requirements vary, so be sure to call to get additional
information. They will refer you to a suitable program. Some health
centers offer limited dental for residents of Eastern Massachusetts.
They also operate an HIV referral and treatment program.

Developmentally Disabled Program
250 Washington St.
Boston, MA 02108-4619
617-624-0606
This program offers dental care for individuals who are mentally
retarded, have cerebral palsy, and those who are physically disabled.
Call for additional information.

Dentistry for All
Massachusetts Dental Society
83 Speen St.
Natick, MA 07160
508-651-7511
www.massdental.org
The *Dentistry for All Program* is a reduced-fee dental program for
qualified low-income individuals who have no insurance or Medicaid
of any kind. Call to get additional information. You must fill out an
application to be approved for this program.

Dental Schools
Harvard School of Dental Medicine
188 Longwood Ave.
Boston, MA 02115
617-432-1423

Annual patient visits: 32,000.
30,000 faculty; 2,000 teaching practices

School of Graduate Dentistry
Boston University
100 E. Newton St.
Boston, MA 02118
617-638-4671
Annual patient visits: 34,324.

School of Dental Medicine
Tufts University
One Kneeland St.
Boston, MA 02111
617-636-6828
Annual patient visits: 87,522.

Dental Society
Massachusetts Dental Society
83 Speen St.
Natick, MA 01760-4144
508-651-7511
http://www.massdental.org

Michigan
Dental Programs
Department of Public Health
Dental Health Division
3423 N. Martin Luther King Jr., Blvd.
P.O. Box 30195
Lansing, MI 48909
517-335-8898
www.mdca.state.mi.us
There are no direct dental services through the State Health
Department. You must call your local or county health department for
participating clinics and qualifications.

Senior Dent Program
Michigan Dental Association

230 North Washington Square, Suite 208
Lansing, MI 48933
517-372-9070
800-589-2632 (MI only)
www.michigandental.org
Dental care at reduced fees are available to senior citizens who meet
the following guidelines: 1) 65 or older; 2) have no private dental
insurance nor federal, state or other dental health insurance; 3) meet
certain low-income requirements. Fees vary, and procedures covered
include all types of dental care except full dentures. Over 800 dentists
in Michigan participate.

Dental Schools
School of Dentistry
University of Detroit-Mercy
2985 E. Jefferson Ave.
Detroit, MI 48207
313-745-4795
www.udmercy.edu
Annual patient visits: 47,152.

School of Dentistry
University of Michigan
1011 North University
Ann Arbor, MI 48109-1078
734-763-6933
Annual patient visits: 88,035.

Dental Society
Michigan Dental Association
230 Washington Square North, Suite 208
Lansing, MI 48933-1392
517-372-9070
http://www.michigandental.org

Minnesota
Dental Programs
State Health Department
Dental Division

717 Delaware Street SE
Minneapolis, MN 55440
651-281-9895
www.health.state.mi.us
Call your Local Health Clinic to find out who offers dental care on a
reduced-fee scale. Also contact "First Call for Help," 612-224-1133, for
additional information on clinics. Low-income is a major factor in
determining eligibility.

Senior Partners Care Dental Program
Minnesota Senior Federation
Iris Park Place
1885 University Ave. W.
Suite 190
St. Paul, MN 55104
800-365-8765
651-642-1398
www.mnseniors.org
The *Senior Partners Care Dental Program* is designed to bridge the
Medicare gap, with participating dentists agreeing to provide a 20%
discount for all professional dental services. Those eligible must: 1)
join the Minnesota Senior Foundation; 2) be 55 or older and retired; 3)
meet the annual income criteria of less than 200% of poverty
($1290/single or $1726/ couple per month in 1995); 4) have less than
$21,000 in liquid assets (cash savings, stocks, CDs, etc.); 5) NOT be a
part of any dental plan.

Wilder Senior Dental Program
516 Humboldt Ave.
St. Paul, MN 55107
651-220-1807
This program is for those 65 years old and older. It is not income-based
and they will set up payment plans.

Dental School
School of Dentistry
University of Minnesota
515 SE Delaware St.
Minneapolis, MN 55455

612-626-0171
www.umn.edu/dental
Call main number to make all appointments
Annual patient visits: 34,078

Dental Society
Minnesota Dental Association
2236 Marshall Ave.
St. Paul, MN 55104-5792
651-646-7454
http://www.mndental.org

Mississippi
Dental Programs
Low-Cost Denture Referral Program
Mississippi Dental Association
2630 Ridgewood Rd.
Jackson, MS 39216-4920
601-982-0442
Under this denture program, patients and
dentists negotiate the reduced cost for
services based on the patients' ability to
pay. Call for additional information.

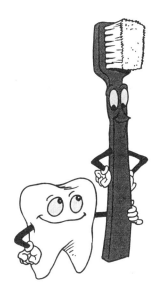

Dental School
School of Dentistry
University of Mississippi
2500 North State St.
Jackson, MS 39216
601-984-6155
www.ums.med.edu
Annual patient visits: 15,097.

Dental Society
Mississippi Dental Association
2630 Ridgewood Rd.
Jackson, MS 39216-4920
601-982-0442

Missouri
Dental Programs
Department of Public Health
Dental Health Division
930 Wildwood
P.O. Box 570
Jefferson City, MO 65109
573-751-6247
Call your nearest health center or clinic for information on reduced fees for dental care. Usually clinics offer a sliding fee scale, and qualifications vary, though low income is a major factor considered. Fluoride Rinse Programs are available through the public school system.

Missouri Elks Program for the Handicapped
Truman Medical Center East
7900 Lee's Summit Rd.
Kansas City, MO 64139
816-373-1486
This program offers dental care for physically challenged, developmentally disabled or mentally retarded adults and children through three mobile units, which provide in-home care for those unable to get out on their own. Call for information on eligibility guidelines.

Dental Care for Senior Citizens
Senior Care Program
Missouri Dental Association
230 W. McCarty
P.O. Box 1707
Jefferson City, MO 65102-1707
800-688-1907
573-634-3436 (in Jefferson City)
This program provides low-cost dental care to seniors who meet the following eligibility requirements: 1) 60 years or older; 2) income no more than $15,000 (single) or $20,000 (for married couples); 3) you cannot be currently receiving dental care through any public aid program or insurance plan. Participating dentists have agreed to

provide a minimum of a 25% discount on services; however, the dentist may charge the usual fee for the initial office visit and examination.

Dental School
School of Dentistry
University of Missouri
650 E. 25th St.
Kansas City, MO 64108-2795
816-235-2100
www.umlcc.edu/dentistry
Annual patient visits: 7,500.

Dental Society
Missouri Dental Association
230 W. McCarty
P.O. Box 1707
Jefferson City, MO 65102-1707
573-634-3436
http://www.modental.org

Montana
Dental Programs
Health Services Division
Dental Department
Health and Environment Sciences
O.O. Box 202951
Cogswell Building
1400 Broadway
Helena, Montana 59620-2951
406-444-0276
Through the Maternal and Child Health department, counties can choose how they wish to use funds for dental care, so call your county health department to find out about treatments. Also Fluoride and Mouthrinse Programs are available for those who are in need. Contact Chau Seed; cseed@state.mt.us.

Dental Society
Montana Dental Association
P.O. Box 1154

Helena, MT 59624-1154
406-443-2061
http://www.mtdental.com
They can help you locate a dentist.

Nebraska
Dental Programs
Health Department
Dental Health Division
3140 N. St.
Lincoln, NE 68510
402-441-8015
www.ci.lincoln.ne.us/city/health/dental
Call your local Clinic to find out if they offer dental care. Low-income
is a major factor in determining eligibility, and fees are usually based
on a sliding scale. Children are a first priority.

Senior Dent Program
Nebraska Dental Association
3120 O Street
Lincoln, NE 68510-1599
402-476-1704
The *Senior Dent Program* offers dental care at a reduced fee for senior
citizens. There are eligibility requirements that include being at least 65
years of age. Cal to find out additional information.

Dental Schools
School of Dentistry
Creighton University
2802 Webster St.
Omaha, NE 68178
402-280-2865
www.creightondental.edu
Annual patient visits: 61,218.

College of Dentistry
University of Nebraska Medical Center
40th and Holdrege Sts.
Lincoln, NE 68583

402-472-1333 (adult)
402-472-1305 (children)
www.info.unmc.edu
Annual patient visits: 17,599.

Dental Society
Nebraska Dental Association
3120 O St.
Lincoln, NE 68510-1599
402-476-1704

Nevada

Dental Programs
Nevada Health Department
Family Services
505 East King St., Room 201
Carson City, NV 89710-4797
775-684-4200
www.state.nv.us
Call your County Health Department to see if they offer dental. Only very limited, low-cost dental care is available to adults other than possibly extractions due to pain. Most often, programs are only for children. Clark County Dental Society keeps a list of dentists who offer discounts to senior citizens. Call 702-255-7873 to get a referral.

Senior Center Bldg.
1155 East 9th St.
Reno, NV 89502
775-328-2575
This center does referrals only to dentists who treat senior and handicapped citizens. Call for discounts.

Dental Society
Nevada Dental Association
6889 W. Charleston #B
Las Vegas, NV 89117
775-255-4211
http://www.nvda.org

Medicaid dentists are part of this association. They provide referrals to their member dentists.

Southern Nevada Dental Society
702-733-8700
House emergency on-call dentists.

New Hampshire
Dental Programs
Department of Health and Human Services
Dental Division
6 Hazen Dr.
Concord, NH 03301
603-271-4685
www.state.nh.us/dental
New Hampshire has a very limited dental care program for those of low-income. Children are a first priority. Call the toll-free Helpline at 800-852-3345, ext. 4238 to find out about other possible dental assistance. Some state technical colleges offer dental Hygiene Programs.

Denture Program
New Hampshire Dental Society
23 South State St.
P.O. Box 2229
Concord, NH 03302-2229
603-225-5961
The *Denture Program* offers dentures to anyone who needs them at a reduced rate. There are financial guidelines that need to be met, but the program is for all ages. Call the above number for additional information.

Dental Society
New Hampshire Dental Society
23 South State St.
P.O. Box 2229
Concord, NH 03302-2229
603-225-5961
www.nhdental.com

New Jersey
Dental Programs
Department of Health
Dental Health Division
P.O. Box 364
50 E. State St., 5th Floor
Trenton, NJ 08625-0364
609-292-1723
Some area hospitals offer dental care on a sliding fee scale based on income, but most services offered are for children. Only limited care is available for adults. Also a limited number of clinics in some towns offer dental care, also using a sliding fee scale.

Senior Dent
New Jersey Dental Association
One Dental Plaza
P.O. Box 6020
North Brunswick, NJ 08902-6020
732-821-9400
www.njda.org
The *Senior Dent* program offers increase access to Dental Care for senior citizens by offering at least a 15% discount on services. Those eligible: 1) you must have a PAA (Pharmacy) card; 2) be age 65 or older; 3) have annual income of less than $15,700 (single) or $19,250 (married couple; 4) have no dental insurance or Medicaid benefits. Call the State Division on Aging for additional information at 800-792-8820.

Donated Dental Services
One Dental Plaza
North Brunswick, NJ 08902-4313
732-821-2977
Donated Dental Services offers comprehensive dental care for handicapped individuals. Those eligible: 1) the mentally or physically disabled including mental retardation, cerebral palsy, MS or other disabilities; 2) New Jersey residents; 3) each patient is screened to find those in most need. Limited income due to disability is a major factor in determining eligibility.

Dental School
New Jersey Dental School
University of Medicine and Dentistry
150 Bergen St.
Newark, NJ 07103
973-972-4300
Annual patient visits: 58,615.

Dental Society
New Jersey Dental Association
One Dental Plaza
P.O. Box 6020
North Brunswick, NJ 08902-6020
732-821-9400

New Mexico
Dental Programs
Department of Health
Dental Division
1190 Saint Francis Dr.
Santa Fe, NM 87502-6110
505-827-2389
www.state.nm.us
The legislature has provided money for the dental director to have
contract with health clinics, so call your nearest Community Health
Center or Clinic for information on reduced fees for dental care. Most
clinics will charge according to ability to pay, and children are usually
a priority. Carrie Tingley Hospital treats mentally disadvantaged and
disabled; call 505-843-7493 for additional information. There are also
some Indian Health Centers that offer dental care to tribal members.

Community Dental Services, Inc.
2116 Hinkle SE
Albuquerque, NM 87102
505-765-5683
Community Dental Services takes only Medicaid or university hospital
cards. Low fees available for low-income earners.

Dental Society
New Mexico Dental Association
3736 Eubank Blvd., NE, #1A
Albuquerque, NM 87111-3556
505-294-1368
They are currently establishing Donated Dental Services to provide free dental services for seniors.

New York
Dental Programs
Oral Health Programs and Policies
Health and Hospital Corp.
299 Broadway, Suite 500
New York, NY 10013
212-978-5540
Clinics throughout the city boroughs offer free or reduced cost dental care to children, ages 2 years to 21 years. Call the above number to get additional information about services offered.

Dental Schools
School of Dental and Oral Surgery
Columbia University
630 W. 168th St.
New York, NY 10032
212-305-6726
Annual patient visits: 53,255.

College of Dentistry
New York University
345 E. 24th St.
New York, NY 10010
212-998-9800
www.nyu.eduGeriatric Clinic: 212-998-9767
Annual patient visits: 269,095.

School of Dental Medicine
State University of New York at Stony Brook
Rockland Hall
Health Science Center

Stony Brook, NY 11794
516-632-8989
516-632-8967 (children)
516-632-8974 (adults)
516-632-9245 (geriatric clinic)
Annual patient visits: 15,321.

School of Dental Medicine
State University of New York at Buffalo
325 Squire
3435 Main St.
Buffalo, NY 14212-3008
716-829-2821
716-829-2723 (children)
716-829-2720 (adults)
http://sdm.buffalo.edu
Annual patient visits: 78,000.

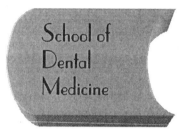

Dental Society
Dental Society of New York
7 Elk St.
Albany, NY 12207
518-465-0044
http://www.dssny.org

North Carolina
Dental Programs
Health and Natural Resources Environment
Dental Health Department
P.O. Box 29598
Raleigh, NC 27626-0598
919-733-3853
Call your nearest County Health Clinic to see if they offer dental care at
a reduced cost. When offered, it is usually on a sliding fee scale and
most often for children. Prevention and education are the main focus
with *Fluoride and Sealant Programs* throughout the various public
school systems.

Dental School
School of Dentistry
University of North Carolina
211 H Brauer Hall
Chapel Hill, NC 27514
919-966-1161
www.dent.unc.edu/
Annual patient visits: 30,395.

Dental Society
North Carolina Dental Society
P.O. Box 12047
Raleigh, NC 27605-2047
918-272-9313

North Dakota
Dental Programs
Health Department
Maternal and Child Health Department
600 E. Blvd. Ave.
Bismarck, ND 58505-0200
701-328-2493
Crippled Children Services offers dental and health care for those in
need. Some Indian Health Centers offer dental for tribal members. The
Fargo Homeless Project offers emergency dental work for the
homeless. No programs other than Medicaid offer dental care, and no
clinics offer dental care.

Senior Dent
North Dakota Dental Association
Box 1332
Bismarck, ND 58502
701-223-8870
The *Senior Dent* program makes a full range of Dental Services
available to financially eligible North Dakotans age 55 or older at a
reduced fee. Those eligible must: 1) be 55 or older; 2) Not be covered
by medical assistance or enrolled in a dental insurance plan; 3) have
income that is 125% or less of federal poverty guidelines. Fees vary,
but dentists have agreed to offer at least a 33% discount off their

regular fees. Contact your local Senior Citizen Center for more information.

Dental Society
North Dakota Dental Association
P.O. Box 1332
Bismarck, ND 58502-1332
701-223-8870

Ohio
Dental Programs
State Health Department
Dental Health Division
246 North High
Columbus, OH 43266-0588
614-466-4180
www.odh.state.oh.us
Ohio offers a *Sealant and Fluoride Mouthrinse Program* through the public school system.

Access to Dental Care Programs
Ohio Dental Association
1370 Dublin Rd.
Columbus, OH 43215-1098
800-MY-SMILE
888-765-6789
The Ohio Dental Association offers the Options Program, a partnership with the Ohio Department of Health. It matches low-income patients who qualify with dentists who offer discounts.

Dental Services for the Handicapped
Donated Dental Services
635 W. 7th St.
Cincinnati, OH 45203
513-621-2517
Free and low-cost dental care is available to the handicapped and elderly is they meet the following guidelines: 1) Mentally or physically disabled including mental retardation, cerebral palsy, MS or other disabilities; 2) individuals may also be elderly living on a fixed income;

3) each patient is screened to find those in most need. Limited income due to handicap is a major factor in determining eligibility.

Greater Cincinnati Oral Health Council
635 W. Seventh St.
Cincinnati, OH 45203
513-621-0248
A charter agency of the United Way, the Public Dental Service Society's dental care programs help special groups such as children from low-income families, the homeless, the aging and those with disabling conditions. 1) *Dental Sealant Program*: sealants are applied to low-income and handicapped children of Cincinnati. 2) *Homeless Program*: provides dental care for homeless adults and children. 3) *Dental Registry for the Elderly and Handicapped:* a computerized referral service matches patients with special needs with a dentist who can accommodate these needs.

Dental Schools
College of Dentistry
Ohio State University
305 W. 12th Ave.
Columbus, OH 43210
614-292-2751
www.dent.ohio-state.edu
Annual patient visits: 51,476.

School of Dentistry
Case Western Reserve University
2123 Abington Rd.
Cleveland, OH 44106
216-368-3200
Annual patient visits: 86,630.

Dental Society
Ohio Dental Association
1370 Dublin Rd.
Columbus, OH 43215-1098
614-486-2700
www.oda.org

Oklahoma
Dental Programs
State Department of Health
Dental Health Services
1000 Northeast Tenth St.
Oklahoma City, OK 73117-1299
405-271-5502
Call your local Health Center or hospital to see if dental is offered.
When offered, it is usually on a sliding fee scale, and in some instances
only for children.

Care-Dent Program
Oklahoma Dental Society
629 West I-44 Service Rd.
Oklahoma City, OK 73118
800-876-8890
www.okdentassoc.org
Care-Dent offers savings to those who need denture service. Dentists
also provide a thorough examination. Call for a participating dentist
and more information.

Senior Dent Program
Oklahoma Dental Society
629 West I-44 Service Rd.
Oklahoma City, OK 73118
800-876-8890
405-848-8873
www.okdentassoc.org
The *Senior Dent Program* offers complete, professional dental care at a
reduced fee to those seniors who meet the following guidelines: 1) 65
or older; 2) have no dental insurance; 3) income no more than
$8,000/single or $12,000 for a married couple. Dentists offer a 20%
discount to qualifying senior citizens. Call for more information.

Disabled Program
4500 North Lincoln Blvd., Suite 101
Oklahoma City, OK 73105-5220
800-522-9510
405-424-8092

The *D-Dent Program* offers free dental care for the physically disabled. You must apply, and applicants are carefully screened.

Dental School
College of Dentistry
University of Oklahoma
Health Sciences Center
1001 Stanton L. Young Blvd.
P.O. Box 26901
Oklahoma City, OK 73190-3044
405-271-6056
www.ouhsc.com
Annual patient visits: 45,615.

Dental Society
Oklahoma Dental Association
629 W. Interstate 44 Service Rd.
Oklahoma City, OK 73118-6032
405-848-8873
www.okdentassoc.org

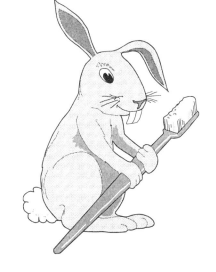

Oregon
Dental Programs
Department of Health
Dental Health Division
800 NE Oregon St.
Portland, OR 97232
503-731-4098

Low-Cost Denture Program
2300 Oakmont Way, Suite 110
Eugene, OR 97401
541-686-1175
Under this program, residents of Lane County, 55 years or older, and who meet the following guidelines may be eligible to receive low-cost denture care, including full upper and lower dentures, partials, reclines and repairs: 1) receive no public assistance; 2) income no more than $7,500 (single) or $10,500 (married couples). Call for additional qualifications and information.

Dental Care for Senior Citizens
Senior Smile Dental Service
Multnomah Dental Society
1618 Southwest
Suite 317
Portland, OR 97201
503-774-3898
Under this program, low income seniors over 60 years old, who live in Multnomah County may be eligible to receive both general and specialized dental care at a 50% reduced fee. Call for more information and to register.

Dental School
School of Dentistry
Sam Jackson Park
Oregon Health Sciences University
611 SW Campus Dr.
Portland, OR 97201
503-494-8867
www.ohsu.edu
Annual patient visits: 44,900.

Dental Society
Oregon Dental Association
17898 SW McEwan Rd.
Portland, OR 97224-7798
503-620-3230

Pennsylvania
Dental Programs
Department of Public Health
Dental Health Division
500 South Broad Street
Philadelphia, PA 19146
215-875-5666
The Dental Program offers reduced-rate dental care through your nearest clinic. Insurance is accepted and fee set according to financial situation. Anyone with low income is eligible, but children are first priority.

Dental Care for Senior Citizens
Access to Care Program
P.O. Box 3341
Harrisburg, PA 17105-3341
800-692-7256
Under this program, individuals 65 or over can receive at least a minimum of 15% discount on dental care through 1,700 participating dentists across PA. To be eligible, you must: 1) have no private dental insurance nor federal, state or other dental health assistance; 2) have income no more than $14,000 (single) or $17,200 (married couples). Call the PA Counsel on Aging at 800-692-7256 for more program information.

Dental Care for Handicapped (Philadelphia only)
Donated Dental Services
Fidelity Bank Bldg.
123 S. Broad St., 22nd Floor
Philadelphia, PA 19109-1022
215-546-0300
Certain low-income mentally or physically handicapped residents of Philadelphia may qualify to receive free or low-cost dental care. Each patient is screened to find those most in need: limited income due to handicap is a major factor.

Dental Schools
School of Dentistry
Temple University
3223 N. Broad St.
Philadelphia, PA 19140
215-707-2900
www.temple.dental.edu
Annual patient visits: 77,665.

School of Dental Medicine
University of Pennsylvania
4001 Spruce St.
Philadelphia, PA 19104
215-898-8961
www.upenn.edu
Annual patient visits: 85,000.

School of Dental Medicine
University of Pittsburgh
3501 Terrace St.
Salk Hall
Pittsburgh, PA 15261
412-648-8760
www.dental.pitt.edu
Annual patient visits: 59,570.

Dental Society
Pennsylvania Dental Association
3501 N. Front St.
P.O. Box 3341
Harrisburg, PA 17110
717-234-5941
www.padental.org

Rhode Island
Dental Programs
Department of Public Health
Oral Health Division
3 Capital Hill
Providence, RI 02908-5097
401-222-2588
The dental program offers reduced-fee basic dental care (not crowns or bridges, for example). Call your nearest clinic for more information. Most insurance are accepted and the pay schedule is according to situation. Anyone with low-income can qualify.

Travelers Aide Society for the Homeless
177 Union St.
Providence, RI 02903
401-521-2255
The Travelers Aide Society offers free dental care for the homeless.

Dental Care for Handicapped
Independence Square
500 Prospect St.
Pawtucket, RI 02860

401-728-9448
Through the *Donated Dental Services Program*, free and low-cost dental care is available to the handicapped that meet the following guidelines: 1) mentally or physically disabled including mental retardation, cerebral palsy, MS, or other disabilities; 2) live in Rhode Island; 3) each patient must be screened to find those in most need. Limited income due to handicap is a major factor in determining eligibility.

South County
Health Center of South County
One River St.
Wakefield, RI 02879
401-782-0853
Basic dental treatments for all ages are available. Discounts are based on income.

Dental Society
Rhode Island Dental Association
200 Centerville Rd.
Warwick, RI 02886-4339
401-732-6833
www.ndental.com

South Carolina
Dental Programs
Department of Health and Environmental Control
2000 Hampton St.
Columbia, SC 29201
803-929-6343
The will refer you to local health clinics for low income adults.

Primary Care Center
P.O. Box 6923
Columbia, SC 29260
803-738-9881
Some Primary Care Clinics or Centers offer dental on a sliding fee scale based on income. Call to get additional information.

Senior Care Dental Program
P.O. Box 1776
Beaufort, SC 29901
843-524-1787
Participating dentists will offer at least a 10% discount for seniors. Call the local council on aging in your county for more information.

Dental School
College of Dental Medicine
Medical University of South Carolina
171 Ashley Ave.
Charleston, SC 29425
843-792-2611
www.musc.edu
Annual patient visits: 25,315.

Dental Society
South Carolina Dental Association
120 Stonemark Ln.
Columbia, SC 29210-3841
803-750-2277
www.scda.org

South Dakota
Dental Programs
Department of Health
Anderson Building
600 E. Capitol Ave.
Pierre, SD 57501
605-773-3361
www.state.sd.us/doh

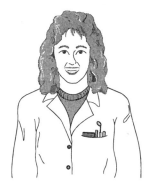

Indian Health Program
Indian Health Services
Federal Building
115 4th Ave. SE
Aberdeen, SD 57401
605-226-7501

Dental care is available at no charge for Indians enrolled in a tribe. Call the office above for additional information and find out locations for treatment.

Dental Society
South Dakota Dental Association
P.O. Box 1194
Pierre, SD 57501-1194
605-224-9133

Tennessee
Dental Programs
Department of Health
Oral Health Services
Cordell Hull Bldg. 5th Floor
425 5th Ave. North
Nashville, TN 37247
615-741-7213
Contact your Local Health Center or Clinic to find out if they offer reduced-fee dental services. Low income is a major factor in determining eligibility, and a sliding fee scale is most often used. Qualifications vary, and care is primarily for children. Emergency care is offered to adults to alleviate pain. Although there are no special programs for the elderly or disabled, they will be treated based on the above income criteria.

Dental Schools
School of Dentistry
Meharry Medical College
1005 D.B. Todd Blvd.
Nashville, TN 37208
615-327-6669
http://patton.mmc.edu/
Annual patient visits: 7,972.

College of Dentistry
University of Tennessee
875 Union Ave.
Memphis, TN 38163

901-448-6257
Annual patient visits: 52,551.

Dental Society
Tennessee Dental Association
P.O. Box 120188
Nashville, TN 37212-0188
615-383-8962
www.tenndental.org

Texas
Dental Programs
www.tdh.state.tx.us/dental/dental.htm
In Texas, several regional offices of the Texas Public Health Office
have additional information on reduced-fee dental care in their regions.
Dental services are provided in public health clinics, private dentists
and in mobile dental units. Call or write the appropriate region to get
additional information.

Region 1
Texas Public Health
1109 Kemper St.
Lubbock, TX 79403
806-744-3577
dale.drennan@tdh.state.tx.us

Regions 2 and 3
1351 E. Bardin
Arlington, TX 76018
817-264-4410
james.belcher@tdh.state.tx.us

Region 4 & 5 North
Texas Public Health
1517 West Front St.
Tyler, TX 75702
903-533-5202
mailto:maureen.weber@tdh.state.tx.us

Region 6
Texas Public Health
5425 Polk Ave, Suite J
Houston, TX 77023-1497
713-767-3470
william.gray@tdh.state.tx.us

Region 7
Texas Public Health
2408 South 37th St.
Temple, TX 76504
254-778-6744
512-467-9875
erwin.heineker@tdh.state.tx.us

Region 8
Texas Public Health
1021 Garnerfield Rd.
Uvalde, TX 78801
830-278-7173
linda.altenhoff@tdh.state.tx.us

Regions 9 and 10
Texas Public Health
6070 Gateway East, Suite 401
El Paso, TX 79995-9428
915-774-6237
douglas.foster@tdh.state.tx.us

Region 11
Texas Public Health
601 West Sesame Drive
Harlingen, TX 78550
956-423-0130
jerry.felkner@tdh.state.tx.us

Dental Schools
Baylor College of Dentistry
3302 Gaston Ave.

Dallas, TX 75246
214-828-8100
www.tamua.edu
Annual patient visits: 75,411.

Health Science Center
Dental Branch
University of Texas
6516 John Freeman Ave.
Houston, TX 77030
713-792-4056
Annual patient visits: 113,153.

Health Science Center
Dental School
University of Texas
7703 Floyd Curl Dr.
San Antonio, TX 78284
210-567-3222
Annual patient visits: 124,783.

Dental Society
Texas Dental Association
P.O. Box 3358
Austin, TX 78764-3358
512-443-3675
www.tda.org

Utah
Dental Society
Utah Dental Association
1151 E. 3900 South, #B160
Salt Lake City, UT 84124
801-261-5315

Vermont
Dental Programs
Island Pond Health Center
P.O. Box 425

HEALTH SCIENCE CENTER

Island Pond, VT 05846-0425
802-723-4300
This nonprofit Health Center in northeastern Vermont offers eligible residents of Essex County and specific surrounding towns dental care for a reduced fee based on a sliding scale based on their income from the previous year. Fees range from 100% to 75% to 50% to 25% coverage for preventive dental services and all other services they provide. No specialty services, such as orthodontics, are available. Call to get additional information and to find out if Health Care Inc. has reduced fee dental care available in your town.

Dental Society
Vermont Dental Society
132 Church St.
Burlington, VT 05401-8401
802-864-0115
www.vsds.org

Virginia
Dental Programs
Health Department
Dental Division
1500 E. Main, Room 239
Richmond, VA 23219
804-786-3556
www.vdh.state.va.us\fhs\dental\dental.htm
Community Health Centers offer dental care at a reduced-fee based on income. Although children are a first priority, adults are treated on an emergency basis. The following treat seniors specially:

MCB School of Dentistry
520 N. 12th St.
Richmond, VA 23298
804-828-9190
Discounts on dental care are available to seniors based on a sliding fee scale.

Donated Dental Services
P.O. Box 6906

Richmond, VA 23230
804-257-9810
You may qualify for free dental services if you are 1) 65 or older; 2) chronically ill, or; 3) permanently disabled.

Dental School
School of Dentistry
Virginia Commonwealth University
Box 980566
Richmond, VA 23298
804-828-9095
www.vcu.edu
Annual patient visits: 61,722

Dental Society
Virginia Dental Association
P.O. Box 6906
Richmond, VA 23230-0906
804-358-4927
www.vadental.org

Washington
Dental Programs
Health Care Authority
Dental Services
P.O. Box 42710
Olympia, WA 98504-2710
360-923-2753
www.wa.gov/hca
Call your nearest Health Department or Clinic to find out if they offer free or discount dental care. When dental care is offered, it is usually for children and senior citizens, with only limited care for adults. A sliding fee scale is used, and low income is a factor in determining what you're charged. Ask to speak with Connie Mix-Clark or Bob Blacksmith to get additional information on these programs. They will refer you to Washington health clinics that offer discount dental care.

Seattle-King County Dental Society
2201 Sixth Ave., Suite 1306

Seattle, WA 98121-1832
206-443-7607
The Seattle-King County Dental Society has a listing of clinics and
programs that offer free or minimal cost dental care. Contact them for a
free copy.

Elderly and Disabled
Washington State Dental Association
2033 Sixth Avenue #333
Seattle, WA 98121
206-448-1914
www.wsda.org
Under the *Access Program for the Elderly and Disabled*, dental care at
a reduced cost is available from participating dentists who meet the
following guidelines: 1) 65 or older; 2) have no dental insurance; 3)
income no more than $15,670/single or $19,765 for a family; 4) for the
disabled, the same criteria for eligibility applies, but there is no age
restriction. Eligibility must be re-certified every 12 months. Fees are
reduced by at least 25% for patients meeting the criteria. Call or write
Angelica Wilkon for an application. They treat Alzheimer's patients on
the same basis as the disabled.

Dental School
School of Dentistry
University of Washington
Health Science Center
Northeast Pacific St.
Seattle, WA 98195
206-543-5830
Annual patient visits: 45,500.

Dental Society
Washington Dental Association
2033 6th Ave., Suite 333
Seattle, WA 98121-2514
206-448-1914
www.wsda.org

West Virginia
Dental Programs
Department of Health and Human Resources
Dental Information
State Capital Complex, Bldg. 6
Charleston, WV 25305
304-926-1700
Very limited dental care is available through the Health Department
other than Medicaid: however, below you'll find other contacts that do
offer reduced-fee services.

Low-Income Adults, Linkline
One United Way Square
Charleston, WV 25301
304-340-3517
Linkline offers reduced-fee dental services for adults 19 to 59, but you
must first apply to the program and be accepted. Low income is a major
factor in determining your eligibility.

Tiskewah Dental Clinic
600 Florida St.
Charleston, WV 25302
304-348-6613
This dental clinic treats children year-round, and senior citizens during
the summer free of charge. Call to find out if you might qualify.

Dental School
School of Dentistry
West Virginia University
The Medical Center
Morgantown, WV 26505
304-598-4810
www.hsc.wvu.edu
Annual patient visits: 27,522.

Dental Society
West Virginia Dental Association
1002 Kanawha Valley Building
300 Capitol St.

Charleston, WV 25301-1794
304-344-5246

Wisconsin
Dental Programs
Bureau of Public Health
1414 E. Washington Ave.
Madison, WI 53703
608-266-5152
www.dhfs.state.wi.us
Very limited reduced-fee dental care is available in Wisconsin. Call
your local Health Center or Clinic to find out if dental is available.

Dental School
School of Dentistry
Marquette University
604 N. 16th St.
Milwaukee, WI 53233
414-288-6500
www.dental.mu.us
Annual patient visits: 48,235.

Dental Society
Wisconsin Dental Association
111 E. Wisconsin Ave.
Suite 1300
Milwaukee, WI 53202-4811
414-276-4520
http://www.wisconsindental.com
They work with donated dental services, 414-276-0370, to provide free
dental care for persons who are 1) 65 or older; 2) have a permanent
disability or chronic illness.

Wyoming
Dental Programs
State Health Department
Dental Division
Hathaway Building, 4th Floor
Cheyenne, WY 82002

307-777-7945

The *Marginal Program* for low-income children provides dental care up to 19 years of age. You must apply and be accepted to be eligible. The *Cleft Palate Clinic* offers free diagnostic treatment and referrals. The *Sealant Program* provides sealant treatment for children of low-income families. The *Elderly Program* offers reduced fees for those low-income adults 65 or older. There is no reduced-fee dental care for those individuals 20 to 64 except through *Title 19 Emergency Care* program.

Dental Society
Wyoming Dental Association
330 S. Center St., Suite 322
Cheyenne, WY 82601-2875
307-634-5878

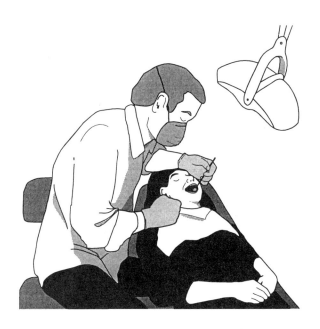

Free Money and Help for People With Disabilities

The Best Places To Start For Help

If you are disabled or handicapped and need help becoming more independent, there are hundreds of sources of free help and money from federal, state, local, private, and non-profit organizations.

The help available ranges from free information services, self-help groups (for specific disabilities and disabilities in general), free legal aid, and independent living programs, to free money for education, job training, living expenses, transportation, equipment and mobility aids. You can even get money to have your home retrofitted to make it more accessible to your specific handicap. And if you're denied any of these programs or services, there are several free sources of legal help to make sure that you get what you're entitled to.

The three best places where you should begin your search for information about services and money programs for the disabled and handicapped are:

★ The Social Security Administration (see page 208)
★ Your State Office of Vocational Rehabilitation (see page 217)
★ Client Assistance Programs (see page 219)

In this section, you'll find descriptions and listings of contacts for these three programs, along with several additional best places for self-help and aid for handicapped or disabled individuals.

Free Money For The Disabled Who Have Worked In The Past

If you're disabled and expect to be so for at least one year, and have worked long enough and recently enough under Social Security, you may be eligible for Social Security Disability Insurance Benefits (DIB). If you are found entitled to DIB, you will receive a monthly check in an amount based on your prior earnings.

If you start back to work after receiving DIB, you have nine months (not necessarily consecutive), to earn as much as you can without affecting your benefits. (The nine months of work must fall within a five-year period before your trial work period can end.) After your trial work period ends, your work is evaluated to see if it is "substantial." This means that your earnings are more than $700. For 36 months after a successful trial work period, if you are still disabled, you will be eligible to receive a monthly benefit without a new application for any month your earnings drop below $700 for people with disabilities or $1110 per month for people who are blind.

If you are still disabled, your Medicare coverage can continue for 39 months beyond the trial work period. If your Medicare coverage stops because of your work, you may purchase it for a monthly premium. For more information on "quarters of coverage" and the trial work period:

Contact:
The Social Security Administration
800-772-1213
TTY 800-325-0778
www.ssa.gov

Extra Benefits for School or Entrepreneuring

Many people with disabilities work, and you're probably one of them. But maybe you need to go back to school before you can get a job. Or, maybe you'd like to start your own business, but you don't have the money. Whatever your work goal may be, a PASS can help you reach it.

A PASS lets you set aside money and/or other things you own to help you reach your goal. For example, you could set aside money to start a business or to go to school or to get training for a job.

Your goal must be a job that will produce sufficient earnings to reduce your dependency on Supplemental 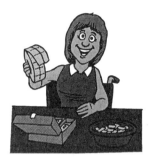 Security Income (SSI) payments. A PASS is meant to help you acquire those items, services or skills you need so that you can compete with able-bodied persons for an entry level job in a professional, business or trade environment. If you have graduated from college or a trade/technical school, you usually are considered able to obtain such a position without the assistance of a PASS. You can contact your local Social Security office to find out whether a PASS is appropriate for you.

How Will a Plan Affect my SSI Benefit?

Under regular SSI rules, your SSI benefit is reduced by the other income you have, but the income you set aside for a PASS doesn't reduce your SSI benefit. This means you can get a higher SSI benefit when you have a PASS, but you can't get more than the maximum SSI benefit for the state where you live.

Money you save or things you own, such as property or equipment, that you set aside for a PASS won't count against the resource limit of $2,000 (or $3,000 for a couple). Under regular SSI rules, you wouldn't be eligible for SSI if your resources are above $2,000, but with a plan, you may set aside some resources so you would be eligible.

Who Can Have a PASS?

You can if:

- ♦ you want to work;
- ♦ you get SSI (or can qualify for SSI) because of blindness or a disability; or
- ♦ you have or expect to receive income (other than SSI) and/or resources to set aside toward a work goal.

What Kind of Expenses
Can a Plan Help Pay For?

A plan may be used to pay for a variety of expenses that are necessary to help you reach your work goal. For example, your plan may help you save for:

- ♦ supplies to start a business;
- ♦ tuition, fees, books and supplies that are needed for school or training;
- ♦ employment services, such as payments for a job coach;
- ♦ attendant care or child care expenses;
- ♦ equipment and tools to do the job;
- ♦ transportation to and from work; or
- ♦ uniforms, special clothing and safety equipment.

These are only examples. Not all of these will apply to every plan. You might have other expenses depending on your goal.

How Will a Plan Affect Other Benefits I Get?

You should check with the agency that is responsible for those benefits to find out if the plan (and the extra SSI) might affect those benefits.

Working While Disabled — How We Can Help

800-772-1213

www.ssa.gov

In many cases, income and resources set aside under a plan will not be counted for food stamps and housing assistance provided through the U.S. Department of Housing and Urban Development. But, it's important that you contact the particular agency to find out how your benefits will be affected.

For more information, ask Social Security for the booklet, *Working While Disabled — How We Can Help* (Publication No. 5-10095).

800-772-1213

www.ssa.gov

Impairment-Related Work Expenses

Certain expenses for items you need for work due to your disability can be deducted when calculating your earnings, which affects your disability insurance benefits. The amount of money you spend on such items is not counted as part of your income when determining your substantial work earnings.

Free and Low-Cost Medical Insurance For the Disabled Who Have Worked In the Past

If you qualify for the Disability Insurance Benefits (DIB) described above, and have been receiving these payments for at least two years, you will also qualify to receive Medicare Part A for free which provides insurance coverage for hospitalization. You can also receive Medicare Part B for a monthly premium

of $45.50. This provides insurance coverage for your doctor visits and testing services. This is the same Medicare coverage those over 65 receive.

Remember, there are deductibles and limits of coverage. For instance, doctor visits are covered after you meet the $100 deductible for the year, after which Medicare will pay 80% of the approved rate, and you are responsible for the other 20%. To apply for this medical insurance or to receive the Medicare Handbook which provides detailed information on coverage:

Contact:
The Medicare Hotline
800-638-6833
www.medicare.gov

Free Help Getting Health Care Benefits For Workers With Disabilities

The United Cerebral Palsy Association of King-Snohomish

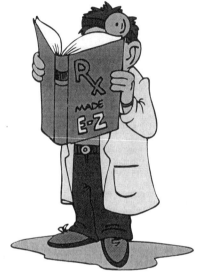

Counties Summit Benefits Counseling Services provides support and advocacy to help people with disabilities retain health care and benefits once they are employed. Clients receive assistance in using Social Security Work Incentives such as PASS Plans or IRWE to continue healthcare. It also provides assistance to get reimbursed for work expenses, and/or save money to reach a vocational goal.

Contact: United Cerebral Palsy Association of King-Snohomish Counties, 14910 1st Ave, NE, Seattle, WA 98155-6898; 206-361-5638 Benefits Counseling; Fax: 206-440-2228; TTY: 205-440-2206; 888-810-0745; Language: Staff bilingual in American Sign Language, {E-mail: mikeh@ucpks.org}; {www.ucpks.org}.

Cash For
Dependents Of the Disabled

If you are eligible for Disability Insurance Benefits (DIB) described above, your dependents (wife, husband, children, or and in some cases, grandchildren) may also be eligible for payments on your record. To find out if your dependent is eligible:

Contact:
Social Security
800-772-1213
TTY 800-325-0778
www.ssa.gov

Money For The Disabled
Who Have Not Worked In The Past

If you are disabled but do not have enough work under Social Security for Disability Insurance Benefits (DIB), you may still be eligible to receive Supplemental Security Income (SSI) benefits if your income and resources are low enough. To see if you are eligible for SSI:

Contact:
The Social Security Administration
800-772-1213
TTY 800-325-0778
www.ssa.gov

WHAT TO DO WHEN BENEFITS ARE DENIED

If you are denied any of the above-mentioned Social Security cash benefits — which often happens regardless of the disability or its severity — you can get free legal help to appeal the Social Security Administration's decision on your application.

Contact your state or local Department of Welfare and request the name and address of the nearest Legal Services Corporation (LSC) program, and also contact your nearest State Client Assistance Program (CAP) office. Both programs offer low-income individuals free legal help and representation in appealing application decisions.

The CAP program will either provide you with free legal help and representation for your appeal or they will help you find such aid. Unlike legal help offered under the Legal Services Corporation, CAP services are not determined by your income. On the chance that neither of these agencies seem to be able to help you,

Contact
The Disability Rights Education
and Defense Fund (DREDF)
415-644-2555 or
415-841-8645
TTY 800-325-0778
www.ssa.gov

Free Money for Education and Job Training

If your disability stops you from being able to keep a full-time job or from being able to competitively look for a job, your state's Office of Vocational Rehabilitation (OVR) can help. OVR can give you up to $6,000 each year for job training or education. You can use this grant money, which you do not have to pay back, to cover any expenses related to your training or education, including tuition and fees, travel expenses, books, supplies, equipment (computers, motorized wheelchairs, etc.), a food allowance, tutoring fees, photocopies, and so on. For more information, contact your state's Office of Vocational Rehabilitation listed below.

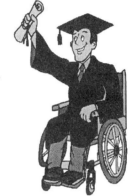

Help For the Handicapped to Find Or Create a Job

Your state Office of Vocational Rehabilitation (OVR) also acts as an employment agency for the disabled and can contact employers for you who have looked favorably on hiring the disabled. OVR will act as a liaison between you and a prospective employer and help them to create a job for you by providing needed disability-related job equipment, providing needed transportation or other mobility equipment, or by providing any other help you might need to be able to work at a job for which you're qualified. For example, OVR has provided books in Braille and Braille-to-speech conversion equipment, and computer-robotics equipment that have allowed disabled individuals to work. For more information, contact your state's Office of Vocational Rehabilitation listed on page 234.

Help For the Handicapped Already On the Job

If you are working and become disabled or handicapped, your state Office of Vocational Rehabilitation (OVR) can provide you with the equipment, transportation, education, training and other help you might need to keep your job.

For example, many times a disability can put someone in a wheelchair. OVR can provide you with a motorized wheelchair so you can continue in your job.

Contact your state Office of Vocational Rehabilitation listed at the end of this section for more information.

MEDICAL HELP FOR THE DISABLED/HANDICAPPED

Your state Office of Vocational Rehabilitation can pay for (or help you pay for) any medical testing or treatment that can be expected to help you, as a handicapped or disabled individual, have a more healthy, prosperous, independent, and fulfilling life. Contact your state Office of Vocational Rehabilitation listed on page 234 for more information.

WHAT TO DO WHEN OVR BENEFITS ARE DENIED

The first place to start when your state Office of Vocational Rehabilitation denies you handicap or disability benefits is your nearest state Client Assistance Program (CAP) office. CAP is a free information, referral, and legal service that helps disabled or handicapped individuals appeal a denial by OVR (or other agency). For a variety of reasons, it is not uncommon for a disabled individual to be turned down for services by OVR even when he/she is in fact eligible to receive them. It is sometimes helpful to get a photocopy of section 103 of Chapter 34 of the *Code of Federal Regulations of the U.S. Department of Education* from your local or county library. These are the federal guidelines that each state OVR must follow when determining eligibility. This part of the code is only a few pages and can help you explain to the Client Assistance Program officer why you believe you are eligible even though you've been denied. CAP can take your appeal process from the first stages and all the way to the U.S. Supreme Court if necessary--and it won't cost you a penny.

It is also sometimes helpful to contact the state Office of Vocational Rehabilitation (OVR) itself and make the executive director aware of your circumstances. When it appears that progress via CAP is stalled or has been dragging on for months, it can also be very helpful to contact the regional commissioner of the Rehabilitation Services Administration (RSA), a branch of the Office of Special Education Programs of the U.S. Department of Education. RSA is responsible for overseeing and funding the state OVR agencies and is generally receptive to a short explanatory phone call and letter from those who believe they can concisely and clearly show that they have been wrongly denied OVR services. If they think you've got a case, they'll contact the OVR in question and make sure that they review your application more favorably.

To get in touch with an RSA official, contact the U.S. Department of Education, Office of Special Education and Rehabilitative Services, RSA, Washington, DC 20202: 202-205-5482, and ask for the address and phone number of the regional commissioner for the ED-OSERS-RSA office serving your area.

Three Important Tips When Appealing an OVR Denial Of Services

1. If your state Office of Vocational Rehabilitation (OVR) denies you services based on other similar cases in which they have denied other prospective clients, it is important and effective to argue that such reasons for denial are not allowable under federal regulations. The 34 Code of Federal Regulations Chapter III section 361.31(b)(1) states clearly that the barriers faced by a disabled individual are unique to each individual and to each individual set of circumstances.

2. If you have previously been accepted by your state Office of Vocational Rehabilitation (OVR) as a client and you have gained employment but your disability has not improved and you lose employment due to no fault of your own, then OVR can again provide you with their services to help you regain employment. For more specifics consult again the 34 Code of Federal Regulations, Chapter III and check under the *Post-Employment Services* sections and *Supported Employment* sections.

3. If you're currently receiving Social Security Disability (SSD), make sure that your state Office of Vocational Rehabilitation (OVR) and Client Assistance Program (CAP) are aware of this fact. Because of the more restrictive SSD definition of what it means to be disabled (compared to OVR), being on SSD almost always automatically qualifies an SSD recipient for

OVR services. It is very hard for OVR to argue otherwise.

Free Legal Help and Information Services For the Handicapped

If you think you've been wrongly denied benefits or discriminated against because of a disability or handicap, the Client Assistance Program (CAP) will help you fight for your rights when you're denied various types of disability benefits from any disability program. They will help you directly and/or put you in contact with the agencies that can help you. Your state CAP office is listed on page 234.

More Free Legal Help for the Disabled

A national non-profit law and policy center, the Disability Rights Education and Defense Fund (DREDF) can provide you with direct legal representation and act as co-counsel in cases of disability-based discrimination. They also educate legislators and policy makers on issues affecting the rights of people with disabilities.

Contact: Disability Rights Education and Defense Fund (DREDF), 2212 Sixth St., Berkeley, CA 94710; 510-644-2555 (Voice/TDD).

Free Legal Help For People With Disabilities

The Disabilities Law Project of the Washington Coalition of Citizens with Disabilities provides free legal advice and representation for severely disabled individuals in cases where their disability is an issue. Special attention is given to the issues of barrier-free buildings, housing and transportation problems, 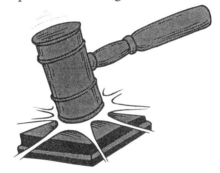 schools and government agencies administering programs for the disabled, and employment discrimination. The project also sponsors law-related and other community education programs on subjects of interest to people with disabilities; prepares handbooks on the rights of people with disabilities; and distributes periodic bulletins on new developments in disabilities laws statewide.

Contact: Washington Coalition of Citizens With Disabilities, 4649 Sunnyside Ave N, #100, Seattle, WA 98103-6900; 206 633-6637; Fax: 206-545-7059; TTY: 206-632-3456. Language: Interpreters will be provided as needed in foreign languages and for persons with hearing impairments, {E-mail: wccd@premier1.net}; {www.premier1.net/~wccd}.

Free On-Line Recorded Books For People With Disabilities

Assistive Media is a non-profit, charitable service that produces RealAudio recordings of literary works for people with disabilities. It is the net's first audio solution designed for persons with print reading/ access barriers.

To access this service you must have a 28.8K modem or better and an installed version of the RealPlayer from RealNetworks Inc. You can download and install the free RealPlayer from Assistive Media's Web site, courtesy of the American Foundation for the Blind. Just click on any icon on this web site and listen to selected literary works from great books and magazines. Contact:

Free Directory Assistance For Customers with Disabilities

US West customers who have difficulty finding or remembering phone numbers can receive directory assistance services at no charge. To apply call and ask for a Directory Assistance Exempt Certificate. It must be signed by your physician and returned to the phone company. Contact: US West - Customer Services, Bell Plaza, 1600 Seventh Ave, Room 2709, Seattle, WA 98191; 206 504-0670 Billing/Service; 206-555-1212 Directory Assistance; 411 Directory Assistance; TTY: 800-223-3131; Toll Free: 800-244-1111; Language: Interpreters available in 21 spoken languages and sign language {www.uswest.com}.

Assistive Media, 400 Maynard St., Suite 404, Ann Arbor MI 48104-2434; {E-mail: info@assistivemedia.org}; {www.assistivemedia.org}.

Information Clearinghouse For All Types Of Disabilities

The Clearinghouse on Disability Information will answer your questions on a wide range of disability topics and send you all kinds of information about services for disabled and handicapped individuals at the national, state, and local levels.

They have several free publications, including *Office Of Special Education and Rehabilitative Services (OSERS) News In Print* newsletter, which describes OSERS programs, research, and topical information on a broad range of disability issues. The *Summary of Existing Legislation Affecting Persons With Disabilities* is available for all federal laws through 1991. The *Pocket Guide to Federal Help For Individuals with Disabilities* is a general, handy beginning reference.

Contact: Clearinghouse On Disability Information, Office Of Special Education and Rehabilitative Services, Communication and Information Services, U.S. Department Of Education, Room 3132 Switzer Bldg., Washington, DC 20202-2524; 202-205-8723, or 205-8241.

Additional Resources

Hiqher Education and Adult Traininq For People With Handicaps

The Higher Education and Adult Training for People with Handicaps (HEATH) Resource Center is a clearinghouse and information exchange center for resources on postsecondary education programs and the disabled. Topics include educational support services, policies, procedures, adaptations, and opportunities on American campuses, vocational-technical schools, adult education programs, 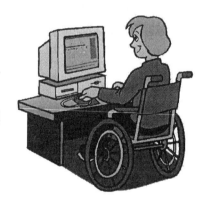 independent living centers, and other training organizations after high school.

Another clearinghouse, National Information Center for Children and Youth with Disabilities, handles the concerns of younger disabled persons through secondary school.

Contact: National Clearinghouse on Postsecondary Education for Individuals with Handicaps, One Dupont Circle, NW, Suite 800, Washington, DC 20036; 202-939-9320 (Voice/TDD), 800-544-3284 (outside DC).

REHABILITATION INFORMATION HOTLINE

The National Rehabilitation Information Center, a library and information center on disability and rehabilitation, collects and disseminates the results of federally funded research projects. NARIC also maintains a vertical file of pamphlets and fact sheets published by other organizations. NARIC has documents on all aspects of disability and rehabilitation including physical disabilities, mental retardation, psychiatric disabilities, independent living, employment, law and public policy and assistive technology.

Their user services include the ABLEDATA database, 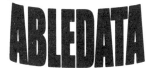 which describes thousands of assistive devices, from eating utensils to wheelchairs. A listing of 50 or fewer products is $5; NARIC charges $10 for 51 to 100 products, and $5 for each additional hundred products.

ABLEDATA also provides an information specialist to answer simple information requests and provide referrals immediately at no cost. Contact: 800-227-0216.

Contact: National Rehabilitation Information Center (NARIC), 1010 Wayne Ave., Suite 800, Silver Spring, MD 20910; 800-346-2742, 301-562-2400, TT: 301-495-5626, Fax: 301-562-2401, {www.naric.com}.

Canine Companions

Several organizations provide companion dogs to people with disabilities. Since 49 million Americans are disabled in some way—and only 3% of the disabled are blind—these animals are more than just "seeing eye dogs." They are trained to help individuals with a host of disabilities. Some organizations provide these dogs for free, while others request a small donation. To learn more about this valuable resource contact any of the following organizations:

* ✳ *Support Dogs, Inc.*, 10755 Indianhead Industrial Blvd., St. Louis, MO 63132; 314-423-1988; {http://members.aol.com/maxidog1/support.htm}; {E-mail: supportdogs@MSN.com}.
* ✳ *Canine Companions for Independence*, National Headquarters, P.O. Box 446, Santa Rosa, CA 95402; 800-572-2275; {www.caninecompanions.org}.
* ✳ *Independence Dogs, Inc.*, 146 State Line Road, Chadds Ford, PA 19317; 610-358-2723; Fax: 610-358-5314; {www.independencedogs.org}; {E-mail: idi@netreach.net}.
* ✳ *Canine Working Companions*, 7453 Morgan Rd., Liverpool, NY 13090; 315-457-2938; {http://members.aol.com/DeMauro5/cwc.htm}.
* ✳ *PAWS WITH A CAUSE*, National Headquarters, 4646 South Division, Wayland, MI 49348; 800-253-PAWS.
* ✳ *Loving Paws Assistance Cogs*, P.O. Box 12005, Santa Rosa, CA 95406; 707-586-0798; Fax: 707-586-0799; {www.lovingpaws.com}; {E-mail: vgpays@lovingpaws.com}.

Free Information for Employers Who Hire the Handicapped

The Job Accommodation Network (JAN) brings together free information about practical ways employers can make accommodations for employees and job applicants with disabilities. The network offers comprehensive information on methods and available equipment that have proven effective for a wide range of accommodations, including names, addresses, and phone numbers of appropriate resources.

Easter Seals in Arizona Offers Free Computers to People With Disabilities

Washington State chapter has a free loan program, and the chapters in Missouri offer computer classes. Contact you local Easter Seals Society to see what they may offer in the way of computers and computer skills for people with disabilities. If you can't find your local office, contact: Easter Seals, 230 West Monroe Street, Suite 1800, Chicago, IL 60606; 800-221-6825; 312-726-6200; Fax: 312-726-1494; {www.seals.com}.

JAN also provides information regarding the Americans with Disabilities Act (ADA) Project Able to find disabled employees. For ADA information, call 800-ADA-WORK (800-232-9675).

Job Accommodation Network (JAN), West Virginia University, P.O. Box 6080, Morgantown, WV 26506-6080; 800-526-7234, 800-526-2262 (Canada), Fax: 304-293-5407, {E-mail: jan@jan.icdi.wvu.edu}, {http://janweb.icdu.wvu.edu}.

Project ABLE is a national resume bank which provides employers an easily accessible applicant pool of qualified job-ready individuals who are ready, willing and very interested in working. The goal is to provide employers convenient access to quality human resources while providing training and employment services to eligible people with disabilities. Further, various tax incentives are available to businesses that hire people with disabilities. You can learn more by contacting the IRS at 800-829-1040.

After the matching process (usually within 24 hours), OPM will respond by forwarding the resumes of qualified individuals. Contact: Project ABLE, Project Leader, Shirley James, 200 Granby St., Room 500, Norfolk, VA 23510; 757-441-3362, Fax: 757-441-3374, {E-mail: projable@opm.gov}.

$$$$$ Money To Buy A Van, A Talking Computer Or Rubber Door Knob Grips

People with disabilities now have a place to turn to learn everything they need to know about how the latest in technology can improve their lives. It can be a specially equipped van, a talking computer, a special kitchen or eating aid, or adaptive toys for children. Or it may be a student with learning disabilities who needs special help getting through school.

A project funded by the U.S. Department of Education, called Technical Assistance Project, has established an office in each state that can provide:

▲ *Information Services*: will help you identify the special products that are available to help you cope with your disability.

▲ *Equipment Loan Program*: allows people to borrow new technology devices for a number of weeks before they purchase them.

▲ *Recycling Program*: matches up people with needs for products with people who want to sell or donate products.

▲ *Funding Information*: collects information on the various sources of funding for this equipment from public and private sources.

▲ *Loans*: many states are offering special loans to help people purchase the necessary equipment; Ohio offers low interest loans up to $10,000, California has loans up to $20,000, North Carolina up to $15,000.

If you have trouble locating your state office, you can contact the office that coordinates all state activities: Rehabilitation Engineering and Assertive Technology Society of North America, (RESNA), 1700 North Moore Street, #1540, Arlington, VA 22209; 703-524-6686; Fax: 703-524-6630; TTY: 703-524-6639; {www.resna.org}. See listing on page 234.

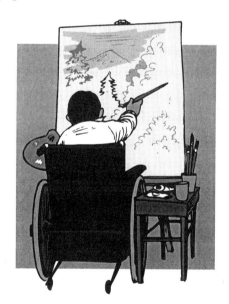

State Client Assistance Program (CAP)

The first place to start when your state Office of Vocational Rehabilitation denies you handicap or disability benefits is your nearest state Client Assistance Program (CAP) office. CAP is a free information, referral, and legal service that helps disabled or handicapped individuals appeal a denial by OVR (or other agency). CAP can take your appeal process from the first stages and all the way to the U.S. Supreme Court if necessary — and it won't cost you a penny.

State Disability Offices

When all else fails the state disability offices are a good place to turn for information on products and services for people with disabilities.

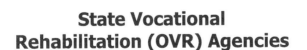

Statewide Technology Assistance Programs

Each state provides information services, equipment loan programs, recycled equipment programs, and funding and grant information.

State Vocational Rehabilitation (OVR) Agencies

These agencies act as an employment agency for the disabled, as well as providing education and training information and funding.

Alabama

Client Assistance Program
Jerry Norsworthy, Director
Client Assistance Program
2125 East South Boulevard
Montgomery, AL 361116-2454
334-281-2276
800-228-3231 (in AL)
E-mail: sacap@hotmail.com
http://members.theglobe.
com/jerlam/

Disability Office
Governor's Committee on
Employment of People with
Disabilities
Department of Rehabilitation
Service
P.O. Box 11586
2129 East South Boulevard
Montgomery, AL 36111-0586
334-281-8780 (Voice/TTY)
334-288-1104 (Fax)
www.personnel.state.al.us

*Technology Assistance
Programs*
Alabama Statewide
Technology Access and
Response Project
(STAR) System For
Alabamians with Disabilities
2125 East South Boulevard
P.O. Box 20752
Montgomery, AL 36120-0752
Project Director: Dr. Tom
Gannaway

334-613-3480
800-STAR656 (In-State)
334-613-3519 (TDD)
334-613-3485 (Fax)
E-mail: jbanks@rehab.
state.al.us
Homepage: www.rehab.
state.al.us

*Vocational Rehabilitation
Offices*
Lamona H. Lucas, Director
Alabama Department of
Rehabilitation Services
2129 East South Boulevard
P.O. Box 11586
Montgomery, AL 36116
334-281-8780
800-441-7607
334-613-2249 (TDD)
334-281-1973 (Fax)
www.rehab.state.al.us

Alaska

Client Assistance Program
Pam Stratton, Director
Client Assistance Program
2900 Boniface Parkway, #100
Anchorage, AK 99504-3195
907-333-2211
907-333-1186 (Fax)

Disability Office
The Governor's Committee on
Employment and Rehabilita-
tion of People with Disabilities

801 W. 10th Street
Suite 200
Juneau, AK 99801
907-465-2814 (Voice/TTY)
907-465-2856 (Fax)
www.educ.state.ak.us/
vocrehab/home.html

*Technology Assistance
Programs*
Assistive Technologies of
Alaska
1016 West 6th
Suite 200
Anchorage, AK 99501
Information and Referral: Rose
Foster
907-563-0138 (V/TDD)
Project Director: Jim Beck
907-269-3569 (V/TDD)
907-269-3632 (Fax)
E-mail: jim_beck@educ.
state.ak.us
Homepage: www.educ.
state.ak.us

*Vocational Rehabilitation
Offices*
Duane French, Director
Division of Vocational
Rehabilitation
801 West 10th St., Suite 200
Juneau, AK 99801-1894
907-465-2814
www.educ.state.ak.us/
vocrehab/home.html
E-mail: stevie.raleigh@
educ.state.ak.us

American Samoa
Client Assistance Program
Minareta Thompson, Director
Client Assistance Program
P. O. Box 3937
Pago Pago, AS 96799
011-684-633-2441
011-684-633-7286 (Fax)
E-mail: opad@samoatelco.com

*Technology Assistance
Programs*
American Samoa Assistive
Technology Service Project
(ASATS)
Division of Vocational
Rehabilitation
Department of Human
Resources
Pago Pago, AS 96799
Project Director: Edmund
Pereira
684-699-1529
684-233-7874 (TDD)
684-699-1376 (Fax)
E-mail: edperei@yahoo.com

*Vocational Rehabilitation
Offices*
Peter P. Galea'i, Director
Division of Vocational
Rehabilitation
Dept. of Human Resources
American Samoa Government
Pago Pago, AS 96799
011684-633-2336
www.ipacific.com/samoa/
samoa.html

Arizona

Disability Office
Governor's Committee on
Employment of People with
Disabilities
1012 E. Willetta
SRI-1Bb
Phoenix, AZ 85006
602-239-4762 (Voice)
602-239-5256 (Fax)
Webpage: None

Technology Assistance Programs
Arizona Technology Access
Program (AZTAP)
Institute for Human
Development
Northern Arizona University
P.O. Box 5630
Flagstaff, AZ 86011
Information and Referral:
ElizBeth Pifer
Director: Daniel Davidson,
Ph.D.
520-523-7035
520-523-1695 (TDD)
520-523-9127 (Fax)
E-mail: daniel.davidson@
nau.edu
Homepage: www.nau.edu

Vocational Rehabilitation Offices
Arizona Rehabilitation
Services Administration
Skip Bingham, Administrator

1789 West Jefferson
2nd Floor, NW
Phoenix, AZ 85007
602-542-3332
602-542-6049 (TDD)
800-563-1221
602-542-3778 (Fax)
www.azrsa.org/vr
E-mail: azrsa@cirs.org

Arkansas

Client Assistance Program
Eddie Miller, Director
Client Assistance Program
Disability Rights Center, Inc.
Evergreen Place
Suite 201
1100 North University
Little Rock, AR 72207
501-296-1775
800-482-1174
501-296-1779 (Fax)
E-mail: panda@
advocacyservices.org
www.advocacyservices.org

Disability Office
Governor's Commission on
People with Disabilities
1616 Brookwood Drive
Little Rock, AR 72202
501-296-1626 (Voice)
501-296-1623 (TTY)
501-296-1655 (Fax)
www.state.ar.us/ars/

Technology Assistance Programs
Arkansas Increasing Capabilities Access Network (ICAN)
Arkansas Department of Workforce Education
Arkansas Rehabilitation Services
2201 Brookwood Dr.
Suite 117
Little Rock, AR 72202
Project Director: Sue Gaskin
501-666-8868 (V/TDD)
800-828-2799 (V/TDD, In-State)
Fax: 501-666-5319
E-mail: sogaskin@ars.state.ar.us
Homepage: www.ars.state.ar.us

Vocational Rehabilitation Offices
Bobby C. Simpson, Director
Division of Vocational Rehabilitation
1616 Brookwood Drive
Little Rock, AR 72203
501-296-1661
Fax: 501-296-1672
www.nchrtm.okstate.edu/rrc/state_brochures/arkansas/statebrochureAR.html
E-mail: Bobby.Simpson@state.ar.us

James C. Hudson, Director
Div. of Services for the Blind

Department of Human Services
522 Main Street
Little Rock, AR 72201
501-682-5463
800-960-9270
501-682-0093 (TTY)
Fax: 501-682-0366

California
Client Assistance Program
Sheila Conlen-Mentkowski, Director
Client Assistance Program
2000 Evergreen St., 2nd Floor
Sacramento, CA 95815
916-322-5066
916-263-7372
800-952-5544
Fax: 916-263-7464
E-mail: smentkow@rehab.cahwnet.gov
www.rehab.cahwnet.gov

Disability Office
The California Governor's Committee for Employment of Disabled Persons
P.O. Box 826880, MIC 41
Sacramento, CA 94280-0001
Street Address:
   800 Capitol Mall
   Room 5078, MIC 41
   Sacramento, CA 95814
916-654-8055 (Voice)
916-654-9820 (TTY)
916-654-9821 (Fax)
www.gcedp.org

*Technology Assistance
Programs*
California Assistive
Technology System
California Department of
Rehabilitation
2000 Evergreen
Sacramento, CA 95815
Mailing Address:
P.O. Box 944222
Sacramento, CA 94244-2220
Information and Referral:
Colin Corby
Project Director: William
Campagna
916-263-8687
916-263-8685 (TTY)
916-263-8683 (Fax)
E-mail: ccorby@rehab.
cahwnet.gov
Homepage: www.rehab.
cahwnet.gov

*Vocational Rehabilitation
Offices*
Director
Department of Rehabilitation
PO Box 944222
Sacramento, CA 94244-2220
916-263-8981
916-263-7477 (TTY)
www.rehab.cahwnet.gov

Colorado
Client Assistance Program
Jeff Peterson, Director
Client Assistance Program

The Legal Center
455 Sherman Street, Suite 130
Denver, CO 80203
303-722-0300
800-288-1376
303-722-0720 (Fax)
E-mail: hn6282@handsnet.org

Disability Office
Colorado Governor's Advisory
Council for People with
Disabilities
c/o Aging and Adult Services
110 16th Street
Denver, CO 80202
303-313-8666 (Voice)
888-887-9135 (In State Only)
303-620-4191 (Fax)

*Technology Assistance
Programs*
Colorado Assistive
Technology Project
University of Colorado Health
Sciences Center
Colorado University Affiliated
Program
The Pavilion
A036/B140
1919 Ogden Street, 2nd Floor
Denver, CO 80218
Project Director: Cathy Bodine
303-864-5100
303-864-5110 (TDD)
303-864-5119 (Fax)
E-mail: cathy.bodine@
UCHSC.edu
Homepage: www.UCHSC.edu

Vocational Rehabilitation Offices
Diana Huerta, Director
Division of Vocational
Rehabilitation
Department of Social Services
110 16th Street, 2nd Floor
Denver, CO 80202
303-620-4152
303-444-9140 (Fax)
http://bcn.boulder.co.us/voc

Connecticut

Client Assistance Program
Susan Werboff, Director
Client Assistance Program
Office of P&A for Persons
with Disabilities
60B Weston Street
Hartford, CT 06120-1551
860-297-4300
860-566-2102 (TDD)
800-842-7303 (statewide)
Fax: 860-566-8714
E-mail: hn2571@handsnet.org
www.state.ct.us/opapd

Disability Office
Governor's Committee on
Employment of People with
Disabilities
Labor Department Building
200 Folly Brook Boulevard
Wethersfield, CT 06109
860-263-6000 (Voice)
860-566-1345 (TTY)
860-566-1629 (Fax)

Technology Assistance Programs
Connecticut Assistive
Technology Project
Dept. of Social Services, BRS
25 Sigourney St., 11th Floor
Hartford, CT 06106
Project Director: John M.
Ficarro
860-424-4881
800-537-2549 (In-State)
TDD: 860-424-4839
Fax: 860-424-4850
E-mail: cttap@aol.com
Homepage: www.tecajct.
uconn.edu

Vocational Rehabilitation Offices
Bureau of Rehabilitation
Services
Department of Social Services
10 Griffin Road, North
Windsor, CT 06095
860-298-2000
860-298-2231 (TDD)
860-298-9590 (Fax)
E-mail: brs.dss@po.state.ct.us
www.dss.state.ct.us/svcs/
rehab.htm

Kenneth Tripp, Director
Board of Education and
Services for the Blind
Vocational Rehabilitation
Division
184 Windsor Avenue
Windsor, CT 06095

860-602-4000
860-602-4002 (TTY)
860-278-6920 (Fax)

Delaware

Client Assistance Program
Theresa Gallagher, Director
Client Assistance Program
United Cerebral Palsy, Inc.
254 E. Camden-Wyoming Ave.
Camden, DE 19934
302-698-9336
800-640-9336
302-698-9338 (Fax)
E-mail: capucp@magpage.com

Disability Office
Governor's Committee on
Employment of People with
Disabilities
DVR, P.O. Box 9969
Wilmington, DE 19809-0969
Street Address:
  4425 North Market Street
  Wilmington, DE 19802
302-761-8275 (Voice)
302-761-6611 (Fax)
www.state.de.us\labor\division\

*Technology Assistance
Programs*
Delaware Assistive
Technology Initiative (DATI)
Center for Applied Science &
Engineering
University of Delaware/duPont
Hospital for Children

1600 Rockland Rd
Room 117E
P.O. Box 269
Wilmington, DE 19899-0269
Director: Beth A. Mineo
Mollica, Ph.D.
302-651-6790
800-870 DATI (3284) (In-
State)
302-651-6794 (TDD)
302-651-6793 (Fax)
E-mail: dati@asel.udel.edu
Homepage: www.asel.udel.edu

*Vocational Rehabilitation
Offices*
Andrea Guest, Director
Division of Vocational
Rehabilitation
PO Box 9969
4425 N. Market Street
Wilmington, DE 19809-0969
302-761-8275
302-761-6611 (Fax)
www.nchrtm.okstate.edu/rrc/
state_brochures/delaware/
statebrochureDE.html

Dedra Walice, Director
Division for the Visually
Impaired
Biggs Building
Health & Social Services
Campus
1901 N. Dupont Highway
New Castle, DE 19720
302-577-4731

District of Columbia
Client Assistance Program
Joseph Cooney, Director
Client Assistance Program
University Legal Services
300 I Street, NE, Suite 202
Washington, DC 20002
202-547-0198
202-547-2083 (Fax)
E-mail: jbrown@uls-dc.com

Disability Office
Mayor's Committee on Persons
with Disabilities
810 First Street, NE
Room 1007
Washington, DC 20002
202-442-8464 (Voice)
202-442-8742 (Fax)

*Technology Assistance
Programs*
University Legal Services AT
Program for the District of
Columbia
Information Specialist: Gil
Shamir
Program Manager: Alicia C.
Johns
300 I Street, NE
Suite 200
Washington, DC 20002
202-547-0198
TDD: 202-547-2657
Fax: 202-547-2662
Email: ajohns@ULS-DC.com
Homepage: www.ULS-
DC.com

*Vocational Rehabilitation
Offices*
D.C. Rehabilitation Services
Administration
800 9th Street, SW
Fourth Floor
Washington, DC 20024-2487
202-645-5883
202-645-5847 (TDD)
202-645-3857 (Fax)
202-645-5798
  (Chinese Speaking)
202-645-5875
  (Spanish Speaking)

Florida
Client Assistance Program
Ann Robinson, CAP Program
Advocacy Center for Persons
with Disabilities
2671 Executive Center
Circle West
Webster Building, Suite 100
Tallahassee, FL 32301-5024
850-488-9071
800-342-0823
800-346-4127 (TDD)
850-488-8640 (Fax)
www.advocacycenter.org

Disability Office
The Governor's Alliance &
The Able Trust
106 E. College Ave.
Suite 820
Tallahassee, FL 32301
850-224-4493 (Voice)

850-924-4496 (Fax)
www.abletrust.org

Technology Assistance Programs
Florida Alliance for Assistive
Service and Technology
1020 E. Lafayette St.
Suite 110
Tallahassee, FL 32301-4546
Project Director: Terry Ward
850-487-3278 (V/TDD)
850-487-2805 (Fax/TDD)
E-mail: faast@faast.org
Homepage: www.faast.org

Vocational Rehabilitation Offices
Tamira Bibb Allen, Director
Division of Vocational
Rehabilitation
Department of Labor and
Employment Security
Building A
2002 Old St. Augustine Road
Tallahassee, FL 32399-0696
850-488-6210
Information & Referral line:
800-451-4327
www.state.fl.us/vocrehab/
mission.html

Randy Touchton, Director
Division of Blind Services
Department of Education
2551 Executive Center Circle
Tallahassee, FL 32399
800-342-1330
850-488-1330

Georgia
Client Assistance Program
Charles Martin, Director
Client Assistance Program
123 N. McDonough
Decartur, GA 30030
404-373-3116
404-373-4110 (Fax)
E-mail: GaCAPDirector@
theOmbudsman.com
www.theOmbudsman.
com/CAP/

Disability Office
Georgia Committee on
Employment of Persons with
Disabilities
Division of Rehabilitation
Services
2 Peachtree St., NW
35rd Floor
Atlanta, GA 30303-3166
404-657-3023 (Voice)
404-657-3086 (Fax)

Technology Assistance Programs
Georgia Tools for Life
Division of Rehabilitation
Services
2 Peachtree Street NW
Suite 35-413
Atlanta, GA 30303-3166
Project Director: Joy Kniskern
404-657-3084
800-479-8665 (In-State)
404-657-3085 (TDD)
404-657-3086 (Fax)

E-mail: 102476.1737@
compuserve.com

*Vocational Rehabilitation
Offices*
Peggy Rosser, Director
Division of Rehabilitation
Services
Georgia Department of Human
Resources
2 Peachtree St., NW
35th Floor
Atlanta, GA 30303-3142
404-657-3000
404-657-3086 (Fax)
E-mail: Gradye@gomail.
doas.state.ga.us
www.doas.state.ga.us/
Departments/DHR/rehab.html

Guam
Client Assistance Program
Fidela Limtiacho, President of
the Board
Client Assistance Program
Parent Agencies Network
P.O. Box 23474
GMF, Guam 96921
671-649-1948
Fax: 671-472-2568

Disability Office
Governor's Commission on
Persons with Disabilities
1313 Central Avenue
Tiyan, Guam 96913
671-475-4646 (Voice)
671-477-2892 (Fax)

*Technology Assistance
Programs*
Guam System for Assistive
Technology (GSAT)
University Affiliated Program-
Developmental Disabilities
303 University Drive
University of Guam
UOG Station
Mangilao, Guam 96923
Principal Investigator: Heidi E.
Farra-San Nicolas, Ph.D.
Project Director: Ben Servino
671-735-2490-3
671-734-8378 (TDD)
671-734-5709 (Fax)
E-mail: gsat@ite.net

*Vocational Rehabilitation
Offices*
Nobert Ungacto, Director
Department of Vocational
Rehabilitation
Government of Guam
122 Harmon Plaza
Room B201
Harmon Industrial Park, Guam
96911
011-671-646-9468
www.gov.gu/

Hawaii
Client Assistance Program
Executive Director
Client Assistance Program
Protection & Advocacy
Agency

1580 Makaloa St.
Suite 1060
Honolulu, HI 96814
808-949-2922
808-949-2928 (Fax)
E-mail: pahi@pixi.com
www.pixi.com/~pahi

Disability Office
Commission on Persons with
Disabilities
919 Ala Moana Blvd.
Suite 101
Honolulu, HI 96814
808-586-8121 (Voice/TTY)
808-586-8129 (Fax)
www.hawaii.gov\health\
cpd_index.htm

*Technology Assistance
Programs*
Hawaii Assistive Technology
Training and Services
(HATTS)
414 Kuwili Street
Suite 104
Honolulu, HI 96817
Information and Resource:
Judith Clark
808-532-7114
Project Director: Barbara
Fischlowitz-Leong, M.Ed.
808-532-7110 (V/TDD)
800-645-3007 (V/TDD, In-
State)
808-532-7120 (Fax)
E-mail: hatts@hatts.org
Homepage: www.hatts.org

*Vocational Rehabilitation
Offices*
Neil Shim, Administrator
Division of Vocational
Rehabilitation & Services for
the Blind
Department of Human Services
Bishop Trust Bldg.
1000 Bishop St., Room 615
Honolulu, HI 96813
808-586-5366
808-586-5377 (Fax)
www.nchrtm.okstate.edu/rrc/
state_brochures/hawaii/
statebrochure.hi.html

Idaho
Client Assistance Program
Shawn DeLoyola, Director
Client Assistance Program
Co-Ad, Inc.
4477 Emerald, Suite B-100
Boise, ID 83706
208-336-5353
800-632-5125
208-336-5396 (Fax)
E-mail: coadinc@
cyberhighway.net
http://users.moscow.com/co-ad

Disability Office
Governor's Committee on
Employment of People with
Disabilities
Department of Employment
317 Main Street
Boise, ID 83735

208-334-6469 (Voice)
208-334-6424 (TTY)
208-334-6300 (Fax)

Technology Assistance Programs
Idaho Assistive Technology Project
129 W. Third Street
Moscow, ID 83844-4401
Information and Referral:
Michelle Doty
208-885-3630
Project Director: Ron Seiler
208-885-3559 (V/TDD)
208-885-3628 (Fax)
E-mail: seile861@uidaho.edu
Homepage: www.uidaho.edu

Vocational Rehabilitation Offices
F. Pat Young, Administrator
Division of Vocational Rehabilitation
P.O. Box 83720
650 W. State St.
Room 150
Boise, ID 83720-0096
208-334-3390
208-334-5305 (Fax)
www.state.id.us/dvr/
dvrhome.htm
E-mail: pyoung@idvr.
state.id.us

F. Pat Young, Director
Idaho Commission for the Blind

Division of Vocational Rehabilitation
Len B. Jordan Building
Room 150
Boise, ID 83702
208-334-3390
www.nchrtm.okstate.edu/rrc/
state_brochures/idaho/
statebrochureID.html

Illinois
Client Assistance Program
Cynthia Grothaus, Director
Client Assistance Program
100 N. First Street, 1st Floor
Springfield, IL 62702
217-782-5374
800-641-3929
217-524-1790 (Fax)
www.state.il.us/agency/
dhs/cap.htm

Disability Office
James R. Thompson Center
Department of Rehabilitative Services
100 W. Randolph St.
Suite 8-100
Chicago, IL 60601
312-814-5081 (Voice)
312-814-5000 (TTY)
312-814-5949 (Fax)

Technology Assistance Programs
Illinois Assistive Technology Project (1989)

1 W. Old State Capitol Plaza
Suite 100
Springfield, IL 62701
Project Director: Wilhelmina
Gunther
217-522-7985
217-522-9966 (TDD)
217-522-8067 (Fax)
E-mail: gunther @midwest.net

Vocational Rehabilitation
Offices
Department of Human Services
Office of Rehabilitation
Services
Carl Suter, Associate Director
623 East Adams, 3rd Floor
P.O. Box 19429
Springfield, IL 62794
800-843-6154
800-447-6404 (TTY)
www.state.il.us/agency/dhs

Indiana
Client Assistance Program
Amy Ames
Client Assistance Program
Indiana Protection and
Advocacy Services
4701 N. Keystone Ave.
Suite 222
Indianapolis, IN 46204
317-722-5555
800-622-4845
317-722-5564 (Fax)
E-mail: tgallagher@ipas.state.
in.us

Disability Office
Governor's Commission on
Planning for People with
Disabilities
143 West Market Street
Indianapolis, IN 46204
317-232-7773 (Voice)
317-233-3712 (Fax)
www.state.in.us\gpcpd

Technology Assistance
Programs
Indiana ATTAIN (Accessing
Technology Through
Awareness in Indiana) Project
1002 North First
Vincennes University
Social Sciences Building
Vincennes, IN 47591
Project Manager: Cris Fulford
317-921-8766
800-528-8246 (In-State)
800-743-3333 (TDD,
National)
317-921-8774 (Fax)
E-mail: cfulford@indian.
vinu.edu
Homepage: www.indian.
vinu.edu

Vocational Rehabilitation
Offices
Division of Disability, Aging
& Rehabilitative Services
Bureau of Vocational
Rehabilitation
Rita Martin, Deputy Director
402 West Washington Street

Room W-451
P.O. Box 7083
Indianapolis, IN 46207-7083
317-232-1147
800-545-7763
800-962-8408 (TDD, Indiana)
www.ai.org/fssa/HTML/PROG
RAMS/2b.html

Iowa

Client Assistance Program
Harlietta Helland, Director
Client Assistance Program
Division on Persons with
Disabilities
Lucas State Office Building
Des Moines, IA 50310
515-281-3957
800-652-4298
515-242-6119 (Fax)
E-mail: helland@willinet.net

Disability Office
Iowa Commission of Persons
with Disabilities
Lucas State Office Building
321 East 12th Street
Des Moines, IA 50319
515-242-6334 (Voice)
888-219-0471 (Toll Free)
515-242-6119 (Fax)
www.iowaaccess.org/dhr

*Technology Assistance
Programs*
Iowa Program for Assistive
Technology
Iowa University Affiliated
Program

University Hospital School
100 Hawkins Drive
Iowa City, IA 52242-1011
Information and Referral: Amy
Hanna
319-356-1514
Co-Directors: Mary Quigley,
319-356-4402
Jane Gay, 319-356-4463
800-331-3027 (V/TDD;
National)
Fax: 319-356-8284
E-mail: mary-quigley@
uiowa.edu
E-mail: jane-gay@uiowa.edu
Homepage: www.uiowa.edu/
infotech/InfoTech.htm

*Vocational Rehabilitation
Offices*
Iowa Division of Vocational
Rehabilitation Services
Marge Knudsen, Administrator
510 East 12th Street
Des Moines, IA 50319
515-281-4311 (Voice/TDD)
800-532-4703 (Iowa only)
515-281-4703 (Fax)
www.dvrs.state.ia.us
E-mail:dvrsdesk@
mail.dvrs.state.ia.us

Kansas

Client Assistance Program
Mary Reyer, Director
Client Assistance Program
2914 S.W. Plass Court

Topeka, KS 66611
785-266-8193
800-432-2326
785-266-8574 (Fax)
www.ink.org/public/srs/
srsrehabcomm.html#vr
E-mail: mreyer5175@aol.com

Disability Office
Kansas Commission on
Disability Concerns
1430 SW Topeka Blvd.
Topeka, KS 66612-1877
800-295-5232 (Toll-free
Voice)
877-340-5874 (Toll-free TTY)
785-296-1722 (Voice)
785-296-5044 (TTY)
785-296-0466 (Fax)
www.adabbs.hr.state.ks.us/dc

Technology Assistance Programs
Assistive Technology for
Kansans Project
2601 Gabriel
P.O. Box 738
Parsons, KS 67357
Project Director: Charles R.
Spellman
316-421-6550, ext. 1890
E-mail: chuck@parsons.lsi.
ukans.edu
Co-Director: Sara Sack
Project Coordinator: Sheila
Simmons
316-421-8367
800-KAN DO IT

316-421-0954 (Fax/TDD)
E-mail: ssack@parsons.
isi.ukans.edu
Homepage: www.parsons.isi.
ukans.edu

Vocational Rehabilitation Offices
Kansas Department of Social
& Rehabilitation Services
Rehabilitation Services
3640 SW Topeka Blvd.
Suite 100
Topeka, KS 66611
785-267-5301
800-432-2326
www.ink.org/public/srs/srsreha
bcomm.html
E-mail:wfd.vocrehab@
mail.state.ks.us

Kentucky
Client Assistance Program
Gerry Gordon-Brown,
Consumer Advocate
Client Assistance Program
209 St. Clair, 5th Floor
Frankfort, KY 40601
502-564-8035
800-633-6283
502-564-2951 (Fax)
E-mail: dianehigh@uky.
campus.mci.net

Disability Office
Kentucky Committee on
Employment of People with
Disabilities

CHR Bldg., Second - West
275 E. Main Street
Frankfort, KY 40621
502-564-2918 (Voice/TTY)
502-564-7452 (Fax)

Technology Assistance
Programs
Kentucky Assistive
Technology Services Network
Charles McDowell
Rehabilitation Center
8412 Westport Road
Louisville, KY 40242
Information and Referral: Jim
Syme
Project Director: J. Chase
Forrester
502-327-0022
800-327-5287 (V/TDD, In-
State)
502-327-9974 (Fax)
502-327-9855 (TDD)
E-mail: katsnet@iglou.com

Vocational Rehabilitation
Offices
Department of Vocational
Rehabilitation
Sam Serraglio, Commissioner
209 St. Clair Street
Frankfort, KY 40601
800-372-7172 (V/TDD,
Kentucky only)
502-564-4440
502-564-6742 (TDD)
www.ihdi.uky.edu/projects/dvr
/dvrhome.htm

Louisiana
Client Assistance Program
Susan Howard, CAP Director
Client Assistance Program
Advocacy Center for the
Elderly and Disabled
225 Baronne
Suite 2112
New Orleans, LA 70112-2112
504-522-2337
800-960-7705
504-522-5507 (Fax)
E-mail: simplo@advocacyLA.
org

Disability Office
Governor's Office of Disability
Affairs
Office of the Governor
P.O. Box 94004
Baton Rouge, LA 70806-9004
225-922-2003 (Voice)
225-342-9739 (Fax)

Technology Assistance
Programs
Louisiana Assistive
Technology Access Network
P.O. Box 14115
Baton Rouge, LA 70898-4115
Executive Director: Julie
Nesbit
225-925-9500 (V/TDD)
800-270-6185 (V/TDD)
225-925-9560 (Fax)
E-mail: latanstate@aol.com

Vocational Rehabilitation Offices
Louisiana Rehabilitation Services
May Nelson, Director
8225 Florida Boulevard
Baton Rouge, LA 70806
504-925-4131
800-737-2958
504-925-4484 (Fax)
504-925-4481 (Fax)
www.dss.state.la.us/
offlrs.index.htm
E-mail: webmaster@
dss.state.la.us

Maine

Client Assistance Program
Steve Beam, Director
Client Assistance Program
CARES, Inc.
4-C Winter Street
August, ME 04330
207-622-7055
800-773-7055
207-621-1869 (Fax)
E-mail: capsite@aol.com

Disability Office
Governor's Committee on
Employment of People with
Disabilities
35 Anthony Avenue
Augusta, ME 04330
207-624-5307 (Voice)
207-624-5302 (Fax)

Technology Assistance Programs
Maine Consumer Information
and Technology Training
Exchange (MAINE CITE)
Maine CITE Coordinating
Center
UMS Network for Ed. & Tech.
Services
46 University Drive
Augusta, ME 04330
Project Director: Kathy Powers
207-621-3195 (V/TDD)
207-621-3193 (Fax)
E-mail: kpowers@maine.
maine.edu
Homepage: www.mecite.
doe.k12.me.us/

Vocational Rehabilitation Offices
Maine Bureau of
Rehabilitation Services
Department of Labor
John G. Shattuck
150 State House Station
Augusta, ME 04333-0150
207-287-5100
800-698-4440 (V/TTY)
207-287-5166 (Fax)
http://janus.state.me.us/
labor/brs/vr.htm
E-mail: brs.me@state.me.us

Maryland
Client Assistance Program
Peggy Dew, Director

Client Assistance Program
MD Rehabilitation Center
Division of Rehabilitation
Services
2301 Argonne Drive
Baltimore, MD 21208
410-554-9358
800-638-6243
410-554-9362 (Fax)

Disability Office
Governor's Committee on
Employment of People with
Disabilities
1 Market Center, Box 10
300 West Lexington Street
Baltimore, MD 21201
800-637-4113
410-333-2263 (Voice/TTY)
410-333-6674 (Fax)
www.mdtap.org/oid.html

*Technology Assistance
Programs*
Maryland Technology
Assistance Program
Governor's Office for
Individuals with Disabilities
300 W. Lexington St., Box 10
Baltimore, MD 21201
Information Specialist: Patrick
McCurdy
Project Director: Paul Rasinski
410-502-9519 (V/TDD)
410-333-6674 (Fax)
E-mail: rasinski@clark.net

*Vocational Rehabilitation
Offices*
Maryland State Department of
Education
Division of Rehabilitation
Services
Robert Burns, Assistant State
Superintendent
2301 Argonne Drive
Baltimore, MD 21218-1696
410-554-9100
888-200-7117
800-735-2258 (TTY)
410-554-9412 (Fax)
www.dors.state.md.us
E-mail: dors@msde.
state.md.us

Massachusetts
Client Assistance Program
Barbara Lybarger
Client Assistance Program
Massachusetts Office on
Disability
One Ashburton Place
Room 1305
Boston, MA 02108
617-727-7440
800-322-2020
617-727-0965 (Fax)
E-mail: blybarger@modi.
state.ma.us
www.state.ma.us/mod/
MSCAPBRO.html

Disability Office
Governor's Commission on
Employment of People with
Disabilities
Department of Employment
and Training Policy Office
19 Stanford Street, 4th Floor
Boston, MA 02114
617-626-5190 (Voice)
617-727-8014 (Fax)
www.detma.org

Technology Assistance
Programs
Massachusetts Assistive
Technology Partnership
MATP Center
Children's Hospital
1295 Boylston St., Suite 310
Boston, MA 02115
Information and Referral:
Patricia Hill
Project Dir.: Marylyn Howe
617-355-7167 (TDD)
800-848-8867 (V/TDD, In-
State)
617-355-7153
617-355-7301 (TDD)
617-355-6345 (Fax)
E-mail: howe_m@a1.tch.
harvard.edu
Homepage: www.al.tch.
harvard.edu

Vocational Rehabilitation
Offices
Massachusetts Rehabilitation
Commission

Elmer C. Bartels,
Commissioner
Fort Point Place
27-43 Wormwood Street
Boston, MA 02210-1616
617-204-3600
800-245-6543 (V/TDD)
617-727-1354 (Fax)
www.state.ma.us/mrc
E-mail:scher@mediaone.net

Michigan
Client Assistance Program
Amy Maes, Director
Client Assistance Program
Michigan P&A Service
106 West Allegan, Suite 300
Lansing, MI 48933
517-487-1755
800-292-4150 (CAP only)
517-487-0827 (Fax)
E-mail: ebauer@mpas.org
www.mpas.org

Disability Office
Michigan Commission on
Disability Concerns
P.O. Box 30659
Lansing, MI 48909
Street Address:
   320 N. Washington Square
   Suite 250
Lansing, MI 48933
517-334-8000 (Voice/TTY)
517-334-6637 (Fax)
www.mfia.state.mi.us/
mcdc.htm

Technology Assistance Programs
Michigan Tech 2000
Michigan Assistive
Technology Project
740 W. Lake Lansing Rd.
Suite 400
East Lansing, MI 48823
Project Director: Sheryl Avery-Meints
Project Manager: Roanne Chaney
517-333-2477 (V/TDD)
800-760-4600 (In-State)
517-333-2677 (Fax)
E-mail: roanne@match.org
Homepage: www.match.org

Vocational Rehabilitation Offices
Michigan Department of
Career Development
Rehabilitation Services
Robert E. Davis, State Director
608 West Allegan
P.O. Box 30010
Lansing, MI 48909
517-373-3390
800-605-6722
888-605-6722 (TTY)
www.mrs.state.mi.us
E-mail:michab@edu.gte.net

Minnesota
Client Assistance Program
Pamela Hoopes, Director
Client Assistance Program

Minnesota Disability Law
Center
430 First Avenue North
Suite 300
Minneapolis, MN 55401-1780
612-332-1441
800-292-4150
612-334-5755 (Fax)
E-mail: hn0518@handsnet.org

Disability Office
Minnesota State Council on
Disability
121 E. 7th Place
Suite 107
St. Paul, MN 55101
651-296-1743 (Voice)
651-296-5935 (Fax)
www.disability.state.mn.us

Technology Assistance Programs
Minnesota STAR Program
300 Centennial Building
658 Cedar Street
St. Paul, MN 55155
Acting Executive Director:
Rona Linforth
800-657-3862 (In-State)
800-657-3895 (TDD In-State)
651-296-2771
651-296-9478 (TDD)
651-282-6671 (Fax)
E-mail: rona.linroth@
state.mn.us
Homepage: www.state.mn.us

*Vocational Rehabilitation
Offices*
Michael T. Coleman, Ed.D.
Department of Economic
Security
Rehabilitation Services Branch
390 North Robert Street
St. Paul, MN 55101
651-296-5616
800-328-9095
651-296-3900 (TTY)

Richard C. Davis
Minnesota Department of
Economic Security
State Services for the Blind
2200 University Ave. W. #240
St. Paul, MN 55114-1840
651-642-0508
800-652-9000
E-mail: Richard.Davis@
state.mn.us

Mississippi
Client Assistance Program
Presley Posey, Director
Client Assistance Program
Easter Seal Society
3226 N. State Street
Jackson, MS 39216
601-982-7051
601-981-1951 (Fax)
E-mail: pposey8803@aol.com

Disability Office
Mississippi Department of
Rehabilitation Services

P.O. Box 1698
Jackson, MS 39215-1698
Street Address:
  1281 Highway 51, North
  Madison, MS 39110
601-853-5100 (Voice)
800-443-1000 (In State Only)
601-853-5325 (Fax)
www.mdrs.state.ms.us.

*Technology Assistance
Programs*
Mississippi Project START
P.O. Box 1698
Jackson, MS 39215-1000
Information and Referral:
Albert Newsome
601-987-4872
Project Dir.: Stephen Power
601-987-4872
800-852-8328 (V/TDD; In-
State)
601-364-2349 (Fax)
E-mail: spower@netdoor.com
Homepage: none

*Vocational Rehabilitation
Offices*
Mississippi Department of
Rehabilitation Services
Office of Vocational
Rehabilitation
Gary Neely, Director
P.O. Box 1698
Jackson, MS 39215-1698
601-853-5321
601-853-5325 (TTY)
601-853-5310 (Fax)

www.mdrs.state.ms.us
E-mail: gneely@
mdrs.state.ms.us

Missouri
Client Assistance Program
Cecilia Callahan, Director of
Advocacy
Client Assistance Project
Missouri P&A Services
925 S. Country Club Drive
Unit B-1
Jefferson City, MO 65109
573-893-3333
800-392-8667
573-893-4231 (Fax)
E-mail: mopasjc@socket.net
http://members.socket.net/
~mopasjc/MOP&A.htm

Disability Office
Missouri Governor's Council
on Disability
P.O. Box 1668
3315 West Truman Boulevard
Jefferson City, MO 65102
573-751-2600 (Voice/TTY)
573-526-4109 (Fax)
www.dolir.state.mo.us/gcd

*Technology Assistance
Programs*
Missouri Assistive Technology
Project
4731 South Cochise
Suite 114

Independence, MO 64055-
6975
Project Director: Diane
Golden, Ph.D.
800-647-8557 (In-State)
816-373-5193
816-373-9315 (TDD)
816-373-9314 (Fax)
E-mail: matpmo@qni.com
Homepage: www.dolir.state.
mo.us/matp/

*Vocational Rehabilitation
Offices*
Ronald Vessell, Director
Missouri Division of
Vocational Rehabilitation
3024 West Truman Boulevard
Jefferson City, MO 65109
573-751-3251
800-735-2466
573-751-0881
800-735-2966 (TTY)
http://services.dese.state.mo.us/
divvocrehab

Missouri Rehabilitation
Services for the Blind
P.O. Box 88
Jefferson City, MO 65103-
0088
573-751-4249
800-592-6004
573-751-4984 (Fax)
www.dss.state.mo.us/dfs/
rehab/vr.htm
E-mail: mmerrick@mail.
state.mo.us

Montana
Client Assistance Program
Lynn Wislow, Director
Client Assistance Project
Montana Advocacy Program
316 N. Park, Room 211
P.O. Box 1680
Helena, MT 59624
406-444-3889
800-245-4743
Fax: 406-444-0261
E-mail: advocate@mt.net
www.mt.net/~advocate
www.mtadv.org

Disability Office
Governor's Advisory Council
on Disability
State Personnel Division
Department of Administration
P.O. Box 200127
Helena, MT 59620-0127
Street Address:
  125 Roberts Street
  Helena, MT 59620
406-444-3794 (Voice)
800-243-4091 Montana State
Relay
406-444-0544 (Fax)

*Technology Assistance
Programs*
MONTECH
Rural Institute on Disabilities
The University of Montana
634 Eddy Avenue
Missoula, MT 59812

Project Director.: Gail
McGregor
406-243-5676
800-732-0323 (TDD,
National)
406-243-4730 (Fax)
E-mail: montech@
selway.umt.edu
Homepage: www.
ruralinstitute.umt.edu

*Vocational Rehabilitation
Offices*
Joe Matthews, Administrator
Department Of Social and
Rehabilitation Services
Rehabilitation/Visual Services
111 North Sanders
Helena, MT 59620
P.O. Box 4210
Helena, MT 59604-4210
406-444-2590
406-444-2590 (TDD)
406- 444-3632 (Fax)
www.dphhs.mt.gov/whowhat/
dsd.htm

Nebraska
Client Assistance Program
Victoria L. Rasmussen,
Director
Client Assistance Program
Division of Rehabilitation
Services
Nebraska Department of
Education

301 Centennial Mall South
Lincoln, NE 68509
402-471-3656
800-742-7594
402-471-0117 (Fax)
E-mail: Vicki_r@nde4.nde.
state.ne.us

Disability Office
Governor's Committee on
Employment of People with
Disabilities
Nebraska Job Service
Department of Labor
550 South 16th Street
Box 94600
Lincoln, NE 68509
402-471-2776 (Voice)
402-471-2318 (Fax)

*Technology Assistance
Programs*
Nebraska Assistive
Technology Partnership
5143 S. 48th St., Suite C
Lincoln, NE 68516-2204
Information and Referral:
Kathryn Kruse
Project Director: Mark
Schultz;
402-471-0735 (V/TDD)
402-471-0734 (V/TDD)
888-806-6287 (In-State)
402-471-6052 (Fax)
E-mail: mschultz@nde4.
nde.state.ne.us
Homepage: www.nde.state.ne.
us/ATP/TECHome.html

*Vocational Rehabilitation
Offices*
Director, Frank C. Lloyd
Vocational Rehabilitation
Services
301 Centennial Mall South
P.O. Box 94987
Lincoln, NE 68509
402-471-3644
800-742-7594
402-471-0788 (Fax)
http://nde4.nde.state.ne.us/
VR/VocRe.html

Pearl VanVandt, Director
Services for Visually Impaired
Department Of Public
Institutions
4600 Valley Road
Suite 100
Lincoln, NE 68510-4844
402-471-2891

Nevada
Client Assistance Program
William E. Bauer, Director
Client Assistance Program
2450 Wrondel Way
Suite E
Reno, NV 89502
775-688-1440
800-633-9879
Fax: 775-688-1627
E-mail:wbauer@govmail.
state.nv.us
http://members.delphi.com/
nvcap

Disability Office
Governor's Committee on
Employment of People with
Disabilities
4001 S. Virginia Street
Reno, NV 89502
775-688-1111 (Voice/TTY)
775-688-1113 (Fax)
www.state.nv.us\b&i\etd\
index.html

*Technology Assistance
Programs*
Nevada Assistive Technology
Collaborative
Rehabilitation Division
Community Based Services
711 South Stewart Street
Carson City, NV 89710
Project Administrator: Donny
Loux
702-259-0789
775-687-3388 (TDD)
775-687-3292 (Fax)
E-mail: pgowins@govmail.
state.nv.us
Homepage: None

*Vocational Rehabilitation
Offices*
Maynard Yasmer,
Administrator
Department of Employment,
Training and Rehabilitation
Rehabilitation Division
Bureau of Vocational
Rehabilitation
505 E. King St., #501

Carson City, NV 89701-3704
775-684-4070
775-684-4186 (Fax)
www.state.nv.us/detr/rehab/
reh_vorh.htm

New Hampshire
Client Assistance Program
Michael D. Jenkins, Executive
Director
Client Assistance Program
Governor's Commission on
Disability
57 Regional Drive
Concord, NH 03301-9686
603-271-2773
603-271-2837 (Fax)
E-mail: bhagy@gov.state.nh.us
www.state.nh.us/disability/
caphomepage.html

Disability Office
Governor's Commission on
Disability
57 Regional Drive
Concord, NH 03301-8518
603-271-2773 (Voice/TTY)
603-271-2837 (Fax)
www.gov.state.nh.us

*Technology Assistance
Programs*
New Hampshire Technology
Partnership Project
Institute on Disability/UAP
#14 Ten Ferry Street
The Concord Center

Concord, NH 03301
Project Director: Jan Nisbet,
(603) 862-4320
Co-Project Director: Therese
Willkomm
603-528-3060
800-427-3338 (V/TDD; In-
State)
603-224-0630 (V/TDD)
603-226-0389 (Fax)
E-mail: twillkomm@
nhaat.mv.com
Homepage: http://iod.unh.edu

***Vocational Rehabilitation
Offices***
Paul K. Leather, Director
Division of Vocational
Rehabilitation
78 Regional Drive
Concord, NH 03301-9686
603-271-3471
800-299-1647
www.state.nh.us/doe/VRWEB/
Copy%20of%20Primary/
E-mail: cfairneny@ed.state.
nh.us

New Jersey
Client Assistance Program
Ellen Lence, Director
Client Assistance Program
New Jersey P&A, Inc.
210 S. Broad Street, 3rd Floor
Trenton, NJ 08608
609-292-9742
800-922-7233

609-777-0187 (Fax)
E-mail: advoca@njpanda.org
www.njpanda.org

Disability Office
New Jersey Division of
Vocational Rehabilitation
Services
CN 398
Trenton, NJ 08625
609-292-7959 (Voice)
609-292-8347 (Fax)
www.wnjpin.state.nj.us\
onestocareercenter\
otherinformation\
divocrehabservices\

***Technology Assistance
Programs***
New Jersey Technology
Assistive Resource Program
(TARP)
New Jersey Protection and
Advocacy, Inc.
210 S. Broad St., 3rd Floor
Trenton, NJ 08608
Project Director: Ellen Lence
609-777-0945
Program Manager: Tim
Montagano
609-292-7498
E-mail: Lav42prg@
concentric.net
800-342-5832 (In-State)
609-633-7106 (TDD)
609-777-0187 (Fax)
E-mail: packr@njpanda.org
Homepage: www.njpanda.org

Vocational Rehabilitation Offices
Thomas G. Jennings, Director
135 East State Street
P.O. Box 398
Trenton, NJ 08625-0398
609-292-5987
609-292-8347 (Fax)
609-292-2919 (TTY)
E-mail: mford@dol.state.nj.us

Jamie Casabianca-Hilton,
Director
Commission for the Blind and
Visually Impaired
Department of Human Services
153 Halsey Street, 6th Floor
P.O. Box 47017
Newark, NJ 07101
201-648-2324
www.state.nj.us/
humanservices/dhsbvi1.html
E-mail: ddaniels@dhs.state.
nj.us

New Mexico
Client Assistance Program
Barna Dean, CAP Coordinator
Protection & Advocacy, Inc
1720 Louisiana Blvd., NE
Suite 204
Albuquerque, NM 87110
505-256-3100
800-432-4682
505-256-3184 (Fax)
E-mail: hn5412@earthlink.net
www.nmprotection-advocacy.
com

Disability Office
Governor's Committee on
Concerns of the Handicapped
Lamy Building - Room 117
491 Old Santa Fe Trail
Santa Fe, NM 87501
505-827-6465 (Voice)
505-827-6329 (TTY)
505-827-6328 (Fax)

Technology Assistance Programs
New Mexico Technology
Assistance Program
435 St. Michael's Dr., Bldg. D
Santa Fe, NM 87505
Information and Referral:
Carol Cadena
Project Director: Alan Klaus
800-866- 2253
505-954-8539 (V/TDD)
505-954-8562 (Fax)
E-mail: nmdvrtap@aol.com
Homepage: www.nmtap.com

Vocational Rehabilitation Offices
Terry Brigance, Director
Division of Vocational
Rehabilitation
435 St. Michael's Drive
Building D
Santa Fe, NM 87505
505-954-8500
800-224-7005
505-954-8562 (Fax)
www.state.nm.us/dvr
E-mail: SKelley@state.nm.us

New York
Client Assistance Program
Michael Peluso, Director
Client Assistance Program
NY Commission on Quality of
Care for the Mentally Disabled
401 State Street
Schenectody, NY 12305-2397
518-381-7098
800-624-4143 (TDD)
518-381-7095 (Fax)
www.cqc.state.ny.us
E-mail: michealp@cqc.state.
ny.us

Disability Office
New York State Office of
Advocate for Persons with
Disabilities
One Empire State Plaza
Suite 1001
Albany, NY 12223-1150
518-473-4129 (Voice)
800-522-4369 (In State Only)
518-473-4231 (TTY)
518-473-6005 (Fax)
www.state.ny.us/
disabledadvocate

*Technology Assistance
Programs*
New York State Triad Project
Office of Advocate for Persons
with Disabilities
One Empire State Plaza
Suite 1001
Albany, NY 12223-1150
Project Dir.: Deborah Buck

518-474-2825
800-522-4369 (V/TDD; In-
State)
518-473-4231 (TDD)
518-473-6005 (Fax)
E-mail: dbuck@nysnet.net
Homepage: www.state.ny.us/
disabledadvocate

*Vocational Rehabilitation
Offices*
John A. Johnson,
Commissioner
Department of Social Services
Commission for the Blind and
Visually Handicapped
40 North Pearl Street
Albany, NY 11243-0001
518-474-7079 (Voice)
518-474-7501 (TTY)
518-486-5819 (Fax)
www.dfa.state.ny.us/cbvh/
default.htm
E-mail: CBVH@dfa.state.ny.us

North Carolina
Client Assistance Program
Kathy Brack, Director
Client Assistance Program
NC Division of Vocational
Rehabilitation Services
P. O. Box 26053
Raleigh, NC 27611
919-733-6300
800-215-7227
919-715-2456 (Fax)
E-mail: kbrack@dhr.state.nc.us

Disability Office
The North Carolina
Employment Network
P.O. Box 26053
Raleigh, NC 27611
919-733-3364 (Voice)
919-715-0616 (Fax)
www.dhhs.state.nc.us

*Technology Assistance
Programs*
North Carolina Assistive
Technology Project
Department of Health and
Human Services
Division of Vocational
Rehabilitation Services
1110 Navaho Drive, Suite 101
Raleigh, NC 27609-7322
Project Director: Ricki Cook
919-850-2787 (V/TDD)
919-850-2792 (Fax)
E-mail: rickic@
mindspring.com

*Vocational Rehabilitation
Offices*
Bob Philbeck, Director
Division of Vocational
Rehabilitation Services
805 Ruggles
Raleigh, NC 27603
919-733-3364
919-733-7968 (Fax)
www.dhhs.state.nc.us/docs/
divinfo/dvr.htm

John DeLuca, Director
Div. of Services for the Blind

309 Ashe Avenue
Raleigh, NC 27606
919-733-9822
919-733-9769 (Fax)
E-mail: jdeluca@dhr.state.
nc.us
www.dhhs.state.nc.us/docs/
divinfo/dsb.htm

North Dakota
Client Assistance Program
Dennis Lyon, Director
Client Assistance Program
600 South 2nd Street, Suite 1B
Bismarck, ND 58504-4038
701-328-8947
800-207-6122
701-328-8969 (Fax)
E-mail: solyod@state.nd.us

Disability Office
Governor's Committee on
Employment of People with
Disabilities
600 South 2nd Street
Bismarck, ND 58504
701-328-8952 (Voice)
701-328-8969 (Fax)

*Technology Assistance
Programs*
North Dakota Interagency
Program for Assistive
Technology (IPAT)
P.O. Box 743
Cavalier, ND 58220
Director: Judie Lee

701-265-4807 (V/TDD)
701-265-3150 (Fax)
E-mail: lee@pioneer.
state.nd.us
Homepage: www.ndipat.org

Vocational Rehabilitation
Offices
Gene Hysjulien, Director
ND Disability Services
Division
Vocational Rehabilitation
600 South 2nd Street, Suite 1B
Bismarck, ND 58504
701-328-8950
800-755-2745
701-328-8968 (TDD)
701-328-8969 (Fax)

N. Marianas Islands
Client Assistance Program
Client Assistance Program
Northern Marianas
Protection and Advocacy
System, Inc.
P.O. Box 3529 C.K.
Saipan, MP 96950
011-670-235-7274/3
011-670-235-7275 (Fax)
E-mail: lbarcinasp&a@
saipan.com

Technology Assistance
Programs
Commonwealth of the
Northern Mariana Islands
Assistive Technology Project

Governor's Developmental
Disabilities Council
Systems of Technology-
Related Assistance for
Individuals with Disabilities
P.O. Box 2565 CK
Saipan, MP 96950
Project Director: Thomas J.
Camacho
670-322-3014(V/TDD)
670-322-4168 (Fax)
E-mail: dd.council@
saipan.com

Ohio
Client Assistance Program
Caroline Knight, Director
Client Assistance Program
Ohio Legal Rights Service
8 East Long Street, 5th Floor
Columbus, OH 43215
614-466-7264
800-282-9181
614-644-1888 (Fax)
E-mail: cknight@mail.olrs.
ohio.gov
www.state.oh.us/olrs/

Disability Office
Ohio Governor's Council on
People with Disabilities
400 East Campus View Blvd.
Columbus, OH 43235-4604
614-438-1393 (Voice)
614-438-1274 (Fax)
800-282-4536, ext. 1391
(Statewide)
www.state.oh.us/gcpd

*Technology Assistance
Programs*
Ohio TRAIN
Ohio Super Computer Center
1224 Kinnear Road
Columbus, OH 43212
Executive Director: Douglas
Huntt
614- 292-2426 (V/TDD)
800-784-3425 (V/TDD, In-
State)
614-292-3162 (TDD)
614-292-5866 (Fax)
E-mail: huntt.1@osc.edu
Homepage: www.osc.edu

*Vocational Rehabilitation
Offices*
Robert L. Rabe, Administrator
Ohio Rehabilitation Services
Commission
400 E. Campus View Blvd.
Columbus, OH 43235-4604
800-282-4536 (Ohio only)
614-438-1200
614-438-1257 (Fax)
www.state.oh.us/rsc/

Oklahoma
Client Assistance Program
Helen Kutz, Director
Client Assistance Program
Oklahoma Office of
Handicapped Concerns
2712 Villa Prom
Oklahoma City, OK 73107
405-521-3756

800-522-8224
405-943-7550 (Fax)

Disability Office
Governor's Committee on
Employment of the
Handicapped
Office of Handicapped
Concerns
Shepherd Mall
2712 Villa Prom
Oklahoma City, OK
73107-2423
405-521-3756 (Voice/TTY)
405-943-7550 (Fax)

*Technology Assistance
Programs*
Oklahoma Able Tech
Oklahoma State University
Wellness Center
1514 W. Hall of Fame Road
Stillwater, OK 74078-2026
Project Manager: Linda Jaco
405-744-9864
405-744-9748
800-257-1705 (V/TDD)
405-744-2487 (Fax)
E-mail: okway.okstate.edu
Homepage: www.okstate.edu

*Vocational Rehabilitation
Offices*
Linda Parker, Director
Department of Rehabilitation
Services
3535 N.W. 58th St.
Suite 500

Oklahoma City, OK 73112-
4815
405-951-3400
405-951-3529 (Fax)
www.onenet.net/~drspiowm/
vremp.htm
E-mail: drspiowm@onenet.net

Oregon
Client Assistance Program
Kim Marks, Director
Client Assistance Program
OR Disabilities Commission
610 SW Alder Ave., Suite 915
Portland, OR 97205
503-721-0135
800-746-7398
503-916-4003 (Fax)
E-mail: ocap@teleport.com

Disability Office
Oregon Disabilities
Commission
1257 Ferry St., S.E.
Salem, OR 97310
503-378-3142 (Voice/TTY)
503-378-3599 (Fax)

*Technology Assistance
Programs*
Oregon Technology Access for
Life Needs Project (TALN)
c/o Access Technologies Inc.
3070 Lancaster Drive NE
Salem, OR 97305-1396
Project Director: Byron
McNaught

800-677-7512 (In-State)
503-361-1201 (V/TDD)
503-370-4530 (Fax)
E-mail: ati@orednet.org
Homepage: www.taln.ncf.com

*Vocational Rehabilitation
Offices*
Gary K. Weeks, Director
Vocational Rehabilitation
Division
Administration Office
500 Summer Street NE
Salem, OR 97310-1012
503-945-5880
503-945-5894 (TTY)
503-945-8991 (Fax)
http://vrdnet.hr.state.or.us/
VRDweb/Default.htm
E-mail: dhr.info@state.or.us

Charles Young, Administrator
Commission for the Blind
535 SE 12th Avenue
Portland, OR 97214
503-731-3221
Toll Free: 1-888-202-5463
www.cfb.state.or.us
E-mail: ocbmail@state.or.us

Pennsylvania
Client Assistance Program
Stephen Pennington, Executive
Director
Client Assistance Program
Center for Disability Law &
Policy

1617 J.F.K. Blvd.
Suite 800
Philadelphia, PA 19103
215-557-7112
888-745-2357
215-557-7602 (Fax)
E-mail: capcdkt@trfn.
clpgh.org
ww.netslink.com/dislaw

Disability Office
Governor's Committee on
Employment of People with
Disabilities
Labor and Industry Building
7th and Forster Streets
Room 1315
Harrisburg, PA 17120
717-787-5232 (Voice)
717-783-5221 (Fax)

Technology Assistance
Programs
Pennsylvania's Initiative on
Assistive Technology
Institute on Disabilities/UAP
Ritter Annex 423
Philadelphia, PA 19122-6090
Project Director: Amy
Goldman
800-204-PIAT (7428)
800-750-PIAT (TT) (TDD)
215-204-9371 (Fax)
E-mail: piat@astro.ocis.
temple.edu
Homepage: www.astro.ocis.
temple.edu

Vocational Rehabilitation
Offices
Susan L. Aldrete, Executive
Director
Office of Vocational
Rehabilitation
Labor & Industry Building
7th and Forster Streets
Harrisburg, PA 17602
800-442-6351 (Voice)
800-233-3008 (TTY)
www.dli.state.pa.us/ovr/
index.htm
E-mail: ovr@dli.state.pa.us

Rose Putric, Acting Director
Bureau of Blindness & Visual
Services
Department of Public Welfare
1401 North 7th Street
P.O. Box 2675
Harrisburg, PA 17105
717-787-6176
http://trfn.clpgh.org/srac/bvs/
brochure.html

Puerto Rico
Client Assistance Program
David Cruz, Director
Client Assistance Program
Office of the Governor
Ombudsman for the Disabled
P. O. Box 4109
San Juan, PR 00902-4234
787-721-4299
787-725-3606

800-981-4125
Fax: 787-721-2455
E-mail: mromero@prtc.net

Disability Office
Governor's Committee on
Employment of Persons with
Disabilities
Office of the Ombudsman for
Persons with Disabilities
P.O. Box 4234
San Juan, PR 00902-4234
Street Address:
  670 Ponce De Leon Avenue
  Miramar, San Juan 00902
787-725-2333, ext. 2021
(Voice)
787-725-4014 (TTY)
787-721-2455 (Fax)

Technology Assistance Programs
Puerto Rico Assistive
Technology Project
University of Puerto Rico
Medical Sciences Campus
College of Related Health
Professions
Office of Project Investigation
and Development
Box 365067
San Juan, PR 00936-5067
Project Director: Maria I.
Miranda, B.A.
800-496-6035 (National)
800-981-6033 (In PR)
787-758-2525, ext. 4413

787-754-8034 (TDD/Fax)
E-mail: pratp@coqui.net

Republic of Palau
Client Assistance Program
Client Assistance Program
Bureau of Public Health
Ministry of Health
P.O. Box 6027
Koror, Republic of Palau
96940
011-680-488-2813
011-680-488-1211 (Fax)
E-mail: phpa@palaunet.com

Rhode Island
Client Assistance Program
Ted Mello, Director
Client Assistance Program
Rhode Island Disability Law
Center Inc.
349 Eddy Street
Providence, RI 02903
401-831-3150
401-831-5335 (TDD)
800-733-5332
401-274-5568 (Fax)
E-mail: hn7384@handsnet.org

Disability Office
Governor's Commission on the
Handicapped
Building 51, 3rd Floor
555 Valley Street
Providence, RI 02908-5686
401-222-3731 (Voice/TTY)

401-222-2833 (Fax)
www.gcd.state.ri.us

Technology Assistance Programs
Rhode Island Assistive
Technology Access
Partnership
Office of Rehabilitation
Services
40 Fountain Street
Providence, RI 02903
Project Director: Susan Olson
401-421-7005, ext. 310
800-752-8088, ext. 2608 (In-State)
401-421-7016 (TDD)
401-421-9259 (Fax)
E-mail: solson@atap.state.ri.us
Homepage: www.atap.
state.ri.us

Vocational Rehabilitation Offices
Raymond A. Carroll,
Administrator
Office of Vocational
Rehabilitation Services
Department of Human Services
40 Fountain Street
Providence, RI 02908
401-421-7005
401-421-7016 (TDD)
401-421-9259 (Fax)
800-752-8088, ext. 2300
E-mail: rcarroll@ors.state.
ri.us.
www.ors.state.ri.us/

South Carolina
Client Assistance Program
Larry Barker, Director
Client Assistance Program
Office of the Governor
Division of Ombudsman &
Citizen Services
P.O. Box 11369
Columbia, SC 29211
803-734-0457
800-868-0040
803-734-0546 (Fax)
E-mail: mbutler@govoepp.
state.sc.us

Disability Office
Governor's Committee on Employment of the Handicapped
Vocational Rehabilitation
Department
1410 Boston Avenue
P.O. Box 15
West Columbia, SC
29171-0015
803-939-0224
803-896-6621 (Voice)
803-896-6877 (Fax)

Technology Assistance Programs
South Carolina Assistive
Technology Program
USC School of Medicine
Center for Developmental
Disabilities
Columbia, SC 29208
Project Director: Evelyn Evans
803-935-5263

803-935-5263 (V/TDD)
803-935-5342 (Fax)
E-mail:scatp@scsn.net
Homepage: www.public.usit.
net\jjendron\

Vocational Rehabilitation
Offices
Vocational Rehabilitation
Department
State Office Building
1410 Boston Avenue
P.O. Box 15
West Columbia, SC 29171-
0015
803-896-6500
www.scvrd.net/scvrinfo.htm
E-mail:scvrpi@infoave.net

South Dakota
Client Assistance Program
Nancy Schade, Director
Client Assistance Program
South Dakota Advocacy
Services
221 South Central Avenue
Pierre, SD 57501
605-224-8294
800-658-4782
605-224-5125 (Fax)
E-mail: sdas@sdadvocacy.com
www.sdadvocacy.com

Disability Office
Governor's Advisory
Committee on Employment of
People with Disabilities

Department of Human Services
221 South Central
Suite 34 A
Pierre, SD 57501
605-945-2207 (Voice)
605-945-2422 (Fax)
www.tie.net/dakotalink

Technology Assistance
Programs
South Dakota Assistive
Technology Project
(DAKOTALINK)
221 S. Central
Pierre, SD 57501
Project Director: Dave Vogel
605-224-5336
800-224-5336 (V/TDD, In-
State)
605-224-8320 (Fax)
E-mail: dvogel@tie.net
Homepage: www.tie.net/
dakotalink

Vocational Rehabilitation
Offices
David Miller, Director
Division of Rehabilitation
Services
East Highway 34
Hillsview Plaza
c/o 500 East Capitol Avenue
Pierre, SD 57501
605-773-3195
605-773-5483 (Fax)
E-mail: infors@dhs.state.sd.us
www.state.sd.us/dhs/drs/vr.htm

Grady Kickul, Director
Division of Service to the
Blind and Visually Impaired
Hillsview Plaza, E. Hwy 34
c/o 500 East Capitol
Pierre, SD 57501-5070
605-773-4644
605-773-5483 (Fax)
E-mail: infosbvi@dhs.state.
sd.us
www.state.sd.us/state/
executive/dhs/sbvi/homepage/
sbvi.htm

Tennessee

Client Assistance Program
Dann Suggs, Director
Client Assistance Program
Tennessee P&A, Inc.
P. O. Box 121257
Nashville, TN 37212
615-298-1080
800-342-1660
615-298-2046 (Fax)
E-mail: shirleys@tpainc.org

Disability Office
Tennessee Committee for
Employment of People with
Disabilities
Division of Rehabilitation
Services
Citizens Plaza Building
Room 1100
400 Deaderick Street
Nashville, TN 37219
615-313-4891 (Voice)

615-313-5695 (TTY)
615-741-6508 (Fax)
www.state.tn.us

*Technology Assistance
Programs*
Tennessee Technology Access
Project (TTAP)
Cordell Hull Bldg., 5th Floor
425 5th Avenue North
Nashville, TN 37247-4850
Project Dir.: Jacque Cundall
615-741-8530/0310
615-741-1063 (Fax)
E-mail: jcundall@mail.
state.tn.us
Homepage: www.state.tn.us

*Vocational Rehabilitation
Offices*
Carl Brown, Assistant
Commissioner
Tennessee Department of
Human Services
Division of Rehabilitation
Services
400 Deaderick St., 11th Floor
Nashville, TN 37248-6000
615-313-4891 (V/TTY)
www.state.tn.us/humanserv
E-mail:carlbrown@
mail.state.tn.us

Texas
Client Assistance Program
Judy Sokolow, Coordinator
Client Assistance Program

Advocacy, Inc.
7800 Shoal Creek Blvd.
Suite 171-E
Austin, TX 78757
512-454-4816
800-252-9108
512-323-0902 (Fax)
E-mail: infoai@
advocacyinc.org
www.advocacyinc.org

Disability Office
Governor's Committee on
People with Disabilities
P.O. Box 12428
Austin, TX 78711
Street Address:
    1100 San Jacinto, Room 300
    Austin, TX 78701
512-463-5742 (Voice)
512-463-5746 (TTY)
512-463-5745 (Fax)
www.governor.state.tx.us/
disabilities/disabilities_index.
html

Technology Assistance Programs
Texas Assistive Technology
Partnership
University of Texas at Austin
Texas University Affiliated
Program
SZB252-D5100
Austin, TX 78712-1290
Information and Referral: John
Moore
800-828-7839

Project Dir.: Susanne Elrod
512-471-7621
512-471-1844 (TDD)
512-471-7549 (Fax)
E-mail: s.elrod@mail.
utexas.edu
Homepage: www.utexas.edu

Vocational Rehabilitation Offices
Vernon M. Arrell,
Commissioner
Texas Rehabilitation
Commission
4900 North Lamar Blvd
Austin, TX 78751
512-424-4410
512-424-4417 (TDD)
800-628-5115
www.rehab.state.tx.us/
p_vrpgm.html

Terry Murphy, Executive Dir.
Texas Commission for the
Blind
4800 North Lamar
Austin, TX 78756-3175
512-459-2500
800-252-5204 (Voice or TDD)
512-459-2685 (Fax)
www.tcb.state.tx.us/

Utah
Client Assistance Program
Nancy Friel, Director
Client Assistance Program
Disability Law Center

455 East 400 South, Suite 410
Salt Lake City, UT 84111
801-363-1347
800-662-9080
801-363-1437 (Fax)
E-mail: dlcall@
disabilitylawcenter.org
www.disabilitylawcenter.org

Disability Office
Utah Governor's Committee on
Employment of People with
Disabilities
c/o BOOST
4490 South 2700 East
Salt Lake City, UT 84124
801-538-7522 (Voice)
800-473-7530 (Voice)
801-538-2434 (Fax)
www.usor.state.ut.us

***Technology Assistance
Programs***
Utah Assistive Technology
Program
Center for Persons with
Disabilities
6588 Old Main Hill
Logan, UT 84322-6588
Project Director: Marvin
Fifield, Ed.D.
435-797-1982
Project Coordinator: Martin
Blair
435-797-3886
435-797-1981 (V/TDD)
Fax: 435-797-2355
E-mail: marv@cpd2.usu.edu

***Vocational Rehabilitation
Offices***
Blaine Petersen, Executive
Director
Vocational Rehabilitation
Services
250 North 1950 West
Suite B
Salt Lake City, UT 84116-
7902
801-323-4374
801-323-4396 (Fax)
www.usor.state.ut.us/

Vermont
Client Assistance Program
Laura Phillips, Director
Client Assistance Program
Vermont Disability Law
Project
Box 1367
Burlington, VT 05402
802-863-2881
802-863-7152 (Fax)
E-mail: lphillips@vtlegalaid.
org

Disability Office
Governor's Committee on
Employment of People with
Disabilities
c/o Vermont D.D. Council
103 South Main Street
Waterbury, VT 05671-0206
802-241-2612 (Voice/TTY)
802-241-2979 (Fax)
www.ahs.state.vt.us/vtddc

Technology Assistance Programs
Vermont Assistive Technology Project
103 South Main Street
Weeks Building, First Floor
Waterbury, VT 05671-2305
Project Dir.: Lynne Cleveland
802-241-2620 (V/TDD)
802-241-2174 (Fax)
E-mail: lynnec@dad.state.vt.us
Homepage: www.ahs.state.vt.us/vtddc

Vocational Rehabilitation Offices
Diane P. Dalmasse, Director
Division of Vocational Rehabilitation
103 South Main Street
Waterbury, VT 05671-2303
802-241-2186
www.dad.state.vt.us/dvr
802-241-2210
802-241-3359 (Fax)
E-mail: steve@dad.state.vt.us
www.dad.state.vt.us/dbvi

Virginia
Client Assistance Program
Mary Hart, Manager
Client Assistance Program
Department for Rights of Virginians with Disabilities
Ninth Street Office Bldg.
202 North 9th Street, 9th Floor
Richmond, VA 23219

804-225-2042
800-552-3962
804-225-3221 (Fax)
E-mail: fergusst@drvd.state.va.us
www.cns.state.va.us/drvd

Disability Office
The Virginia Board for People with Disabilities
202 North 9th St., 9th Floor
Richmond VA 23219
804-786-0016(Voice/TTY)
800-846-4464 (Voice/TTY)
(In State Only)
804-786-1118 (Fax)
www.vbpd.state.da.us

Technology Assistance Programs
Virginia Assistive Technology System
8004 Franklin Farms Drive
Richmond, VA 23288-0300
Information and Referral: 800-435-8490
Project Director: Kenneth Knorr
804-662-7000
804-662-9040 (V/TDD)
804-662-9532 (Fax)
E-mail: vatskhk@aol.com
Homepage: www.cns.state.va.us/drs/

Vocational Rehabilitation Offices
Joseph Ashley, Director

Virginia Department of
Rehabilitation Services
8004 Franklin Farms Drive
Richmond, VA 23288
800-552-5019
804-662-7000
800-464-9950 (TTY)
804-662-9533 (Fax)
www.cns.state.va.us/drs
E-mail: DRS@drs.state.va.us

W. Roy Grizzard, Jr.,
Commissioner
Department For the Visually
Handicapped
Commonwealth of Virginia
397 Azalea Avenue
Richmond, VA 23227
804-371-3140
800-622-2155
www.cns.state.va.us/dvh

Virgin Islands
Client Assistance Program
Amelia Headley LeMont
Client Assistance Program
Virgin Islands Advocacy
Agency
7A Whim Street
Suite 2
Frederiksted, VI 00840
340-772-1200
340-776-4303
340-772-4641 (TDD)
Fax: 809-772-0609
E-mail: viadvocacy@
worldnet.atl.net

Disability Office
Governor's Committee on
Employment of the
Handicapped
Administrator Disabilities &
Rehabilitation Services
Department of Human Services
Barbel Plaza South
St. Thomas, VI 00802
340-774-0930, ext. 157
340-774-3466 (Fax)

Technology Assistance Programs
U.S. Virgin Island
Technology-Related
Assistance for Individuals with
Disabilities (TRAID)
University of the Virgin
Islands/UAP
#2 John Brewers Bay
St. Thomas, VI 00801-0990
Executive Director: Dr. Yegin
Habtes
809-693-1323
809-693-1325 (Fax)
E-mail: yhabtey@ uvi.edu
Homepage: www.uvi.edu

Vocational Rehabilitation Offices
Caterine Mall, Administrator
Division of Disabilities and
Rehabilitation Services
Department of Human Services
1403 Hospital Road
St. Thomas, VI 00802
340-774-0930

Washington

Client Assistance Program
Jerry Johnsen, Director
Client Assistance Program
P. O. Box 22510
Seattle, WA 98122
206-721-5999
800-544-2121
206-721-4537 (Fax)
E-mail: capseattle@
adccomsys.net

Disability Office
Governor's Committee on
Disability Issues and
Employment
State of Washington
Employment Security
Department
P.O. Box 9046
Olympia, WA 98507-9046
Street Address:
    605 Woodland Square Loop
    SE, 3rd Floor
    Lacey, WA 98503
360-438-3168 (Voice)
360-438-3167 (TTY)
360-438-3208 (Fax)
E-mail: algoodwin@
esd.wa.gov

*Technology Assistance
Programs*
Washington Assistive
Technology Alliance
DSHS/DVR
AT Resource Center
Univ. of Washington

Box 357920
Seattle, WA 98195-7920
Project Director: Debbie Cook
206-685-4181
206-685-4181
206-616-1396 (TDD)
206-543-4779 (Fax)
E-mail: uwat@
u.washington.edu
Homepage: www.u.
washington.edu

*Vocational Rehabilitation
Offices*
Jeanne Munro, Director
Division of Vocational
Rehabilitation
Department Of Social &
Health Services
P.O. Box 45340
Olympia, WA. 98504
612 Woodland Sq. Loop SE
Lacey, WA 98503-1044
800-637-5627
360-438-8000
360-438-8007 (Fax)
http://www.wa.gov/dshs/dvr/

Bill Palmer, Acting Director
Department of Services for the
Blind
1400 S. Evergreen Park Drive
Suite 100
P.O. Box 40933
Olympia, WA 98504-0933
360-586-1224
800-552-7103
360-586-7627 (Fax)

360-586-6437 (TDD)
www.wa.gov/dsb/

West Virginia
Client Assistance Program
Susan Edwards, Director
Client Assistance Program
West Virginia Advocates, Inc.
Litton Building
4th Floor
1207 Quarrier Street
Charleston, WV 25301
304-346-0847
800-950-5250
304-346-0867 (Fax)
E-mail: wvadvocates@
newwave.net
www.newwave.net/
~wvadvocates

Disability Office
Division of Rehabilitation
Services
State Capitol Building
P.O. Box 50890
Charleston, WV 25305
304-766-4601 (Voice)
304-766-4965 (TTY)
304-766-4905 (Fax)
www.wvdrs.wvnet.edu

Technology Assistance Programs
West Virginia Assistive
Technology System
University Affiliated Center for
Developmental Disabilities

Airport Research and Office
Park
955 Hartman Run Road
Morgantown, WV 26505
Project Manager: Jack Stewart
304-293-4692 (V/TDD)
800-841-8436 (In-State)
304-293-7294 (Fax)
E-mail: stewiat@
wvnvm.wvnet.edu
Homepage: www.wvnvm.
wvnet.edu

Vocational Rehabilitation Offices
Jim Jeffers, Director
West Virginia Department of
Education and the Arts
Division of Rehabilitation
Services
State Capitol
P. O. Box 50890
Charleston, W V 25305-0890
800-642-8207
304-766-4600
800-642-8207
304-766-4690 (Fax)
E-mail: Charley@mail.wvdrs.
wvnet.edu
www.wvdrs.wvnet.edu

Wisconsin
Client Assistance Program
Linda Vegoe
Department of Health &
Family Services
Client Assistance Program

P. O. Box 7850
Madison, WI 53707-7850
608-267-7422
800-362-1290
608-267-0949 (Fax)
E-mail: vegoeli@
dhfs.state.wi.us

Disability Office
Governor's Committee for
People with Disabilities
P.O. Box 7850
Madison, WI 53707-7850
Street Address:
  1 West Wilson #558
  Madison, WI 53707-7850
608-266-5451 (Voice/TTY)
608-264-9832 (Fax)
www.dhfs.state.wi.us/
disabilities/physical/facts.htm

*Technology Assistance
Programs*
WISTECH
Wisconsin Assistive
Technology Program
Division of Supportive Living
P.O. Box 7852
2917 International Lane
3rd Floor
Madison, WI 53707
Project Director: Judi Trampf
608-243-5674 (V/TDD)
608-243-5681 (Fax)
E-mail: trampju@dwd.
state.wi.us
Homepage: www.dwd.
state.wi.us

*Vocational Rehabilitation
Offices*
Tom Dixon, Administrator
Division of Vocational
Rehabilitation
2917 International Lane
Suite 300
P.O. Box 7852
Madison, WI 53707-7852
608-243-5600
608-243-5601 (TTY)
800-442-3477
608-243-5680 or
608-243-5681 (Fax)
www.dwd.state.wi.us/dvr

Wyoming
Client Assistance Program
Kriss Smith, Director
Client Assistance Program
Wyoming P&A System
2424 Pioneer Ave., Suite 101
Cheyenne, WY 82001
307-638-7668
307-632-3496
800-821-3091 (Voice/TDD)
800-624-7648
307-638-0815 (Fax)
E-mail: wypanda@vcn.com
http://wind.uwyo.edu/WILDD/
P&A_Home_Page.htm

Disability Office
Governor's Committee on
Employment of People with
Disabilities
1st Floor - East Wing

Herschler Bldg., Room 1126
Cheyenne, WY 82002
307-777-7191 (Voice/TTY)
307-777-5939 (Fax)
www.state.wy.us

Technology Assistance Programs
Wyoming's New Options in
Technology (WYNOT)
University of Wyoming
1465 N. 4th St., Suite 111
Laramie, WY 82072
Project Director: Rich Gannon
307-766-2095
307-766-2084 (V/TDD)

307-721-2084 (Fax)
E-mail: wynot.uw@uwyo.edu
Homepage: www.uwyo.edu

Vocational Rehabilitation Offices
Gary W. Child, Administrator
Division of Vocational
Rehabilitation
Department of Employment
1100 Herschler Building
Cheyenne, WY 82002
307-777-7389
http://wydoe.state.wy.us/
vocrehab/

Free Care For Children With Disabilities

A portion of the same federal funds for pregnant women and children also provides help for disabled children. Blind or disabled children under the age of 18 who qualify for Supplemental Security Income must receive access to rehabilitation services; and others may qualify for assistance as well. How one qualifies and the amount of assistance a child receives varies from state to state. Parents may need to advocate on the child's behalf. Some of the services that may be covered include:

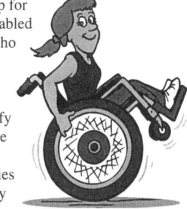

- lab services
- appliances and assistive technology
- transportation reimbursement
- physical, speech, language, and occupational therapy
- special dental or orthodontic services
- medical care
- hospitalization, and more

For more information from your state contact:

Alabama
Children's Rehabilitation
Service
Alabama Department of
Rehabilitation Services
2129 East South Blvd.
P.O. Box 11586
Montgomery, AL 36111
334-281-8780
http://www.rehab.state.al.us/
children.html

Alaska
Alaska Department of Health
and Social Services
Special Needs Services Unit
1231 Gambell St.
Anchorage, AK 99501
907-269-3400
800-799-7570
http://www.hhs.state.ak.us

Arizona
Arizona Department of Health
Services
411 North 24th St.
Phoenix, AZ 85008
602-220-6572
http://www.hs.state.az.us

Arkansas
Children's Medical Services
Arkansas Department of
Human Services
P.O. Box 1437
Slot No. 526
Little Rock, AR 72203

501-682-8224
http://www.state.ar.us/dhs

California
Children's Medical Services
Branch
California State Department of
Health Services
714 P St.
Sacramento, CA 95814
916-654-0499
http://www.dhs.cahwnet.gov

Colorado
Health Care Program for
Children with Special Health
Needs
Family and Community Health
Services Division
Colorado Department of Public
Health and Environment
4300 Cherry Creek Dr., South
Denver, CO 80222
303-692-2389
http://www.state.co.us/gov_dir/
cdphe_dir/cdphehom.html

Connecticut
Family Health Services
Division
Bureau of Community Health
Connecticut Department of
Public Health
410 Capitol Ave., MS11FHS
P.O. Box 340308
Hartford, CT 06134
860-509-8074
http://www.state.ct.us/dph

Delaware
Family Health Services
Delaware Health and Social
Services
Division of Public Health
P.O. Box 637
Dover, DE 19903
302-739-3111
http://www.sate.de.us/govern/
agencies/dhss/irm/dhss.htm

District of Columbia
Office of Maternal and Child
Health
Commission of Public Health
800 9th St., SW, Third Floor
Washington, DC 20024
202-645-5615

Florida
Florida Department of Health
Children's Medical Services
Program
Building 6, Room 130
1317 Winewood Blvd.
Tallahassee, FL 32399
850-487-2690
http://www.state.fl.us/health

Georgia
Division of Public Health
Child and Adolescent Health
Unit
Georgia Department of Human
Resources
2600 Skyland Dr., NE
Lower Level
Atlanta, GA 30319

404-679-0546
http://www2.state.ga.us/
Department/DHR

Hawaii
Hawaii Department of Health
741 Sunset Ave.
Honolulu, HI 96816
808-586-9070
http://www.hawaii.gov/health

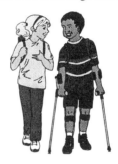

Idaho
Idaho Department of
Health/Welfare
Children's Special Health
Program
405 West State St.
P.O. Box 83720
Boise, ID 83720
208-334-5962
http://www.state.id.us/dhw/
hwgd_www/home.html

Illinois
Illinois Department of Human
Services
Office of Rehabilitation
Services

623 E. Adams
P.O.Box 19429
Springfield, IL 62794
217-785-0234
http://www.state.il.us/agency/
dhs

Indiana
Division of Services for
Children with Special Health
Care Needs
Indiana State Department of
Health
2 North Meridian St.
Suite 700
Indianapolis, IN 46204
317-233-5578
http://www.ai.org/doh/
index.html

Iowa
Iowa Child Health Specialty
Clinics
247 Hospital School
University of Iowa
Iowa City, IA 52242
319-356-1118

Kansas
Bureau for Children, Youth,
and Families
Kansas Department of Health
and Environment
Landon State Office Building
900 SW Jackson
Topeka, KS 66612
785-296-1313

http://www.state.ks.us/public/
kdhe/index.html

Kentucky
Commission for Children with
Special Health Care Needs
Cabinet for Health Services
982 Eastern Parkway
Louisville, KY 40217
502-595-4459
http://cfc-chs.state.ky/
chshone.htm

Louisiana
Office of Public Health
Louisiana Department of
Health and Hospitals
1201 Capitol Access Rd.
P.O. Box 629
Baton Rouge, LA 70821
504-342-9500
http://204.58.127.20/dhh/

Maine
Maine Department of Human
Services
11 State House Station
Augusta, ME 04333
207-287-5139
http://www.state.me.us/dhs/

Maryland
Office of Child Health and
Children's Medical Services
Maryland Department of
Health/Mental Hygiene
201 W. Preston St.

Baltimore, MD 21201
410-767-6749
http://www.charm.net/~epi9/

Massachusetts
Bureau of Family and
Community Health
Massachusetts Department of
Public Health
250 Washington St.
Boston, MA 02108
617-624-6060
Children's Medical Security
Plan - 800-909-2677
http://www.state.ma.us/dph/dp
hhome.htm

Michigan
Bureau of Child and Family
Services
Michigan Department of
Community Health
3423 North Logan/Martin
Luther King Jr. Blvd.
P.O. Box 30195
Lansing, MI 48909
517-335-8969
http://www.mdch.state.mi.us

Minnesota
Minnesota Department of
Health
717 Delaware St., SE
P.O. Box 9441
Minneapolis, MN 55440
800-728-5420
612-623-5140
http://www.health.state.mn.us

Mississippi
Children's Medical Program
Mississippi Department of
Health
421 Stadium Circle
P.O. Box 1700
Jackson, MS 39215
601-987-3965
http://www.msdh.state.ms.us

Missouri
Division of Maternal, Child
and Family Health
Missouri Department of Health
930 Wildwood
P.O. Box 570
Jefferson City, MO 65102
573-526-5520
http://www.health.state.mo.us

Montana
Family and Community Health
Bureau
Health Policy Services
Division
Montana Department of Public
Health and Human Services
1400 Broadway, Room C314
Cogswell Bldg.
Helena, MT 59620
406-444-4740
http://www.dphhs.state.mt.us

Nebraska
Special Services for Children
and Adults
Nebraska Department of
Health and Human Services

301 Centennial Mall South
5th Floor
P.O. Box 95026
Lincoln, NE 68509
402-471-9345
http://www.hhs.state.ne.us

Nevada
Bureau of Family Health
Services
Nevada State Health Division
505 East King St.
Room 200
Carson City, NV 89710
702-687-4885
http://www.state.nv.us/health/
home.htm

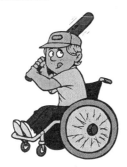

New Hampshire
Department of Health and
Human Services
Office of Family Service
Bureau of Special Medical
Services
6 Hazen Dr.
Concord, NH 03301
603-271-4596
http://www.state.nh.us/dhhs

New Jersey
Special Child and Adult Health
Services
New Jersey Department of
Health and Senior Services
50 East State St., CN 364
Trenton, NJ 08625
609-984-0755
http://www.state.nj.us/health

New Mexico
Public Health Division
Children's Medical Services
New Mexico Dept. of Health
1190 St. Francis Dr.
P.O. Box 26110
Santa Fe, NM 87505
505-827-2350
http://www.state.nm.us/state/
doh.html

New York
New York State Department of
Health
Center for Community Health
Empire State Plaza
Corning Tower Building
Albany, NY 12237
518-473-8389
http://www.health.state.ny.us

North Carolina
Children and Youth Section
Division of Women's and
Children's Health
North Carolina Department of
Environment, Health, and
Natural Resources

P.O. Box 29597
Raleigh, NC 27626
919-733-3816
http://www.dhr.state.nc.us/
DHR/

North Dakota
Children's Special Health
Services
Department of Human Services
State Capitol Bldg.
600 East Boulevard Ave.
Bismarck, ND 58505
701-328-2436

Ohio
Ohio Department of Health
Bureau for Children with
Medical Handicaps
246 N. High St.
Columbus, OH 43215
614-466-1652
http://www.state.oh.us/health

Oklahoma
Family Support Services
Division
Oklahoma State Department of
Human Services
P.O. Box 25352
Oklahoma City, OK 73125
405-521-3076
405-521-3679
http://www.onenet.net/okdhs

Oregon
Child Development/
Rehabilitation Center

Oregon Health Sciences
University
P.O. Box 574
Portland, OR 97207
503-494-8362
http://www.ohsu.edu/cdrc

Pennsylvania
Division of Special Health
Services
Pennsylvania Department of
Health
Health and Welfare Bldg.
P.O. Box 90
Harrisburg, PA 17108
717-783-5436
800-692-7254
http://www.pa.us/PA_Exec/
Health/overview.html

Puerto Rico
Commonwealth of Puerto Rico
Department of Health
P.O. Box 70184
San Juan, PR 00936
787-274-5660

Rhode Island
Rhode Island Department of
Health
Three Capitol Hill
Providence, RI 02908
401-222-1185

South Carolina
South Carolina Department of
Health and Environmental
Control

Division of Children's
Rehabilitative Services
Mills/Jarrett Complex
Box 101106
Columbia, SC 29211
803-737-4050
http://www.state.sc.us/dhec

South Dakota
Children's Special Health
Services
South Dakota Department of
Health
415 E. Fourth St.
Pierre, SD 57501
605-773-3737
800-738-2301
http://www.state.sd.us/doh/
Famhlth/child.htm

Tennessee
Health Promotion and Disease
Control
Tennessee Department of
Health
426 Fifth Ave., North
Cordell Hull Bldg.
Nashville, TN 37247
615-741-0310
http://www.state.tn.us/health

Texas
Bureau of Children's Health
Texas Department of Health
1100 West 49th St.
Austin, TX 78756
512-458-7700
http://www.tdh.state.tx.us

Utah
Division of Community and
Family Health Services
Utah Department of Health
Box 144410
Salt Lake City, UT 84114
801-538-6161
801-538-6869
http://161.119.100.19

Vermont
Vermont Department of Health
108 Cherry St.
P.O. Box 70
Burlington, VT 05402
802-863-7338
http://www.state.vt.us/health

Virginia
Office of Family Health
Services
Division of Children's
Specialty Services
Virginia Department of Health
1500 E. Main St.
P.O. Box 2448
Richmond, VA 23218
804-786-3693
http://www.vdh.state.va.us

Virgin Islands
U.S. Virgin Islands
Department of Health
Charles Harwood Hospital
3500 Richmond
St. Croix, VI 00820
809-773-1311

Washington
Division of Community and
Family Health
Department of Health
P.O. Box 47830
Olympia, WA 98504
360-236-3508
http://www.doh.wa.gov

West Virginia
Bureau of Public Health
Division of Handicapped
Children's Services
West Virginia Department of
Health
1141 Virginia St., E
Charleston, WV 25301
304-558-3071
http://www.wvdhhr.org

Wisconsin
Wisconsin Division of Health
Department of Health and
Family Services
1414 E. Washington Ave.
Madison, WI 53703
608-266-3674
http://www.dhfs.state.wi.us

Wyoming
Division of Public Health
Children's Health Services
Wyoming Department of
Health
Hathaway Building, 4th Floor
Cheyenne, WY 82002
307-777-7941
http://wdhfs.state.wy.us/WDH

Help is Just a Phone Call Away

No child — no matter if its parents are rich or poor- should be denied a healthy start to life. Under Title V of the Social Security Act, all families with young children and expecting mothers whose incomes fall near the federal poverty guidelines receive Medicaid. Poverty thresholds for 1999 were $8,240 for one person, $11,060 for two, $13,880 for three, and $16,700 for a family of four. In addition, many prenatal and infant care services often are available to these low-income families. These include:

- ★ Prenatal care clinics
- ★ Home visiting services
- ★ Translation services and other culturally focused services
- ★ Parenting classes
- ★ Programs for smoking cessation
- ★ Male support programs
- ★ Substance abuse treatment programs
- ★ Help obtaining assistance such as Medicaid, food stamps, and WIC (supplemental food program for Women, Infants, and Children)

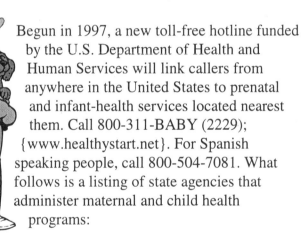

Begun in 1997, a new toll-free hotline funded by the U.S. Department of Health and Human Services will link callers from anywhere in the United States to prenatal and infant-health services located nearest them. Call 800-311-BABY (2229); {www.healthystart.net}. For Spanish speaking people, call 800-504-7081. What follows is a listing of state agencies that administer maternal and child health programs:

Alabama
Bureau of Family Health
Services
Alabama Department of Public
Health
434 Monroe St., Room 314
Montgomery, AL 36130
334-242-5661

Alaska
Alaska Department of Health
and Social Services

Section of Maternal, Child and
Family Health
1231 Gambell St.
Anchorage, AK 99501
907-269-3400

Arizona
Arizona Department of Health
Services
411 North 24th St.
Phoenix, AZ 85008
602-220-6550

Arkansas
Section of Maternal and Chile
Health
Arkansas Department of
Human Services
4815 West Markham
Slot N. 41
Little Rock, AR 72205
501-661-2199

California
Maternal and Child Health
Branch
California State Department of
Health Services
714 P St.
Sacramento, CA 95814
916-657-1347

Colorado
Maternal and Child Health
Family and Community Health
Services Division
Colorado Department of Public
Health and Environment

4300 Cherry Creek Dr., South
Denver, CO 80222
303-692-2315

Connecticut
Family Health Services
Division
Bureau of Community Health
Connecticut Department of
Public Health
410 Capitol Ave.
MS11FHS
P.O. Box 340308
Hartford, CT 06134
860-509-8066

Delaware
Family Health Services
Delaware Health and Social
Services
Division of Public Health
P.O. Box 637
Dover, DE 19903
302-739-3111

District of Columbia
Office of Maternal and Child
Health
Commission of Public Health
800 9th St., SW, Third Floor
Washington, DC 20024
202-645-5624

Florida
Florida Department of Health
Family Health Services
Building 6, Room 130
1317 Winewood Blvd.

Tallahassee, FL 32399
904-487-1321

Georgia
Family Health Branch
Georgia Department of Human
Resources
8th Floor, Room 113
2 Peachtree St., SW
Atlanta, GA 30303
404-657-2850

Hawaii
Hawaii Department of Health
741 Sunset Ave.
Honolulu, HI 96816
808-733-9022

Idaho
Idaho Department of
Health/Welfare
Clinical Preventive Services
450 West State St.
P.O. Box 83720
Boise, ID 83720
208-334-0670

Illinois
Division of Family Health
Illinois Dept. of Public Health
535 West Jefferson St.
Springfield, IL 62794
217-782-2736

Indiana
Indiana State Department of
Health
CSHCS/MHC/WIC

2 North Meridian St.
Suite 700
Indianapolis, IN 46204
317-233-1240

Iowa
Bureau of Family Services
Division of Family and
Community Health
Iowa Department of Public
Health
Lucas State Office Building
Des Moines, IA 50319
515-281-4911

Kansas
Bureau for Children, Youth,
and Families
Kansas Department of Health
and Environment
Landon State Office Building
900 SW Jackson
Topeka, KS 66612
913-296-1310

Kentucky
Department for Public Health
Division for Maternal and
Child Health
Health Services Building-2R
275 East Main St.
Frankfort, KY 40621
502-564-4830

Louisiana
Office of Public Health
Louisiana Department of
Health and Hospitals

325 Loyola Ave.
New Orleans, LA 70112
504-568-5073

Maine
Maine Department of Human
Services
Division of Community and
Family Health
Bureau of Health
11 State House Station
Augusta, ME 04333
207-287-5180

Maryland
Office of Child Health and
Children's Medical Services
Maryland Department of
Health/Mental Hygiene
201 W. Preston St.
Baltimore, MD 21201
410-767-6749

Massachusetts
Bureau of Family and
Community Health
Massachusetts Department of
Public Health
250 Washington St.
Boston, MA 02108
617-624-6060
Children's Medical Security
Plan - 800-909-2677

Michigan
Bureau of Child and Family
Services
Michigan Department of
Community Health

3423 North Logan/Martin
Luther King Jr. Blvd.
P.O. Box 30195
Lansing, MI 48909
517-335-8932

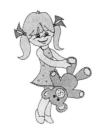

Minnesota
Minnesota Department of
Health
Division of Family Health
717 Delaware St., SE
P.O. Box 9441
Minneapolis, MN 55440
612-623-5167

Mississippi
Office of Personal Health
Services
Mississippi State Department
of Health
2423 North State St.
P.O. Box 1700
Jackson, MS 39215
601-960-7464

Missouri
Division of Maternal, Child
and Family Health
Missouri Department of Health
930 Wildwood

P.O. Box 570
Jefferson City, MO 65102
573-526-5520

Montana
Family and Community Health
Bureau
Health Policy Services
Division
Montana Department of Public
Health and Human Services
1400 Broadway, Room C314
Cogswell Bldg.
Helena, MT 59620
406-444-4740

Nebraska
Section of Family Health
Nebraska Dept. of Health
301 Centennial Mall South
3rd Floor
P.O. Box 95007
Lincoln, NE 68509
402-471-3980

Nevada
Bureau of Family Health
Services
Nevada State Health Division
505 East King St., Room 200
Carson City, NV 89710
702-687-4885

New Hampshire
Division of Public Health
Services
Bureau of Maternal and Child
Health

6 Hazen Dr.
Concord, NH 03301
603-271-4516

New Jersey
Maternal and Child Health
Services
New Jersey Department of
Health and Senior Services
50 East State St., CN 364
Trenton, NJ 08625
609-292-5656

New Mexico
Public Health Division
Children's Medical Services
New Mexico Dept. of Health
1190 St. Francis Dr.
P.O. Box 26110
Santa Fe, NM 87505
505-827-2350

New York
New York State Department of
Health
Division of Family and Local
Health
Empire State Plaza
Corning Tower Building
Albany, NY 12237
518-473-4441

North Carolina
Children and Youth Section
Division of Maternal and Child
Health
North Carolina Department of
Environment, Health, and
Natural Resources

P.O. Box 29597
Raleigh, NC 27626
919-733-3816

North Dakota
Division of Maternal and Child
Health
North Dakota Department of
Health
State Capitol Bldg.
600 East Boulevard Ave.
Bismarck, ND 58505
701-328-2493

Ohio
Ohio Department of Health
Bureau for Maternal and Child
Health
246 N. High St.
Columbus, OH 43215
614-466-1652

Oklahoma
Child Health and Guidance
Service
Oklahoma State Department of
Health
1000 NE 10th St., Room 506
Oklahoma City, OK 73117
405-271-4471

Oregon
Center for Child and Family
Health
Oregon State Health Division
800 NE Oregon St.
Portland, OR 97232
503-731-4398

Pennsylvania
Division of Special Health
Services
Pennsylvania Dept. of Health
Health and Welfare Bldg.
P.O. Box 90
Harrisburg, PA 17108
717-787-7192

Puerto Rico
Commonwealth of Puerto Rico
Department of Health
P.O. Box 70184
San Juan, PR 00936
787-274-5660

Rhode Island
Rhode Island Department of
Health
Division of Family Health
Three Capitol Hill
Providence, RI 02908
401-277-2312

South Carolina
South Carolina Department of
Health and Environmental
Control
Mills/Jarrett Complex
Box 101106
Columbia, SC 29211
803-737-4190

South Dakota
Health, Medical and
Laboratory Services
South Dakota Department of
Health

445 East Capitol
Pierre, SD 57501
605-773-3737

Tennessee
Tennessee Department of
Health
426 Fifth Ave., North
Cordell Hull Bldg.
Nashville, TN 37247
605-741-0323

Texas
Bureau of Children's Health
Texas Department of Health
1100 West 49th St.
Austin, TX 78756
512-458-7700

Utah
Division of Community and
Family Health Services
Utah Department of Health
Box 144410

Salt Lake City, UT 84114
801-538-6161
801-538-6869

Vermont
Vermont Department of Health
108 Cherry St.
P.O. Box 70
Burlington, VT 05402
802-863-7270

Virginia
Division of Women's and
Infants' Health
Virginia Department of Health
1500 E. Main St.
P.O. Box 2448
Richmond, VA 23219
804-786-5916

Virgin Islands
U.S. Virgin Islands
Department of Health
Charles Harwood Hospital

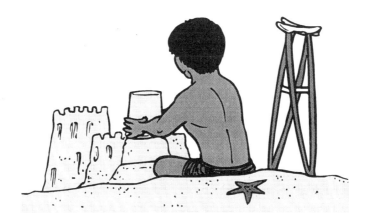

3500 Richmond
St. Croix, VI 00820
809-773-1311

Washington
Division of Community and
Family Health
Department of Health
P.O. Box 47830
Olympia, WA 98504
360-753-7021

West Virginia
West Virginia Department of
Health
1141 Virginia St., E
Charleston, WV 25301
304-558-5388

Wisconsin
Wisconsin Division of Health
Department of Health and
Family Services
Bureau of Public Health
1414 E. Washington Ave.
Madison, WI 53703
608-266-5818

Wyoming
Division of Public Health
Children's Health Services
Wyoming Department of
Health
Hathaway Building, 4th Floor
Cheyenne, WY 82002
307-777-7941

Free Summer Camp For People With Health Problems

If you were lucky enough to go to summer camp — some
time away from school and family — you know how it
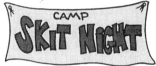 made you change. You found
out a little bit more about who
you were and what you could
do without your mom
hovering in the distance. Changes
are, you have at least a few vivid
memories of that childhood
place.

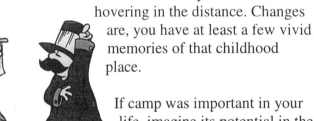

If camp was important in your
life, imagine its potential in the
lives of children whose
disabilities can make even simple tasks more complicated.
Fortunately, a number of national organizations such as the
American Cancer Society, the American Kidney Fund and
the American Lung Association have recognized that the
camp experience can change the lives of disabled children,
too. If you are looking for such an experience for your
child, contact the local chapter of one of the national not-
for-profit support groups or call the national headquarters.
The camps listed below will give you some idea of what's
available.

Camp Wheezeaway Is Free For Kids With Asthma

Every year, about 80 kids with asthma, between 8 and 12 years of age, can go to summer camp for free in Jackson Cap, Alabama. For information on how to apply, contact American Lung Association of Alabama, 900 South 18th St., Birmingham, AL 35205; 205-933-8821.

For more information on other camps for children with asthma, or other questions concerning asthma, contact The American Lung Association, 1740 Broadway, New York, NY 10019; 212-315-8700; 800-LUNG-USA; {www.lungusa.org}.

Free Trips and Free Summer Camps For Kids With Kidney Disease

Each year, the American Kidney Fund (AKF) invites children with kidney disease from across the United States to submit drawings of their favorite things to AKF's "KID"ney Kid Calendar Contest. The art work of the lucky 13 winners graces the pages of the annual AKF Calendar. The lucky 13 and their parents are also treated to a weekend in Washington, DC where they meet AKF staff and tour the national capital. The AKF "KID"ney Calendar is available for a donation of $5.23.

Children with kidney disease can also go to summer camp with the help of AKF's Pediatric Campership Grants. This program provides financial aid for camp tuition, transportation or camping supplies. For many KIDney Kids, this is their first opportunity to experience the freedom, and independence that healthy children take for granted. Pediatric kidney patients are eligible for all of AKF's Patient Aid Programs and AKF Camperships.

Contact: American Kidney Fund, 6110 Executive Boulevard, Suite 1010, Rockville, MD 20852; 800-638-8299; 301-881-3052; Fax: 301-881-0898; {E-mail: helpline@akfinc.org}; {www.akfinc.org}.

Free Summer Camp for Kids With Cancer

In some areas, the American Cancer Society sponsors camps for children who have, or have had, cancer. These camps are equipped to handle the special needs of children undergoing treatment. The American Cancer Society offers patients, their families, their caregivers, and the community the full range of emotional and practical help from the time of diagnosis throughout one's life to life's end. In 1996, almost one million cancer patients were helped through the programs of the American Cancer Society.

Contact: American Cancer Society, 1599 Clifton Rd., NE, Atlanta, GA 30329; 800-ACS-2345; {www.cancer.org}.

Free Camp for Kids With Life-Threatening Illnesses

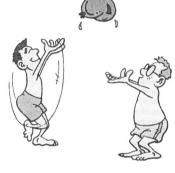

Children ages 7-17 with life-threatening illnesses can experience swimming, boating, fishing, hiking, arts and crafts, special activities, water balloon tosses, dancing, and much more at a special camp in Florida. The Boggy Creek Gang Camp is a permanent, year-round center where young people with life-threatening illnesses can come at no charge to them or their families. Transportation to and from the camp are typically the family's responsibility; however, many local health organizations will help with the cost and coordination of travel plans.

The Boggy Creek Gang provides a safe and exciting camp experience for children with: arthritis, asthma, cancer & related blood disorders, craniofacial disorders, diabetes, epilepsy, heart disease, hemophilia, rheumatic disease, kidney disease, immunodeficiencies including HIV/AIDS, sickle cell anemia, disorders requiring ventilator assistance. The camp medical staff and facility accommodates many kinds of special needs, from bandaging a minor cut to administering chemotherapy.

Contact: The Boggy Creek Gang, 30500 Brantley Branch Road, Eustis, FL 32736; 352-483-4200; Fax: 352-483-

0358; {E-mail: info@boggycreek.org}; {www.boggycreek.
org/admissions.html}.

FinanciaL HeLp, Counseling and Even Free Summer Camps For Families in Need

Financial assistance, counseling, casework and other
services to help strengthen and unify the family unit is
available from the Salvation Army. Counseling by
Salvation Army staff assists with child/parent relationships,
marital problems, adolescent problems, unmarried mother
situations, and unemployment. Christmas activities and
summer camp holidays are an important part of the
Salvation Army's family programs.

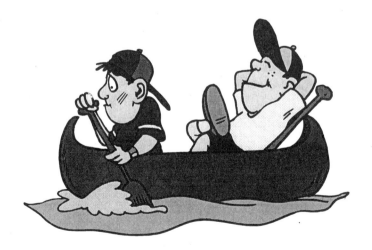

Contact: The Salvation Army National Headquarters
Commissioner Robert A. Watson, National Commander
615 Slaters Lane, P.O. Box 269, Alexandria, VA 22313;
703-684-5500; Fax: 703-684-3478; {www.
salvationarmyusa.org}.

Free Summer Camp For Kids and Seniors

Thousands of children from low-income families enjoy
fresh air, exercise, and new friendships at annual Salvation
Army summer and day camp programs. Children learn new
skills and self-reliance. Trained counselors are on hand
who understand their emotional needs and problems while
helping them mature. Often, entire families receive the
benefits from these camping experiences through expanded
services.

Seniors also find recreation at camp sessions. Plus, many
camps sponsored by The Salvation Army are winterized for
year-round use by other groups of young people and adults.
Contact: The Salvation Army National Headquarters
Commissioner Robert A. Watson, National Commander
615 Slaters Lane, P.O. Box 269, Alexandria, VA 22313;
703-684-5500; Fax: 703-684-3478; {www.
salvationarmyusa.org}; {www.salvationarmyusa.org/
disfol/disast2.htm}.

Free Help With Pregnancy and Childbirth

You are bringing a new life into the world and it will cost you a fortune over your lifetime. Here are some free and cheap resources you can use to help you through the pregnancy and newborn stages. Put the savings into some high yield fund for college!

Is Your Baby Smoking?

You know that smoking isn't good for you. And if you are pregnant or have a newborn, you are putting the child at risk as well. The Office on Smoking and Health has free information to help you learn about the dangers of smoking and how to quit. *Is Your Baby Smoking?* and *Pregnant? That's Two Good Reasons To Quit Smoking* will get you on your way to independence from cigarettes.

For more information, contact the Office on Smoking and Health, National Center for Chronic Disease Prevention and Health Promotion, Centers for Disease Control and

Prevention, Mail Stop K-50, 4770 Buford Hwy. NE,
Atlanta, GA 30341; 800-CDC-1311;
{www.cdc.gov/tobacco}.

The Power of
Positive Pregnancy

What do folic acid supplements, Group B strep screening,
and proper safety belt positioning have in common? The
Coalition for Positive Outcomes in Pregnancy counts all
three as important items towards improving your odds of
having a healthy baby.

In the free brochure, *12
Ways to Achieve a
More Positive
Pregnancy*, you'll find
information about the
types of over-the-
counter and
prescription
medications to avoid—
including antihis-
tamines, ibuprofen and
tetracycline—before
you even become
pregnant. And, once
you're pregnant, you'll
benefit from the tips on
proper sleep positions,

Just For Fun

Once Junior has arrived,
send a birth announce-
ment to the White House.
If you include your name
and address, the White
House will send a
"welcome to the world
card" to your newborn.
It's not everyone's baby
that gets a Presidential
Seal of Approval.

Send the information to
Greetings Office, The
White House, Washington,
DC 20500.

avoiding dehydration and over-exertion, and staying alert to signs of pregnancy complications. Contact: The Coalition for Positive Outcomes in Pregnancy, 711 Second St., NE, Suite 200, Washington, DC 20002; 202-544-7499.

Lessening the Risk of Spina Bifida

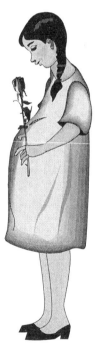

Spina bifida, one of the most common and most devastating of the neural tube defects, is also one of the most preventable. Studies have shown that if all women of childbearing age were to consume 0.4mg of folic acid before becoming pregnant and during the first trimester of pregnancy, the incidence of spina bifida would decrease by up to 75%.

In this free brochure produced by the Spina Bifida Association, find out about the connection between spina bifida and folic acid and how to be sure you're getting enough folic acid in your diet. A supplemental pamphlet is provided with lists of foods rich in folic acid and the portions necessary to meet your daily requirements.

Contact Spina Bifida Association of America, 4590 MacArthur Blvd., NW, Suite 250, Washington, DC 20007; 800-621-3141.

Don't Lose Your Lunch

Pregnancy can be a time of extreme joy, but for some it can also be a time of extreme — even excessive — nausea. Many mothers find the first months of pregnancy a little rocky, but if you're one of the few women who vomits so much that you're losing weight and can't keep anything down, you may be suffering from hyperemesis gravidarum, or excessive nausea.

Fortunately, help is on the way. The Center for Health Promotion offers a free pamphlet with dietary tips, a

---

Mothering the Mother

New mothers go through lots of physical and emotional changes during pregnancy, but there are still more changes to come after delivery.

In *New Mother Care*, some of the most common experiences new mothers face are highlighted, as are their various causes and potential cures. For example, engorged breasts can be helped with heat or ice, perineal discomforts may be soothed with ice and warm tub soaks, and sciatica pain may respond well to heat and acetaminophen. Also included are exercises for helping pelvic muscles return to normal and special instructions for moms who've had cesarean births.

Contact HealthPartners, Center for Health Promotion, MOD C 3105 East 80th St., Bloomington, MN 55440; 612-883-6713.

---

sample menu plan and other treatment options, including herbal teas and liquid nutritional supplements, that may help keep you standing up!

Contact: HealthPartners, Center for Health Promotion, MOD C 3105 East 80th St., Bloomington, MN 55440; 612-883-6713.

Preventing Preterm Birth

While no pregnant woman wants to face the possibility of pre-term labor, it's important to know if you're at risk and how to lessen the likelihood of having a premature birth if you are.

Preventing Preterm Birth

Preventing Preterm Birth, a free booklet, lists several medically related risk factors for pre-term labor as well as some lifestyle risk factors. Methods for minimizing stress and checking for contractions are included, as well as information about early pre-term labor warning signs and how to respond to them. Also included are resources for managing bed rest, a publication guide for more comprehensive reading, and a list of support services.

Contact: HealthPartners, Center for Health Promotion, MOD C 3105 East 80th St., Bloomington, MD 55440; 612-883-6713.

The Journey of Pregnancy

For every journey in life, a guidebook can be a useful item to take along. The same holds true of pregnancy.

In *Expecting the Best: The Journey Toward a Healthy Pregnancy*, a free comprehensive guidebook, you'll learn about the important milestones of pregnancy, the detours and potential hazards, and how to ensure you reach your destination safely. Chapters include information on selecting and developing a relationship with your health care provider; the physical, emotional and sexual changes you'll experience; lifestyle changes that can affect your baby, such as nutrition, exercise and medications; and what to do when something goes wrong — miscarriage or pre-term labor.

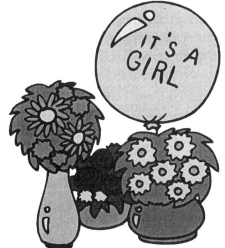

This valuable resource has space for you to jot down your questions and concerns and evaluate your diet, as well as a useful worksheet in case of pre-term labor. A reading list is also included. Contact: HealthPartners, Center for Health Promotion, MOD C 3105 East 80th St., Bloomington, MN 55440; 612-883-6713.

Postpartum Support

With so much of your energy focused on preparing for and having a healthy baby, you've probably given little thought to the emotional changes that may occur following the birth of your baby.

Postpartum Support International can help new mothers navigate what can be a difficult and confusing time.

Dedicated to eliminating denial and ignorance surrounding maternal emotional postpartum health, the organization offers support that is just a phone call away. Postpartum Support International will also hook you up with support groups operating in your area, send you a free

---

EATING FOR TWO

Pickles and ice cream for nine months just won't do! So what should you eat? *All About Eating for Two* focuses on the changing nutritional needs of women during pregnancy and can help you establish a healthy diet for nine months and beyond.

Topics addressed include: how to make sure you're getting enough iron, folic acid, calcium, and protein to ensure healthy fetal development; guidelines for proper weight gain; and how to control and cope with nausea. Charts with recommended daily dietary allowances for women are also included.

For your free copy, contact: Division of Consumer Affairs, Food and Drug Administration, Room 16-75, 5600 Fishers Lane, Rockville, MD 20857; 800-532-4440; {www.fda.gov}.

---

resource guide that includes a bibliography of books, videos and Internet sites, and supply you with a list of telephone support lines. Contact: Jane Homikman, Postpartum Support International, 927 North Kellogg Ave., Santa Barbara, CA 93111; 805-967-7836; {www.iup.edu/an/postpartum/}.

Expectant Fathers

With all the attention being lavished on the mom-to-be, it's easy to lose track of dad. Fathers play an important role throughout a woman's pregnancy, however, and the March of Dimes has a couple of free pamphlets to help dads better understand their role and what to expect as a woman's pregnancy progresses.

In *Dad, It's Your Baby Too: A Guide For Expectant Fathers*, expectant dads learn how their participation and support can make a difference in their partner's pregnancy. Going to childbirth classes, reading about pregnancy, and attending prenatal checkups are just a few of the ideas that can make dads feel more connected to their babies and help their partners feel supported.

In *Men Have Babies Too: A Guide for Fathers-to-Be*, dads learn how their diet and lifestyle affects the health of their baby. For example, while it's long been asserted that women should not drink, smoke or take drugs when they are trying to conceive, recent evidence suggests that a father exposed to any of these risk factors may be influencing his unborn baby as well. The pamphlet offers suggestions on how dads can promote a positive and healthy pregnancy and lists reproductive hazards that dads-to-be (and moms) should avoid.

Contact Health Information Specialist, March of Dimes Birth Defects Foundation, 1275 Mamaroneck Ave., White Plains, NY 10805; 914-428-7100; 888-663-4637; {www.modimes.org}.

Understanding Cesarean Birth

While most moms-to-be don't enter the delivery room thinking they will have a cesarean birth, it's a good idea to educate yourself in advance about the possibility — just in case. In this free pamphlet, you'll learn exactly what a c-section is, how and why it's most often performed, and what risks are involved.

Special sections discuss the necessity of a c-section (it's estimated that more than half of the cesarean sections performed aren't necessary!); how to work with your health care provider to prevent an unnecessary cesarean birth (by choosing a doctor who delivers a large number of babies with a low overall percentage of c-sections); and, should you need a c-section, how to make the delivery the best one possible for you and your baby. Information is also included about how to ensure a speedy recovery from a c-section and how to cope with any emotional issues that may arise.

Contact: Health Information Specialist, March of Dimes Birth Defects Foundation, 1275 Mamaroneck Ave., White Plains, NY 10605; 914-428-7100; 888-663-4637; {www.modimes.org}.

Prenatal Testing

In a high-tech era, and with more women opting to delay childbirth and therefore increasing the risk of some birth defects, it has become increasingly common for doctors to recommend sophisticated prenatal testing during the course of pregnancy. Before having any tests, however, it's important that you know the facts about each procedure and discuss them with your health care provider.

Take A Pill

Did you know that taking folic acid supplements before you try to conceive may improve your baby's health? In *Pre-Pregnancy Planning* find out how folic acid works to prevent neural tube defects, as well as what other things — a pre-pregnancy check-up among them — you can be doing now to prepare for the day you get the big news that you're pregnant. Contact: Health Information Specialist, March of Dimes Birth Defects Foundation, 1275 Mamaroneck Ave., White Plains, NY 10605; 914-428-7100; 888-663-4637; {www.modimes.org}.

The March of Dimes offers free educational fact sheets on some common prenatal tests, including the Chorionic Villus Sampling (CVS), Alpha-Fetoprotein Test, and Amniocentisis. Contact: Health Information Specialist, March of Dimes Birth Defects Foundation, 1275 Mamaroneck Ave., White Plains, NY 10605; 914-428-7100; 888-663-4637; {www.modimes.org}.

SEX
AND THE NEW MOTHER

While a few new mothers want to have sex soon after they've delivered, it's much more likely that you will need several weeks—maybe more—of recovery time before you'll be erotically interested in your beloved again.

In *Sex After the Baby Comes* (50 cents), you'll learn about the sexual adjustment that comes with the birth of a new baby as part of the larger emotional adjustments all new parents make. Several reasons you may not be craving sex are discussed in-depth, such as tiredness, depression, pain and breastfeeding. And solutions for putting you back in the mood are highlighted: how to minimize interruptions from baby, for example, and exercises for putting your pelvic floor muscles back in shape.

Contact: International Childbirth Educational Association, 8060 26th Ave., South, Minneapolis, MN 55425; 612-854-8660; 800-624-4934; {www.icea.org}.

Let's Get Physical

Being pregnant doesn't mean you need to get fat or feel tired all the time. Regular exercise during pregnancy is critical for both your mental and physical health, and will give you the added strength you'll need when baby arrives. Fitness does not require strenuous workout—in fact, you shouldn't exercise strenuously during pregnancy, and before embarking on any exercise program you should check with your doctor.

In *Fitness for the Childbearing Year* (50 cents) you'll learn how to craft a complete workout tailored to you, what kinds of exercises are best during pregnancy, and complete step-by-step instructions for doing proper stretch and strength conditioning

Avoiding Accutane

Among the many drugs physicians warn against taking during pregnancy, accutane may not be one you've heard of. But, if you've had severe acne, and your doctor prescribed accutane, you should be aware that it could potentially cause serious birth defects. In this free fact sheet from the March of Dimes, find out about accutane, the risks it poses during pregnancy and other vitamin-A related drugs that are potentially unsafe during pregnancy. Contact Health Information Specialist, March of Dimes Birth Defects Foundation, 1275 Mamaroneck Ave., White Plains, NY 10605; 914-428-7100; 888-663-4637; {www.modimes.org}.

exercises. You'll also learn what exercises to avoid when you're pregnant and how to begin exercising after delivery. Contact: International Childbirth Educational Association, 8060 26th Ave., South, Minneapolis, MN 55425; 612-854-8660; 800-624-4934; {www.icea.org}.

DIABETES DURING PREGNANCY

Approximately 3-5 percent of all pregnant women in the United States develop gestational diabetes while pregnant. Gestational diabetes disappears after delivery, but careful control of blood sugar levels is necessary in order to manage and prevent complications.

Understanding Gestational Diabetes: A Practical Guide to a Healthy Pregnancy answers questions about diet, exercise, measurement of blood sugar levels, and general medical and obstetric care for women with gestational diabetes. Questions addressed include: Will gestational diabetes hurt your baby? How will it affect labor and delivery? What foods help keep blood sugar levels normal? And how much weight should you gain?

For your free booklet, contact National Institute of Child Health and Human Development, National Institutes of Health, Building 31, Room 2A32, 9000 Rockville, Pike, Bethesda, MD 20892; 301-496-5133; {www.nih.gov/nichd}.

Is Drinking Safe During Pregnancy?

Many women have questions about drinking and drugs during pregnancy, and the National Clearinghouse for Drug and Alcohol Information has answers in several free publications. Did you know that pregnant women who consume between one and two drinks per day are twice as likely as non-drinkers to have a low birth weight baby? Or that women who smoke are more likely than non-smokers to have babies whose physical and intellectual growth is below normal?

For a Strong and Health Baby gives you the facts on alcohol, tobacco, and street drugs. *How to Take Care of Your Baby Before Birth* emphasizes the importance of saying no to alcohol and drugs during pregnancy and offers some helpful do's and don'ts for ensuring a successful pregnancy. *Healthy Women, Healthy Lifestyles* focuses on women and their specific health related risks due to alcohol, tobacco, and illicit drugs and discusses how fetal alcohol syndrome affects newborn babies.

> **15% of Adult TV Characters are identified as parents of minor children, in real life it's 32%**
>
> **34% of Adult TV WOMEN Characters are working for pay, in real life it's 67%**
>
> *Source: National Partnership for Women & Families; {www.womenandfamilies.org}*

Contact: National Clearinghouse for Alcohol and Drug Information, P.O. Box 2345, Rockville, MD 20852; 800-729-6686; {www.health.org}.

Dear Diary

Following your development — and that of your baby — can be fun with this free booklet entitled, *Health Diary: Myself, My Baby.*

Divided into two sections, the "Myself" section provides several pages for documenting your own health history, prenatal care, diet, weight gain and special memories of your pregnancy. Chock-full of information about labor and delivery, there's even a pull-out chart illustrating your baby's week-by-week development from birth to 24 months. You'll find spaces for snapshots of your newborn, information about caring and feeding, and a schedule for taking your baby to the doctor. There's also a section on treating minor problems, as well as spaces to record illnesses and notes following each doctor's visit.

Contact: National Maternal and Child Health Clearinghouse, 2070 Chain Bridge Rd., Suite 450, Vienna, VA 22182; 703-356-1964; {www.nmchc.org}.

PREGNANCY AND HIV

If you're pregnant and have HIV or AIDS, you may pass the virus to your baby. Taking the drug AZT can help lessen the chance that your baby will contract HIV.

Pregnancy and HIV: Is AZT the Right Choice for You and Your Baby? provides you with information about AZT, discusses what researchers know so far about babies and AZT based on a study conducted by the National Institutes of Health, and provides you with a list of questions to ask your health care provider.

Contact: National Maternal and Child Health Clearinghouse, 2070 Chain Bridge Rd., Suite 450, Vienna, VA 22182; 703-356-1964; {www.nmchc.org}.

Be in the Know

The people at the National Women's Health network have a number of free publications ("one-pagers," as they call them) available about pregnancy and childbirth through their women's health clearinghouse. Topics include: choosing the place and attendant for the birth, deciding about technology, labor positions, and information on the physical and emotional aspects of the postpartum time. There's separate information on having a child in mid-life; becoming a parent for the first time; postpartum depression; and cesarean sections.

Because the network seeks to educate women to be information medical consumers, there's also a booklet entitled, *The Pregnant Patient's Bill of Rights* in which the rights of pregnant women under obstetrical care are outlined. Contact: The National Women's Health Network, 514 10th St., NW, Suite 400, Washington, DC 20004; 202-347-1140.

Getting the Facts About Your Ultrasound Exam

For most pregnant women, having an ultrasound exam will be recommended by their doctor as a routine part of prenatal care. But what exactly is an ultrasound exam? Is it safe for you and your baby?

The American Institute of Ultrasound in Medicine has published a pamphlet ($1.50) titled *What You Should Know About Your Obstetric Ultrasound*, to help you understand

---

Ultrasound Information

Why are ultrasounds becoming almost commonplace for pregnancies? For more information on the use of ultrasound in pregnancy and how the information may be used to alter prenatal care to improve the chances of delivering a healthy baby, see *Ultrasound*, a free fact sheet published by the March of Dimes Foundation, 1275 Mamaroneck Ave., White Plains, NY 10605; 914-428-7100; 888-663-4637; or online at {www.modimes.org}.

---

how and why ultrasound is used. Specific sections discuss when and how ultrasound should be used (In pregnancy, doctors recommend ultrasound to determine a due date, rule out multiple fetuses and to evaluate the growth and development of the baby); the safety of sonography (There has been no direct link established between the diagnostic use of ultrasound and any adverse fetal outcomes); and whether or not the ultrasound will hurt (It doesn't, but can be somewhat uncomfortable). Also included is information about who performs the ultrasound, as well as about ultrasound and miscarriage.

Contact: American Institute of Ultrasound in Medicine, 14750 Sweitzer Lane, Suite 100, Laurel, MD 20707; 301-498-4100; {www.aium.org}.

Pre-Pregnancy
Quiz Time

The March of Dimes has put together a couple of free pamphlets to help you think about what you need to know before you even try to get pregnant. In *If You Think You're Ready to Have a Baby, Think Ahead*, put your pre-pregnancy knowledge to the test. Here are a couple of sample true/false questions from the ten item quiz:

★ You don't need to be concerned about your weight before pregnancy, since you'll be putting on pounds anyway. (False).

★ The lifestyle of the father has no impact on the health of his baby. (False).

Contact: Health Information Specialist, March of Dimes Birth Defects Foundation, 1275 Mamaroneck Ave., White Plains, NY 10605; 914-428-7100; 888-663-4637; {www.modimes.org}.

Think Ahead

In *Think Ahead for a Healthy Baby: A Pre-Pregnancy Guide,* begin to plan for the months ahead. Do you have any family history of birth defects in your family? If so, now is the time to take inventory and find out about any genetically inherited problems so you can discuss them with your health care provider. Have you had all your immunizations, including measles and rubella? These diseases can be harmful to your growing baby should you develop them during pregnancy. For other information about diseases to avoid during pregnancy, check out:

- Childhood Illnesses in Pregnancy: Chickenpox and Fifth Disease
- Toxoplasmosis
- Group B Strep Infection

Though it may seem overwhelming learning about all these potentially harmful infections, try not to panic, and remember the old aphorism, "Knowledge is power." Once you know the facts, you can relax and just enjoy your pregnancy. Contact: Health Information Specialist, March of Dimes Birth Defects Foundation, 1275 Mamaroneck Ave., White Plains, NY 10605; 914-428-7100; 888-663-4637; {www.modimes.org}.

THE STORK REPORT

For many moms-to-be, pregnancy can be a time when you find the changes taking place in your body endlessly fascinating. If you want to follow each and every step, the March of Dimes has a free brochure to help.

How Your Baby Grows provides you with a month-by-month diary of your baby's development. Each section discusses baby's development, as well as the myriad changes your body may be experiencing. There's even a handy month-by-month prenatal care guide and several helpful diagrams to assist you in visualizing your little bundle.

Contact: Health Information Specialist, March of Dimes Birth Defects Foundation, 1275 Mamaroneck Ave., White Plains, NY 10605; 914-428-7100; 888-663-4637; {www.modimes.org}.

Midlife Mommies

Many women today are electing to have their babies after age 30. It is estimated that by the year 2000, one in every 12 babies will be born to women age 35 and older.

Advances in medical care help women in their 30s and 40s have safer pregnancies, but women should be aware of the risks associated with delayed childbearing so that they can make informed decisions about when to start their families. In *Pregnancy After Age 30*, find out how age affects fertility; what the risk of miscarriage is as a woman gets older; the risk of birth defects in babies of women over thirty; and whether or not women over 30 have more problems in labor or delivery.

Understanding DNA Testing

When a specific inherited disease occurs within a particular family, parents often want to know if they might develop the same disease or if they might be carriers and pass on an inherited trait to their children. *Understanding DNA Testing* walks you through technology's labyrinth by starting with the basics: What is DNA? What is an inherited trait? How is DNA testing conducted? What are its advantages? And how long will it take? This brochure also lists several diseases that can be diagnosed through DNA testing. Contact: National Maternal and Child Health Clearinghouse, 2070 Chain Bridge Rd., Suite 450, Vienna, VA 22182; 703-356-1964; {www.nmchc.org}.

Contact: Health Information Specialist, March of Dimes
Birth Defects Foundation, 1275 Mamaroneck Ave., White
Plains, NY 10605; 914-428-7100; 888-663-4637;
{www.modimes.org}.

COMPUTERS AND PREGNANCY

Many pregnant women who spend long hours at their
computers wonder if video display terminals (VDTs) and
the electromagnetic field (EMF) produced by them may be
harmful to their unborn child. One 1991 study that analyzed
the risk of EMFs reported that women who work at VDTs
all day have no more risk of miscarriage than women with
similar jobs who do not use VDTs. Still, women concerned
about the issue and unsatisfied with the pace or research
may want to find out what they can do to reduce their risks
of exposure.

VDT Facts, a free fact sheet from the March of Dimes,
provides some helpful information about controlling your
exposure to VDTs as well as controlling some of the
physical discomforts that may come as a result of long
hours at the computer. Sitting an arm's length away from
the computer screen can significantly cut the strength of
EMFs, for example, and taking regular 15-minute breaks
can help reduce the physical stress.

Contact: Health Information Specialist, March of Dimes
Birth Defects Foundation, 1275 Mamaroneck Ave., White
Plains, NY 10605; 914-428-7100; 888-663-4637;
{www.modimes.org}.

Expecting the Unexpected
(Or How to Write a Birth Plan)

Since no two women will have exactly the same labor, there's a limit to how much control you can have over your baby's birth. But many childbirth educators recommend putting together a birth plan — a written plan agreed upon by you and your doctor (or midwife) — detailing your preferences for the procedures and atmosphere surrounding your baby's birth.

In the low-cost pamphlet *Planning Your Baby's Birth* (50 cents), you will learn how to write a birth plan (using the most flexible and communicative language possible) and how to choose options that reflect your philosophy and attitude about birth. Several questions about how to deal with unexpected birth situations are discussed, along with information about how to make informed yet flexible and educated choices. A full-page chart outlining typical medical routines as well as choices for parents more interested in natural childbirth is included, as is a chart for births that may not be routine — such as cesarean births or premature/sick infants.

Contact: International Childbirth Educational Association, 8060 26th Ave., South, Minneapolis, MN 55425; 612-854-8660; 800-624-4934; {www.icea.org}.

Sexually Transmitted Diseases and Pregnancy

A pregnant woman who has a sexually transmitted disease (STD) can pass the disease along to her baby. So if you suspect that you have an STD infection or just want to be certain you don't have one, then go to your doctor and get tested.

In *Protect Yourself and Your Baby from Sexually Transmitted Diseases*, a free pamphlet from the American Social Health Association, find out the most common STDs and how they affect you and your baby. For those STDs

Money For Living Expenses While You're Pregnant

The Crisis Pregnancy Hotline at Catholic Charities will link you up with a nearby Catholic Charities agency that offers supportive services ranging from counseling and parenting information to adoption and help with living expenses during and after pregnancy. Call 1-800-CARE-002 at Catholic Charities USA, 1731 King St., Suite 200, Alexandria, VA 22314; 703-549-1390; Fax: 703-549-1656; {www.catholiccharitiesusa.org}.

that have warning signs, there's a checklist of symptoms that may indicate infection, and information about what to do if you think you have an STD. Contact: American Social Health Association, P.O. Box 13827, Research Triangle Park, NC 27709; 919-361-8400.

Free Help At Your Home, Every Day, For The First 3 Weeks After Childbirth

The Healthy Families America Project operates 300 programs in 40 states. It helps new mothers cope with the pressures of being a new parent by offering volunteer home visitors who come to your home for the first three weeks after birth. They are trained to show you how to deal with the physical, emotional and financial strains of a new baby. First time mothers and older mothers are among those considered for the program.

To see if there is a program in your area and if you qualify, contact National Committee to Prevent Child Abuse, 200 S. Michigan Ave., 17th Floor, Chicago, IL 60604; 312-663-3520; Fax: 312-939-8962; {www.childabuse.org}.

Help Is Just A Phone Call Away

No child, no matter if his parents are rich or poor, should be denied a healthy start to life. Under Title V of the Social Security Act, all families with young children and expecting mothers whose incomes fall near the federal poverty guidelines receive Medicaid. Poverty thresholds for 1999 were $8,240 for one person, $11,060 for two, $13,880 for three, and $16,700 for a family of four.

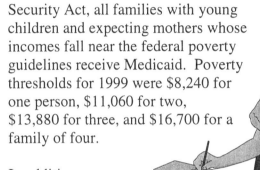

In addition, many prenatal and infant care services are often available to these low income families. These services include:

➡ Prenatal care clinics
➡ Home visiting services
➡ Translation services and other culturally focused services
➡ Parenting classes
➡ Programs for smoking cessation
➡ Male support programs
➡ Substance abuse treatment programs
➡ Help obtaining assistance such as Medicaid, food stamps, and WIC (supplemental food program for Women, Infants, and Children).

Begun in 1997, a new toll-free hotline funded by the U.S. Department of Health and Human Services links callers from anywhere in the United States to prenatal and infant health services located nearest them. Call 800-311-BABY (2229). For Spanish speakers, call 800-504-7081.

How Do I Find An OB/GYN?

The Resource Center of the American College of Obstetricians and Gynecologists (ACOG) can provide a list of ACOG ob/gyn members in your area, as well as subspecialists, if appropriate. The Center has lists of subspecialists in maternal-fetal medicine, reproductive endocrinology, and gynecologic oncology. You can also search for ACOG ob/gyn members by name, zip code, or state on the ACOG home page.

If you have a personal medical question, ACOG Resource Center staff will be happy to provide copies of ACOG pamphlets related to your topic — ACOG publishes more than 100 titles in the ACOG Patient Education Pamphlet series. The Resource Center is not a hotline, so be sure to also consult your own health care provider, who is familiar with your medical situation, and can counsel you on the best options for your care.

Contact: ACOG Resource Center, 409, 12th St. SW, Washington DC 20024; 202-883-2518 (9-5 EST); Fax: 202-484-1595; {E-mail: resources@acog.org}; {www.acog.org}.

Having Your Baby With A Nurse-Midwife

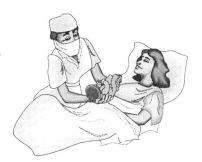

You can call 24-hours a day or go to the Internet to find a nurse-midwife in your area. Certified Nurse-Midwives (CNMs) are registered nurses and licensed health care practitioners educated in the two disciplines of nursing and midwifery. CNMs provide gynecological services and care of mothers and babies throughout the maternity cycle.

Contact: American College of Nurse-Midwives, 818 Connecticut Avenue, NW, Suite 900, Washington, DC 20006; 202-728-9660; 888-MIDWIFE – 24-hour toll free midwife locator; {E-mail: info@acnm.org}; {www.midwife.org}.

BIRTH CENTERS

Birth centers are places where healthy pregnant women receive prenatal care and deliver their babies, with assistance. They offer the time and place for unhurried, low-tech birth guided by professionals with a standard for safety.

Most birth centers are free-standing, unattached to any other building or institution; a few are attached to hospitals. Most are owned by nurse-midwives or doctors; a smaller number are not-for-profit centers governed by a board of directors. Almost all insurance companies pay for birth centers, including Medicaid and CHAMPUS. Some pay 100 percent, instead of the 80 percent coverage for hospital birth. Check your benefits through your employer. View the Birth Center Safe & Sensitive Care Video on-line at {www.birthcenters.org/customizedguides}.

To learn more about birth centers or to find one in your community, contact: National Association of Childbearing Centers (NACC), 3123 Gottschall Road, Perkiomenville, PA 18074; 215-234-8068; Fax: 215-234-8829; {E-mail: ReachNACC@BirthCenters.org}; or American College of Nurse-Midwives (ACNM), 818 Connecticut Avenue, NW, Suite 900, Washington, DC 20006; 202-728-9860; {E-mail: info@acnm.org}; {www.midwife.org}.

Are You Worried About Breastfeeding?

La Leche League Leaders are experienced mothers who are accredited by La Leche League International to help mothers and mothers-to-be with all aspects of breastfeeding. To locate an LLL Leader near you, look first in your local telephone directory. There is also an index of La Leche League Groups on their web site.

To find a La Leche League leader near you, contact: La Leche League International, 1400 N. Meacham Rd., P.O. Box 4079, Schaumburg, IL 60168-4079; 800-LALECHE; 847-519-7730; {www.lalecheleague.org}.

Free Health Insurance For Kids

Are you pregnant or the parent of young children? Do you have a child with special needs? The federal government provides block grants, called Title V, to each state to provide maternal and child (including teens) health care services. Each state has some latitude as to how they spend the money, but 30% must go to providing services for children with special health care needs, and 30% for children and adolescents. The Maternal and Child Health Division of your state Department of Health is responsible for administering the funds. The states are required by Title V to start establishing 800 numbers to provide information regarding services available in the state (see listing on page 336).

Federal law requires that all states provide Medicaid to pregnant women and children through the age of six whose income does not exceed 133% of poverty. Federal poverty thresholds in 1999 were $8,240 for one person, $11,060 for two, $13,880 for three, and $16,700 for four people. The government is going to raise the age level for Medicaid benefits one year at a time until all children are covered to age eighteen. Many states have additional benefits for children and programs for children with special needs.

Free Help For the 10 Million Kids Who Don't Have Health Insurance

Of the 10 million kids not covered, 4 million are eligible for Medicaid coverage and 5 million more are eligible for the new CHIP program. But most of the parents of these children are either unaware that they qualify or they become discouraged by the cumbersome enrollment process.

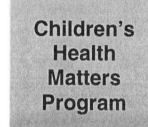

Children's Health Matters Program

There are thousands of advocacy offices around the country that know the laws and requirements for your state and will help you get the health coverage your kid needs and is entitled to. Contact your local Catholic Charities Office listed in your telephone book and ask them about the Children's Health Matters program. Or contact Catholic Charities USA, 1731 King St., Suite 200, Alexandria, VA 22314; 703-549-1390; Fax: 703-549-1656; {www.catholiccharitiesusa.org}.

Low-Cost Or Free Health Insurance For Kids Is Here

You love your children and work hard to help them grow up strong and healthy. But like many parents, you haven't been able to give them health insurance. Now, many families who work hard to make ends meet can get low-cost or free health insurance for their children through 18 years of age. Each state has its own program that makes

Top 10 States With Largest % of Children Without Health Insurance

State	Children Uninsured
Texas	46%
New Mexico	43%
Louisiana	43%
Arkansas	42%
Mississippi	41%
District of Columbia	39%
Alabama	38%
Arizona	38%
Nevada	37%
California	37%
Total US	**33%**

Of the children who lacked insurance, 89% lived in households where the parents worked.

Source: One Out Of Three Kids Without Health Insurance 1995-1996, Families USA Foundation {http://tap.epn.org/families/kwohi.htm}.

health insurance coverage available to children in working families.

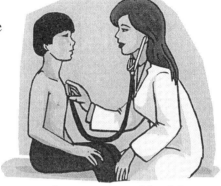

Services covered include regular check-ups and immunizations, school and sports physicals, dental care, vision and hearing testing, medications, hospital visits, and more. Some states may also cover prescription drugs, laboratory and x-ray, mental health, substance abuse, medical equipment and supplies, chiropractic services, foot doctor services, speech therapy, physical therapy, and more.

Eligibility requirements vary from state to state and are typically based on family size and income. In Connecticut, Missouri, and New Hampshire, for example, a family of four can have an annual income up to $49,350 and still qualify for low-cost health insurance for their children. Some states require modest co-payments or nominal monthly premiums based on income. In many states, all services are offered at no cost once you are enrolled in the program.

It is important to remember that eligibility requirements are approximate and may be revised because of changes in the state program or the economy. Always call your state for the most accurate numbers. The best way to find out if your children are eligible is to apply for your state's program.

Don't let your kids go another day without health coverage. Use the information below to access information about children's health insurance in your state. You can also learn more about Children's Health Insurance Program (C.H.I.P.) at the federal website **{http://insurekidsnow.gov/}**. There, you will find links to information about your state's program. By calling toll-free 877-KIDS NOW anywhere in the United States, you will be connected with a local operator who can answer your questions and send you an application. Please note that all of the states prefer that you use this or other listed hotline telephone numbers rather than write them for information.

ALABAMA

The State of Alabama has created ALL Kids in order to provide health insurance to children who are presently uninsured. Covered services include regular check-ups and immunizations, school and sports physicals, prescription drugs, dental care, vision and hearing testing, medications, hospital visits, and more.

For children at 150% federal poverty level and below there are no premiums and no co-payments for any service. For children from 151% FPL through 200% FPL, the premium is $50-$60 annually. There are also small (under $5) co-pays for some services. There are no co-pays for any preventive service. Eligibility requirements are based on size of family and income. For example, a family of four must have an annual income under $32,900 to qualify.

The best way to find out if your children are eligible for ALL Kids is to apply for the program. Applications are available at your county health department, clinics, many doctors' offices, hospitals, and social service agencies. For more information or to apply, contact All Kids Program, P.O. Box 304900, Montgomery, AL 36177-7280; 877-KIDS NOW (543-7669); 888-373-KIDS (5437); {E-mail: allkids@alapubhealth.org}; **{www.alapubhealth.org/chip/ index.htm}.**

ALASKA

The State of Alaska has created Denali KidCare in order to provide health insurance to children and teens through age 18, and for pregnant women who are presently uninsured. With Denali KidCare, children and teens receive the full range of prevention and treatment services such as: doctor's visits, health check-ups & screenings, vision exams & eyeglasses, dental checkups, cleanings & fillings, hearing tests and hearing aids, speech therapy, physical therapy, mental health therapy, substance abuse treatment, chiropractic services, foot doctor services, hospital care, laboratory tests, prescription drugs, and medical transportation. There is no cost for eligible children, teens and pregnant women. However, youth who are 18 years old may be required to share a limited amount of the cost for some services.

Denali KidCare income guidelines are based on family size. For example, if you have four members in your family, and your income does not exceed $41,140, you may qualify for Denali KidCare. It's best to apply, but call Denali KidCare to ask about the income guidelines.

The best way to find out if your children are eligible for Denali KidCare is to apply for the program. For more information or to apply, contact Denali KidCare, P.O. Box 240047, Anchorage, AK 99524-0047; 877-KIDS NOW (543-7669); 888-318-8890; {E-mail: Denali_Kid_Care@ health.state.ak.us}; **{www.hss.state.ak.us/dma/denali.htm}.**

ARIZONA

The State of Arizona has created the KidsCare program in order to provide health insurance to children who are presently uninsured. Covered services include regular check-ups and immunizations, school and sports physicals, immunizations, prescription drugs, dental care, vision and hearing testing, medications, hospital visits, and more.

All services are offered at no cost except non-emergency visits to an emergency room for which there is a co-payment of $5.00. Depending on their income, some families will be required to pay a monthly premium in the $10-$20 range based on their number of children. Eligibility requirements are based on size of family and income. For example, a family of four must have an annual income under $24,675 to qualify.

The best way to find out if your children are eligible for KidsCare is to apply for the program. For more information or to apply, contact KidsCare, Maildrop 500, 920 E. Madison, Phoenix, AZ 85034; 877-KIDS NOW (543-7669); 877-764-KIDS (5437); **{www.kidscare.state.az.us/}.**

ARKANSAS

The State of Arkansas has created ARKids First in order to provide health insurance to children who are presently uninsured. Covered services include regular check-ups and immunizations, school and sports physicals, dental care, vision and hearing testing, medications, hospital visits, and more.

ARKids First

Nominal co-payments are required for prescriptions, office visits, and hospital stays, but well-health and preventative services are provided at no cost. Eligibility requirements are based on size of family and income. For example, a family of four must have an annual income under $32,900 to qualify.

The best way to find out if your children are eligible for ARKids First is to apply for the program. For more information or to apply, contact ARKids Unit, Pulaski County North, DHS Office, 1900 East Washington Ave., P.O. Box 5791, North Little Rock, AR 72119; 877-KIDS NOW (543-7669); 888-474-8275; **{www.ar.medicaid.eds. com/ArkansasMedicaid/dmsprograms/ARKidsFirst/ arkmain.htm}.**

CALIFORNIA

The State of California has created the Healthy Families program in order to provide low-cost health coverage to children who are presently uninsured. Covered services include regular check-ups and immunizations, prescription drugs, dental care, vision and hearing testing, hospital visits, and more.

Depending on the plan you select, you may be required to pay a small fee to receive some services. You are also required to pay a nominal monthly premium based on the plan you select and your category. Eligibility requirements are based on size of family and income. For example, a family of four must have a monthly income under $2,742 to qualify.

The best way to find out if your children are eligible for Healthy Families is to apply for the program. For more information or to apply, contact Managed Risk Medical Insurance Board (MRMIB), 1000 G Street, Suite 450, Sacramento, CA 95814; 877-KIDS NOW (543-7669); 888-747-1222; {E-mail: healthyfamilies@eds.com}; **{www.healthyfamilies.ca.gov}.**

COLORADO

The State of Colorado has created the Child Health Plan Plus (CHP+) program in order to provide health insurance to children who are presently uninsured. Families may be required to pay a monthly premium of not more than $30 and a co-payment per visit and for medication of not more than $5. Covered services include regular check-ups and immunizations, vision and hearing testing, medications, hospital visits, and more.

Although you may be required to pay a small fee to receive some services, many are provided free of charge. You may also be required to pay a nominal monthly premium. Eligibility requirements are based on size of family and income. For example, a family of four must have an annual income under $30,433 to qualify.

The best way to find out if your children are eligible for CHP+ is to apply for the program. For more information or to apply, contact Child Health Plan Plus, P.O. Box 469022, Glendale, CO 80246; 877-KIDS NOW (543-7669); 800-359-1991; **{www.cchp.org/}.**

CONNECTICUT

The State of Connecticut has created The Husky Plan in order to provide health insurance to children who are presently uninsured. Covered services include regular check-ups and immunizations, school and sports physicals, prescription drugs, dental care, vision and hearing testing, hospital visits, and more.

For many families, there will be no premiums or co-payments. Depending on your income and which plan you participate, you may be required to pay a nominal monthly premium (maximum of $50 if under 300% Federal Poverty Level) and nominal co-payments. Eligibility requirements are based on size of family and income. For example, a family of four must have an annual income under $49,350 to qualify.

The best way to find out if your children are eligible for The Husky Plan is to apply for the program. For more information or to apply, contact HUSKY Program, P.O. Box 948, Farmington, CT 06034-9822; 877-KIDS NOW (543-7669); 877-CT-HUSKY (284-8759); TDD/TYY 800-842-4524; {E-mail: webmaster@huskyhealth.com}; **{www.huskyhealth.com}**.

DELAWARE

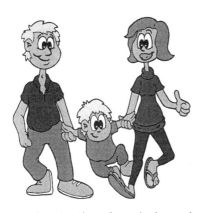

The State of Delaware has created the **Delaware Healthy Children Program** in order to provide health insurance to children who are presently uninsured. Covered services include regular check-ups and immunizations, laboratory and x-ray services, prescription drugs, inpatient and outpatient hospital services, and more.

Some low-income families can receive services at no cost. Based on your family size and income, you may be required to pay a nominal monthly premium between $10-$25. There are no co-payments. Eligibility requirements are based on size of family and income. For example, a family of four must have an annual income under $32,900 to qualify.

The best way to find out if your children are eligible for Healthy Children is to apply for the program. For more information or to apply, contact Delaware Healthy Children Program, University Office Plaza, Bristol Building, 248 Chapman Road, Suite 200, Newark, DE 19720; 877-KIDS NOW (543-7669); 800-996-9969; **{www.childrensdefense. org/signup/states/delaware.html}.**

DISTRICT OF COLUMBIA

The District of Columbia has created the DC Healthy Families program in order to provide health insurance to children who are presently uninsured. Covered services include regular check-ups and immunizations, school and sports physicals, prescription drugs, dental care, vision and hearing care, outpatient and inpatient hospital services, and more.

All services are provided at no cost. Eligibility requirements are based on size of family and income. For example, a family of four must have an annual income under $32,900 to qualify. The best way to find out if your children are eligible for Healthy Families is to apply for the program. For more information or to apply, contact Department of Health, Attn. Healthy Families, 825 North Capitol Street, NE, Washington, DC 20002; 877-KIDS NOW (543-7669); 800-666-2229; **{www.dchealth.com/}.**

FLORIDA

The State of Florida has created the KidCare program in order to provide health insurance to children who are presently uninsured. Covered services include regular check-ups and immunizations, school and sports physicals, vision and hearing testing, medications, hospital visits, and more.

Although you may be required to pay a small fee to receive some services, many are provided free of charge. You may also be required to pay a nominal monthly premium. Eligibility requirements are based on size of family and income. For example, a family of four must have an annual income under $32,900 to qualify.

The best way to find out if your children are eligible for KidCare is to apply for the program. For more information or to apply, contact Florida Healthy Kids, 661 E. Jefferson St., 2nd Fl., Tallahassee, FL 32311; 877-KIDS NOW (543-7669); 888-FLA KIDS (352-5437); {**www.floridakidcare.com/**}.

GEORGIA

The State of Georgia has created the PeachCare for Kids program in order to provide health insurance to children who are presently uninsured. Covered services include regular check-ups and immunizations, school and sports physicals, prescription drugs, dental care, vision and hearing testing, medications, hospital visits, and more.

There are no costs for families whose children are under the age of six. Families with children over the age of six are required to pay a monthly premium of $7.50 for one child and $15 for two or more children. Eligibility requirements are based on size of family and income. For example, a family of four must have an annual income under $32,900 to qualify.

The best way to find out if your children are eligible for PeachCare is to apply for the program. For more information or to apply, contact PeachCare, P.O. Box 2583, Atlanta, GA 30301-2583; 877-KIDS NOW (543-7669); 877-GA-PEACH (427-3224); {E-mail: peachcare@dma. state.ga.us}; **{www.state.ga.us/dma/peachcare/}.**

HAWAII

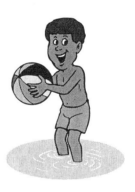

The Hawaii state legislature is still trying to determine how it will use its funds from the new Children's Health Insurance Program (CHIP) to expand health insurance coverage to uninsured children in Hawaii. If Hawaii begins a new CHIP program, the information will be posted online at **{http://insurekidsnow.gov/childhealth/states/fs_hi.asp}.**

For more information, contact Med-Quest Division, Department of Human Services, P.O. Box 339, Honolulu, HI 96809-0339; 877-KIDS NOW (543-7669); 808-586-5391.

IDAHO

The State of Idaho has created the Children's Health Insurance Program in order to provide health insurance to children who are presently uninsured. Covered services include regular check-ups and immunizations, prescription drugs, dental care, vision and hearing testing, medications, hospital visits, and more.

All services are currently provided at no cost. Eligibility requirements are based on size of family and income. For example, a family of four must have a monthly income under $2,056 to qualify. The best way to find out if your children are eligible for Brighter Futures Children's Health Insurance Program is to apply for the program.

For more information or to apply, contact Division of Medicaid Administration, Attn. CHIP Program, Bureau of Medicaid Programs and Resource Management, P.O. Box 83720, Boise, ID 83720-0036; 877-KIDS NOW (543-7669); 800-926-2588; {**www2.state.id.us/dhw/ hwgd_www/oldhome.html**}.

ILLINOIS

The State of Illinois has created the KidCare program in order to provide health insurance to children. Pregnant women who are Illinois residents and meet the income requirements are also eligible. Covered services include doctor and nursing care, immunizations and preventive care, hospital and clinic care, laboratory test and x-rays, prescription drugs, medical equipment and supplies,

medical transportation, dental care, eye care, psychiatric
care, podiatry, chiropractic care, physical therapy, mental
health and substance abuse services. Pregnant women
receive pre-natal care and other medical services.

While most families will receive services at no cost, some
families, based on their income and family size, will be
required to pay a nominal monthly premium (a family of 3
would pay $30). Eligibility requirements are based on size
of family and income. For example, a family of four must
have an annual income under $30,433 to qualify.

The best way to find out if your children are eligible for
KidCare is to apply for the program. For more information
or to apply, contact State of Illinois - KidCare Unit, P.O.
Box 19122, Springfield, IL 68794-9122; 877-KIDS NOW
(543-7669); 800-323 GROW (4769); TTY: 877-204-1012;
{E-mail: aidd2421@mail.idpa.state.il.us};
{www.state.il.us/dpa/kidcare.htm}.

INDIANA

The State of Indiana has created the Hoosier Healthwise
program in order to provide health insurance to children
who are presently uninsured. Covered services include
regular check-ups and immunizations, school and sports
physicals, immunizations, prescription drugs, dental care,
vision and hearing testing, medications, hospital visits, and
more. It also has benefits for children with special health
care needs like asthma or diabetes. All services are
provided at no cost. Eligibility requirements are based on

size of family and income. For example, a family of four must have an annual income under $24,675 to qualify.

The best way to find out if your children are eligible for Healthwise is to apply for the program. For more information or to apply, contact Hoosier Healthwise, P.O. Box 7213, Indianapolis, IN 24207-7213; 877-KIDS NOW (543-7669); 800-889-9949; **{www.state.in.us/chip/}.**

IOWA

The State of Iowa has created the HAWK-I program in

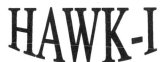 order to provide health insurance to children who are presently uninsured. Covered services include regular check-ups and immunizations, school and sports physicals, immunizations, prescription drugs, dental care, vision and hearing testing, medications, hospital visits, and more.

Based on their income, some families may be required to pay a small premium of $10 per child per month with a maximum of $20. There are no additional costs to receive services except a $25 co-payment for a non-emergency visit to an emergency room. Eligibility requirements are based on size of family and income. For example, a family of four must have an annual income under $30,432 to qualify.

The best way to find out if your children are eligible for HAWK-I is to apply for the program. For more information or to apply, contact HAWK-I, 8435 University Blvd., Suites 5, 6, 7, P.O. Box 71336, Des Moines, IA 50325-9958; 877-KIDS NOW (543-7669); 800-257-8563; {www.hawk-i.org}.

KANSAS

The State of Kansas has created the Health Wave program in order to provide health insurance to children who are presently uninsured. Covered services include regular check-ups and immunizations, school and sports physicals, dental care, vision and hearing testing, medications, hospital visits, and more.

Although there are no co-payments, some families may be required to pay a monthly premium up to $15 based on their income and number of children. Eligibility requirements are based on size of family and income. For example, a family of four must have an annual income under $32,900 to qualify.

The best way to find out if your children are eligible for KidCare is to apply for the program. For more information or to apply, contact Health Wave, P.O. Box 3599, Topeka, KS 66601; 877-KIDS NOW (543-7669); 800-792-4884.

KENTUCKY

The State of Kentucky has created the Kentucky Children's Health Insurance Program (KCHIP) in order to provide health insurance to children who are presently uninsured. Covered services include regular check-ups and immunizations, school and sports physicals, prescription drugs, dental care, vision and hearing testing, medications, hospital visits, and more.

Although you may be required to pay a small fee to receive some services, many are provided free of charge. Eligibility requirements are based on size of family and income. For example, a family of four must have an annual income under $32,900 to qualify. The best way to find out if your children are eligible for KCHIP is to apply for the program. For more information or to apply, contact Kentucky Cabinet for Health Services, 275 East Main Street, Frankfort, KY 40621; 877-KIDS NOW (543-7669); 800-635-2570; TTY: 800-775-0296; {**http://cfc-chs.chr.state. ky.us/chs/kchip/kchip.htm**}.

LOUISIANA

The State of Louisiana has created LA CHIP in order to provide health insurance to children who are presently uninsured. Covered services include regular check-ups and immunizations, school and sports physicals, dental care, vision and hearing testing, medications, hospital visits, and more. All services are provided at no cost. Eligibility requirements are based on size of family and income. For example, a family of four must have an annual income under $21,888 to qualify.

The best way to find out if your children are eligible for LA CHIP is to apply for the program. For more information or to apply, contact LA CHIP Processing Office, P.O. Box 91278, Baton Rouge, LA 70821; 877-KIDS NOW (543-7669); 877-252-2447 (2- LA CHIP).

MAINE

The State of Maine has created Cub Care in order to provide health insurance to children who are presently uninsured. Covered services include regular check-ups and immunizations, school and sports physicals, prescription drugs, dental care, vision and hearing testing, hospital visits, and more.

For low-income families, these services are provided at no cost. Depending on their income and number of children, a family may be required to pay a monthly premium ranging from $5 - $30. Eligibility requirements are based on size of family and income. For example, a family of four must have an annual income under $30,432 to qualify.

The best way to find out if your children are eligible for Cub Care is to apply for the program. For more information or to apply, contact CHIP Coordinator, Department of Human Services, 11 State House Station, Augusta, ME 04333-0011; 877-KIDS NOW (543-7669); 800-432-7338; {E-mail: jerry.mccarthy@state.me.us}; {www.state.me.us/dhs/main/cc_menu.htm}.

MARYLAND

The State of Maryland has created the Maryland Children's Health Program in order to provide health insurance to children who are presently uninsured. Covered services include regular check-ups and immunizations, school and sports physicals, prescription drugs, dental care, vision and hearing care, outpatient and inpatient hospital services, and more. All services are offered at no cost. Prescriptions may require a nominal co-payment. Eligibility requirements are based on size of family and income. For example, a family of four must have an annual income under $32,900 to qualify.

The best way to find out if your children are eligible for Maryland Children's Health Program is to apply for the program. For more information or to apply, contact HealthChoice, Maryland Department of Health and Mental Hygiene, 201 West Preston Street, Room L, Baltimore, MD 21201; 877-KIDS NOW (543-7669); 800-456-8900; TDD: 800-735-2258; {E-mail: healthchoice@dhmh.state.md.us}; **{www.dhmh.state.md.us/healthchoice/html/fact2.htm}.**

MASSACHUSETTS

The State of Massachusetts has expanded MassHealth in order to provide health insurance to children who are presently uninsured. Covered services include regular check-ups and immunizations, school and sports physicals, prescription drugs, dental care, vision and hearing testing, hospital visits, and more. Some low income families can receive services at no cost. For others, there is a monthly premium of $10, $20, or $30 for one, two, or three children. Some services require an additional co-payment, but cost sharing will not exceed 5% of a family's annual income. Eligibility requirements are based on size of family and income. For example, a family of four must have an annual income under $32,900 to qualify.

The best way to find out if your children are eligible for MassHealth is to apply for the program. For more information or to apply, contact Division of Medical Assistance, 600 Washington Street, 5th Floor, Boston, MA 02111; 877-KIDS NOW (543-7669); 800-841-2900; {www.state.ma.us/dma/}.

MICHIGAN

The State of Michigan has created the MIChild program in order to provide health insurance to children who are presently uninsured. Covered services include regular check-ups and immunizations, school and sports physicals, immunizations, prescription drugs, dental care, vision and hearing testing, medications, hospital visits, and more.

All services are provided at no cost, but you will be required to pay a nominal monthly premium ($5.00). Eligibility requirements are based on size of family and income. For example, a family of four must have an annual income under $32,000 to qualify. The best way to find out if your children are eligible for MIChild is to apply for the program. For more information or to apply, contact Maximus, 2651 Coolidge Road, East Lansing, MI 48823; 877-KIDS NOW (543-7669); 888-988-6300; {www.mdch.state.mi.us/MSA/mdch_msa/michild.htm}.

MINNESOTA

The State of Minnesota has created the MinnesotaCare program in order to provide health insurance to children who are presently uninsured. Adults are also eligible for this program even if they have no children. Covered services include regular check-ups and immunizations, school and sports physicals, dental care, vision and hearing testing, medications, hospital visits, and more.

Although there are no co-payments for services, families are required to pay a monthly premium ranging from $4 - $423 depending upon their income. Eligibility requirements are based on size of family and income. For example, a family of four must have a monthly income under $3,770 to qualify.

The best way to find out if your children are eligible for MinnesotaCare is to apply for the program. For more information or to apply, contact Minnesota Care, P.O. Box 64838, St. Paul, MN 55164-0838; 877-KIDS NOW (543-

7669); 800-657-3672; **{www.dhs.state.mn.us/HealthCare/ Default.htm}**.

MISSISSIPPI

The State of Mississippi has created the Mississippi Children's Health Insurance Program (CHIP) in order to provide health insurance to children who are presently uninsured. Phase I of this program provides services to children age 15-19 at no cost through Medicaid. Phase II which is currently being setup will provide more comprehensive service to a larger age range. Covered services include regular check-ups and immunizations, school and sports physicals, prescription drugs, dental care, vision and hearing testing, hospital visits, and more.

Eligibility requirements are based on size of family and income. For example, a family of four must have an annual income under $16,450 to qualify. The best way to find out if your children are eligible for CHIP is to apply for the program. For more information or to apply, contact Mississippi Department of Human Services, 750 North State Street, Jackson, MS 39202; 877-KIDS NOW (543-7669); 800-421-2408.

MISSOURI

The State of Missouri has created MC+ For Kids in order to provide health insurance to children who are presently uninsured. Covered services include regular check-ups and immunizations, school and sports physicals, dental care, vision and hearing testing, medications, hospital visits, and more. For many families, services are provided at no cost. Higher income families may be required to pay a small fee to receive some services as well as a nominal monthly premium. Eligibility requirements are based on size of family and income. For example, a family of four must have an annual income under $49,350 to qualify.

The best way to find out if your children are eligible for MC+ For Kids is to apply for the program. For more information or to apply, contact Department of Social Services, Division of Family Services, 221 West High Street, Jefferson City, MO 65101-1516; 877-KIDS NOW (543-7669); 888-275-5908.

MONTANA

The State of Montana has created the Children's Health Insurance Plan (CHIP) in order to provide health insurance to children who are presently uninsured. Covered services include regular check-ups and immunizations, sports and employment physicals, vision and hearing testing, medications, hospital visits, and more.

Although you may be required to pay a small fee to receive some services, many are provided free of charge. You may also be required to pay a nominal enrollment fee. Eligibility requirements are based on size of family and income. For example, a family of four must have an annual income under $24,675 to qualify. The best way to find out if your children are eligible for Children's Health Insurance Plan is to apply for the program. For more information or to apply, contact Healthy Mothers, Healthy Babies, P.O. Box 876, Helena, MT 59601; 877-KIDS NOW (543-7669); 800-421-6667; **{www.dphhs.mt.gov/res/chip.htm}.**

NEBRASKA

The State of Nebraska has created the Kids Connection program in order to provide health insurance to children who are presently uninsured. Covered services include regular check-ups and immunizations, school and sports physicals, dental care, vision and hearing testing, medications, hospital visits, and more. Although you may be required to pay a small fee to receive some services, many are provided free of charge. Eligibility requirements are based on size of family and income. For example, a family of four must have an annual income under $30,432 to qualify.

The best way to find out if your children are eligible for Kids Connection is to apply for the program. For more information or to apply, contact Nebraska Department of Health & Human Services Finance & Support, P.O. Box 95026, Lincoln, NE 68509-5026; 877-KIDS NOW (543-7669); 877-NEB KIDS (632-5437); {E-mail: deb.scherer@ hhss.state.ne.us}; **{www.hhs.state.ne.us/med/ kidsconx.htm}.**

NEVADA

The State of Nevada has created the Nevada Check Up program in order to provide affordable, comprehensive health insurance to children who are presently uninsured. Covered services include regular check-ups and immunizations, prescription drugs, dental care, vision and hearing testing, hospital visits, and more.

Once a family is eligible for Nevada Check Up, the family will be required to pay quarterly premium costs based on their gross annual income (the range for a family of four is $10 - $50 per quarter). Eligibility requirements are based on size of family and income. For example, a family of four must have an annual income under $32,900 to qualify.

The best way to find out if your children are eligible for Nevada Check Up is to apply for the program. For more information or to apply, contact Nevada Check Up, 1100 East William Street, Suite 116, Carson City, NV 89701; 877-KIDS NOW (543-7669); 800-360-6044.

NEW HAMPSHIRE

The State of New Hampshire has created Healthy Kids Gold and Healthy Kids Silver in order to provide health insurance to children who are presently uninsured. Covered services include regular check-ups and immunizations, school and sports physicals, prescription drugs, dental care, vision and hearing testing, hospital visits, and more. Services are provided at no cost to lower income families who participate in the Healthy Kids Gold program. Some families will be required to pay a monthly premium of $20, $40, or $80 based on their family size and annual income. Eligibility requirements are based on size of family and income. For example, a family of four must have an annual income under $49,350 to qualify.

The best way to find out if your children are eligible for Healthy Kids is to apply for the program. For more information or to apply, contact New Hampshire Healthy Kids, 6 Dixon Avenue, Concord, NH 03301; 877-KIDS NOW (543-7669); 877-4NH-CHIP (877-464-2447).

NEW JERSEY

The State of New Jersey has created NJKidCare in order to provide health insurance to children who are presently uninsured. Covered services include regular check-ups and immunizations, school and sports physicals, prescription drugs, dental care, vision and hearing testing, hospital visits, and more.

Premiums and co-payments may have to be paid by some families based on income. For example, a family of four with an annual income under $25,050 would pay $15 per month no matter how many children are on NJ KidCare. They may also be required to pay small co-payments for certain services. Total yearly premiums and co-payments will never exceed 5% of the family's income. Eligibility requirements are based on size of family and income. For example, a family of four must have an annual income under $33,400 to qualify.

The best way to find out if your children are eligible for NJKidCare is to apply for the program. For more information or to apply, contact Office of New Jersey KidCare, Department of Human Services, P.O. Box 712, 7 Quakerbridge Plaza, Trenton, NJ 08625-0712; 877-KIDS NOW (543-7669); 800-701-0710; TTY 1-800-701-0720; **{www.state.nj.us/humanservices/kcintro.html}.**

NEW MEXICO

Your children can receive the medical services they need through the New Mexikids program. Covered services include regular check-ups and immunizations, school and **Mexikids** sports physicals, vision and hearing testing, medications, hospital visits, and more. All services are provided at no cost. Eligibility requirements are based on size of family and income. For example, a family of four must have an annual income under $38,658 to qualify.

The best way to find out if your children are eligible for New Mexikids is to apply for the program. For more information or to apply, contact Department of Human Services/MED, P.O. Box 2348, Santa Fe, NM 87504-2348; 877-KIDS NOW (543-7669); 888-997-2583.

NEW YORK

The State of New York has created the Child Health Plus program in order to provide health insurance to children who are presently uninsured. Covered services include regular check-ups and immunizations, school and sports physicals, prescription drugs, dental care, vision and hearing services, hospitalization and more. There are no co-payments for services or benefits received. Depending on your gross family income, you may have to pay a family contribution to enroll in Child Health Plus. Eligibility requirements are based on size of family and income. For example, a family of four must have an annual income under $38,477 to qualify.

The best way to find out if your children are eligible for Child Health Plus is to apply for the program. For more information or to apply, contact Department of Health, Attn. Child Health Plus, Corning Tower, Empire State Plaza, Albany, NY 12237; 877-KIDS NOW (543-7669); 800-698-4KIDS; **{www.health.state.ny.us/}** (click on the Child Health logo).

NORTH CAROLINA

The State of North Carolina has created the NC Health Choice for Children program in order to provide health insurance to children who are presently uninsured. Covered services include regular check-ups and immunizations, prescription drugs, dental care, vision and hearing care including glasses, medications, hospital visits, and more.

For many lower income families, no enrollment fee or co-payments will be charged. For those at higher income levels, there will be an annual cost of $50 for one child and $100 for two or more children. There will also be a co-payment levied of $5 per visit, $6 per prescription, and $20 for non-emergency visits to an emergency room. Well child and other preventive health visits are offered at no cost. Eligibility requirements are based on size of family and

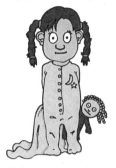

income. For example, a family of four must have an annual income under $ 33,400 to qualify.

The best way to find out if your children are eligible for NC Health Choice for Children is to apply for the program. Applications are available at social services departments, or local health departments in your county. These numbers are usually located in the "Government Services" section of the phone book, or in the Yellow Pages. For more information, contact North Carolina Department of Health and Human Services, Division of Medical Assistance, Attn. NC Health Choice, P.O. Box 29529, Raleigh, NC 27626-0529; 877-KIDS NOW (543-7669); 800-367-2229; **{www.sips.state.nc.us/ DHR/DMA/cpcont.htm}.**

NORTH DAKOTA

The State of North Dakota has created the Healthy Steps Program. Phase I of the Healthy Steps Program expands Medicaid coverage to children through 18 years of age with family income under 100% of the federal poverty level. Prior to this expansion, Medicaid coverage ended after age 17 for children in North Dakota. The services program is called EPSDT (Early and Periodic Screening, Diagnostic and Treatment) and includes regular checkups, immunizations, dental care, vision and hearing testing, medications, hospital visits and more. All the services offered as part of the Healthy Steps Program are provided free of charge. Eligibility requirements are based on size of family, age of children, and income. For example, a family of four with children under age 6 must have a monthly income under $1,823.21 to qualify.

The best way to find out if your children are eligible for North Dakota's Medicaid or Healthy Steps Program is to apply. For more information or to apply, contact Healthy Steps Program, Healthy Steps, North Dakota Department of Human Services, Medical Services Division, 600 E. Boulevard Avenue, Bismarck, ND 58505-0250; 877-KIDS NOW (543-7669); 888-222-2542; **{http://lnotes.state.nd.us/ dhs/dhsweb.nsf}** (search for "healthy steps").

OHIO

Ohio's Healthy Start program was created to provide free health insurance to children who do not have access to comprehensive health coverage. Coverage used to be available to younger children with lower incomes, but now, coverage through Healthy Start is available to all children up to age 19 in families with low to moderate incomes.

Children eligible for Healthy Start will be covered by a comprehensive benefit package. The benefit package is a primary and acute care package that includes coverage for the following: regular check-ups, annual physicals, immunizations, dental, vision, prescriptions, hospital visits, and much more. All services are provided at no cost. Eligibility requirements are based on size of family and income. For example, a family of four must have a monthly income under $2,056 to qualify.

The best way to find out if your children are eligible for Healthy Start is to apply. Applications are available at the Department of Human Services in your county. The number is usually located in the "Government Services" section of the phone book, or in the Yellow Pages. A list of Ohio County Human Services Agencies can be found online at **{www.state.oh.us/odhs/county/cntydir.html}.** For more information, contact Bureau of Consumer and Program Support, Attn. Healthy Start, Ohio Department of Human Services, 30 East Broad Street, 33rd Floor, Columbus, OH 43266-0423; 877-KIDS NOW (543-7669); 800-324-8680; TDD: 800-292-3572; **{www.state.oh.us/odhs/medicaid/flyer01.stm}.**

OKLAHOMA

The State of Oklahoma has a program called SoonerCare that provides health insurance to children who are presently uninsured. Covered services include regular check-ups and immunizations, school and sports physicals, vision and hearing testing, medications, hospital visits, and more.

Some services may require co-payments. Eligibility requirements are based on size of family and income. For example, a family of four must have an annual income under $30,444 to qualify. The best way to find out if your children are eligible for SoonerCare is to apply for the program. Applications are available at the Department of Human Services in your county. The number is usually 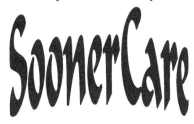 located in the "Government Services" section of the phone book, or in the Yellow Pages. For more information, contact Oklahoma Health Care Authority, 4545 N. Lincoln Blvd., Suite 124, Oklahoma City, OK 73105; 877-KIDS NOW (543-7669); 800-987-7767; {E-mail: web.team@ ohca.state.ok.us}.

OREGON

The Oregon Health Plan has expanded to allow more children to qualify at higher income levels. Covered services include regular check-ups and immunizations, vision and hearing testing, medications, hospital visits, and more. All services are provided at no cost and pregnant women are also eligible. Eligibility requirements are based on size of family and income. For example, a family of four must have a monthly income under $2,330 to qualify.

The best way to find out if your children are eligible for the Oregon Health Plan is to apply for the program. For more information or to apply, contact Oregon Health Plan, P.O. Box 14520, Salem, OR 97309; 877-KIDS NOW (543-7669); 800-359-9517; {www.omap.hr.state.or.us/}.

PENNSYLVANIA

The State of Pennsylvania has created the Children's Health Insurance Program (CHIP) in order to provide health insurance to children who are presently uninsured. Covered services include regular check-ups and immunizations, prescription drugs, emergency care, certain dental, vision and hearing services, mental health services, outpatient and inpatient hospital services, and more. Most children who qualify will get free coverage. Depending on their income, some families will be required to pay monthly rates much lower than insurance usually costs based on their family size and income. For others, CHIP coverage is provided at no cost. Eligibility requirements are based on size of family and income. For example, a family of four qualifies for free CHIP services if their annual income falls below $32,900. If their income falls between $32,901 and $38,658, they still qualify for low-cost CHIP services.

The best way to find out if your children are eligible for the CHIP is to apply for the program. For more information or to apply, contact Children's Health Insurance Plan, 1326 Strawberry Square, Harrisburg, PA 17120; 877-KIDS NOW (543-7669); 800-986-KIDS (5437).

RHODE ISLAND

The State of Rhode Island has expanded RIteCare in order to provide health insurance to children who are presently uninsured. Covered services include regular check-ups and immunizations, school and sports physicals, prescription drugs, dental care, vision and hearing testing, hospital visits, and more. Depending upon your family size and income, you may be required to pay a small monthly premium. You may also be required to pay a small fee to receive some services or a nominal monthly premium. Eligibility requirements are based on size of family and income. For example, a family of four must have an annual income under $41,125 to qualify.

The best way to find out if your children are eligible for RIteCare is to apply for the program. For more information or to apply, contact RIteCare, 600 New London Avenue, Cranston, RI 02920; 877-KIDS NOW (543-7669); 800-346-1004.

SOUTH CAROLINA

The State of South Carolina has created the Partners for Healthy Children program in order to provide health insurance to children who are presently uninsured. Covered services include regular check-ups and immunizations, school and sports physicals, prescription drugs, dental care, vision and hearing testing, medications, hospital visits, and more. All services and prescriptions are offered at no cost. Eligibility requirements are based on size of family and income. For example, a family of four must have an annual income under $24,675 to qualify.

The best way to find out if your children are eligible for Partners For Healthy Children is to apply for the program. For more information or to apply, contact South Carolina Partners for Healthy Children, P.O. Box 100101, Columbia,

SC 29202-3101; 877-KIDS NOW (543-7669); 888-549-0820; {**www.dhhs.state.sc.us/programs.htm**}.

SOUTH DAKOTA

The State of South Dakota has added the Child Health Insurance Program (CHIP) to its Medicaid program in order to provide health insurance to children who are presently uninsured. This expansion raises the allowable income for families with children 6 through 18 to that of the younger children, i.e., standardizing the income level for all children. The services program is called EPSDT (Early and Periodic Screening, Diagnostic and Treatment) and includes regular checkups, immunizations, dental care, vision and hearing testing, medications, hospital visits and more. All the services offered as part of Medicaid/CHIP are provided free of charge. Eligibility requirements are based on size of family and income. For example, a family of four must have a monthly income under $1,824 to qualify.

The best way to find out if your children are eligible for Medicaid/CHIP is to apply. For more information or to apply, contact Department of Social Services, Economic Assistance, 700 Governor's Drive, Pierre, SD 57501; 877-KIDS NOW (543-7669); or call your local Department of Social Services office; {**www.state.sd.us/chip/**}.

TENNESSEE

The State of Tennessee has created the TennCare program in order to provide health insurance to children who are presently uninsured. Coverage for adults is also available through TennCare. Covered services include inpatient and outpatient hospital care, physician services, prescription drugs, lab and x-ray services, medical supplies, home health care, hospice care, and ambulance transportation, and more. Eligibility requirements are based on size of family and income. For example, a family of four must have an annual income under $33,400 to qualify.

The best way to find out if your children are eligible for TennCare is to apply for the program. For more information or to apply, contact TennCare Bureau, 729 Church Street, Nashville, TN 37247-6501, 615-741-0213; 877-KIDS NOW (543-7669); 800-669-1851; 615-741-4800; {**www.state.tn.us/health/tenncare/**}.

TEXAS

The State of Texas has changed the family income limits for teens. Teenagers who are under 19 years old may now qualify for health care coverage through Medicaid, even if they did not qualify before. With Medicaid, teens can receive medical and dental check-ups and treatments. Benefits include medicines, office visits, hospital care, medical equipment and supplies, and many other medically necessary services. Eligibility requirements are based on size of family and income. For example, a family of four must have an annual income under $16,450 to qualify.

The best way to find out if your children are eligible is to apply for the program. Families can call or visit their local Medicaid representative to find out if they qualify and receive information on how to enroll. Call 800-422-2956 to locate your closest Department of Health Services (DHS) office. For more information or to apply, contact Texas Health and Human Services Commission, 4900 North Lamar, 4th Floor, P.O. Box 13247, Austin, TX 78711-3247; 877-KIDS NOW (543-7669); 512-424-6500; TDD: 512-424-6597; **{www.hhsc.state.tx.us/}.**

UTAH

The State of Utah has created a Children's Health Insurance Program in order to provide health insurance to children who are presently uninsured. Covered services include regular checkups, immunizations, vision and hearing testing, medications, hospital visits and more. Although you will be required to pay a small fee to receive some services, many are provided free of charge. Eligibility requirements are based on size of family and income. For example, a family of four must have a monthly income under $2,742 to qualify.

The best way to find out if your children are eligible for the Children's Health Insurance Program is to apply for the program. For more information or to apply, contact Utah CHIP, Utah Department of Health, P.O. Box 141000, Salt Lake City, UT 84114-1000; 877-KIDS NOW (543-7669); 888-222-2542; **{http://hlunix.hl.state.ut.us/chip/ index.html}.**

VERMONT

The State of Vermont has expanded Dr. Dynasaur in order to provide health insurance to children. Covered services include regular check-ups and immunizations, school and sports physicals, prescription drugs, dental care, vision and hearing testing, hospital visits, and more. There are no co-payments required for children. Depending on your family size and income, you may be required to pay a small monthly premium. Eligibility requirements are based on size of family and income. For example, a family of four must have an annual income under $40,956 to qualify.

The best way to find out if your children are eligible for Dr. Dynasaur is to apply for the program. For more information or to apply, contact Health Access Services, 5 Burlington Square, Burlington, VT 05401; 877-KIDS NOW (543-7669); 800-250-8427; 802-2410-2880; **{www.cit.state.vt.us/governor/dynasaur.htm}**.

VIRGINIA

The State of Virginia has created the Children's Medical Security Insurance Plan in order to provide health insurance to children up to and including age 18 who are presently uninsured. Covered services include regular check-ups and immunizations, inpatient and outpatient hospital services, prescription drugs, laboratory and x-ray, dental care, vision and hearing services, mental health, substance abuse, medical equipment and supplies, and more. Currently, services are offered at no cost. However, a cost sharing system is currently under the public comment period. Once that has been reviewed, a cost share may be initiated. Eligibility requirements are based on size of family and income. For example, a family of four must have an annual income under $30,895 to qualify.

The best way to find out if your children are eligible for Children's Medical Security Insurance Plan is to apply for the program. For more information or to apply, contact Department of Medical Assistance Services, 600 East Broad Street, Suite 1300, Richmond, VA 23219; 877-KIDS NOW (543-7669); 877-VA-CMSIP (822-6747); {www.state.va.us/~dmas/chip.htm}.

WASHINGTON

The Washington Basic Health Plan is a state-sponsored health insurance program for any Washington resident who is not eligible for Medicare and not institutionalized at the time of enrollment. Free or low-cost health coverage is now available for Washington children through Medicaid/Healthy Options. Basic Health provides members with an affordable basic package of health benefits through contracts with 10 private health plans. Members pay a monthly premium based on income, age, family size, and the health plan they choose. Washington State helps pay part of the premium for members who meet income guidelines. Eligibility requirements are based on size of family and income. For example, a family of four must have an annual income under $33,400 to qualify.

The best way to find out if your children are eligible for Children's Medical Security Insurance Plan is to apply for the program. For more information, contact Washington Basic Health Plan, P.O. Box 42683, Olympia, WA 98504-2683; 877-KIDS NOW (543-7669); 800-204-6429; TDD: 800-204-6430; **{www.wa.gov/hca/Basic.htm}.**

WEST VIRGINIA

The State of West Virginia has created the West Virginia Children's Health Insurance Program in order to provide health insurance to children who are presently uninsured. The Program is currently available for children age one to five years. Soon this coverage will be available to children up to age 19. Covered services include regular check-ups and immunizations, prescription drugs, dental care, inpatient and outpatient hospital services, and more. All services including prescriptions are provided at no cost. Eligibility requirements are based on size of family and income. For example, a family of four must have an annual income under $24,675 to qualify.

The best way to find out if your children are eligible for West Virginia Children's Health Insurance Program is to apply for the program. For more information or to apply, contact West Virginia Children's Health Insurance Program, Building 6, 1900 Kanawha Boulevard East, Charleston, WV 25305; 877-KIDS NOW (543-7669); 888-

WVFAMILY (983-2645); {E-mail: wvchip@wvdhhr.org};
{www.wvdhhr.org/PAGES/wvchip/default.htm}.

WISCONSIN

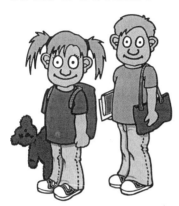

The State of Wisconsin has created BadgerCare in order to provide health insurance to children who are presently uninsured. Covered services include regular check-ups and immunizations, school and sports physicals, dental care, vision and hearing testing, medications, hospital visits, and more. Depending upon your family size and income, you may be required to pay a monthly premium ranging between $35 - $105. Eligibility requirements are based on size of family, age of children, and income. For example, a family of four with children under the age of six must have an annual income under $30,895 to qualify. If their children are under the age of nineteen, their monthly income must not exceed $1,300.

The best way to find out if your children are eligible for BadgerCare is to apply for the program. For more information or to apply, contact Bureau of Managed Health Care Systems, 1 West Wilson Street, Room 237, P.O. Box 309, 1 Wilson Street, Madison, WI 53701; 877-KIDS NOW (543-7669); 608-266-1935; {E-mail: webmaster@dhfs.state.wi.us}; **{www.dhfs.state.wi.us/}.**

WYOMING

Free or low-cost health coverage is now available for Wyoming children through Medicaid. Eligibility requirements are based on size of family and income. For example, a family of four must have an annual income under $22,211 to qualify.

The best way to find out if your children are eligible is to apply for the program. For more information contact Department of Health, Division of Health Care Financing, 17 Hathaway Building, Cheyenne, WY 82002; 877-KIDS NOW (543-7669); 800-251-1269; Cheyenne Area 777-5520.

Free Immunization and Flu Shots

Free Flu Shots

Who should get flu shots? The U.S. Center for Disease Control recommends it for

- adults over 65
- residents of nursing homes
- persons over 6 months of age with chronic cardiovascular or pulmonary disorders, including asthma
- persons over 6 months of age with chronic metabolic diseases including diabetes, renal dysfunction, hemoglobinipathies, immunosupressive or immunodeficiency disorders
- women in their 2nd or 3rd trimester of pregnancy during flu season
- persons 6 months to 18 years receiving aspirin therapy
- groups, including household members and care givers, who can infect high risk persons

Almost anyone can get free or low cost ($10-$15) flu shots from their county health office or other community sources. Some doctors, like Dr. Donald McGee in New Hampshire {www.drmcgee.com}, offer free shots in their office. Medicare Part B also pays for flu shots.

Contact your county office of public health listed in your telephone book or your state Department of Health listed in the Appendix. If you have trouble finding a local low cost source, or would like more information on the flu vaccine contact the National Immunization Information Hotline at 800-232-2522 (English); 800-232-0233 (Spanish); {www.cdc.gov/nip}.

Free Immunizations For Your Kids

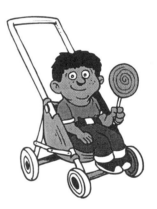

Only 78% of children receive their full recommended vaccinations that protect them against polio, diphtheria, mumps, whooping cough, German measles, tetanus, spinal meningitis, chicken pox, and hepatitis B. An increasing number of children are exposed to diseases in day-care settings and elsewhere.

Almost any child, no matter what their income, can receive free or very low cost immunizations in their local area. Contact your county office of health listed in your telephone book or your State Department of Health listed in the Appendix. If you have trouble, call the National Immunization Information Hotline at 800-232-2522 (English); 800-232-0233 (Spanish); {www.cdc.gov/nip}.

Low Cost Immunizations for Travelers

In order to prevent contracting diseases like yellow fever, cholera or Japanese encephalitis when traveling in other countries, the government's Center for Disease Control recommends that certain vaccines would eliminate your risk of infection. Some local Public Health offices offer these vaccines at a fraction of what you would pay at a doctor's office.

To find your local county office of health, look in your telephone book or contact your state Department of Health listed in the Appendix. For more information about disease and vaccines for travel, contact: Center for Disease Control and Prevention, National Center for Infectious Diseases, Division of Quarantine, 1600 Clifton Road, MS E-03, Atlanta, GA 30333; 404-638-8100; Fax: 404-639-2500; {www.cdc.gov/travel/index.htm}.

Free Hepatitis B Shots To Children

Oswego County Health Department offers free shots for children 18 and younger. The same with Buena-Vista County in Iowa, but people 19 and over are charged $31.75

for the shot. However, you won't be turned away if you cannot pay.

Hepatitis can cause serious liver disease, cancer and even death. About 1 in 20 people in the United States have been infected, and over 4,000 a year die. To find out about services in your area, contact the county office of health listed in your telephone book or your state Department of Health listed in the Appendix.

Free Flights To Get The Care You Need

Cheap Air Fare to See a Sick Relative

Not free, but at least you don't have to pay full price. When a family member is very ill or has died, families have to make last-minute airline reservations. Obviously you lose out on the 21-day advance purchase rates, but almost all

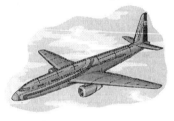

airlines offer *bereavement* or *compassion* fares for domestic travel.

Generally the fares are available to close family members, and the discount on the full-fare rate varies from airline to airline. Many require that you provide the name of the deceased and the name, address and phone number of the funeral home handling arrangements. In the case of a medical emergency, the name and address of the affected family member and the name, address and phone number of the attending physician or hospital are required.

Contact the airline of your choice to learn more about the *"Bereavement/Compassion Fares."* Full fare rates vary from airline to airline, but you could save up to 50%.

Free Transportation
To Medical Appointments For Your Mom

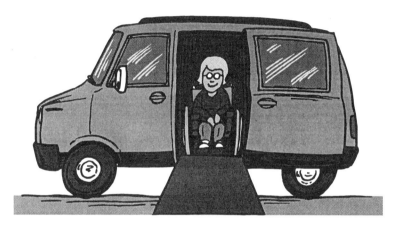

Mom has to get to a doctor's visit in the middle of the day and you can't take her. Or you have a disability that may cause you to miss an appointment if someone else doesn't drive. You may be able to get free transportation and escort services provided by either your local health office or local office on aging. Some communities even provide very low cost door-to-door services for seniors to go anywhere.

If you can't find your local area agency on aging or public health office in your telephone book, contact your state Department of Aging or Health listed in the Appendix. If that fails, contact the Eldercare Locator Hotline at 1-800-677-1116. They are available to help anyone identify services for seniors.

Free Flights To Medical Treatment

The Air Care Alliance is a nationwide league of humanitarian flying organizations dedicated to community service, health care, patient transport, and related kinds of public-benefit flying. Air Care Alliance member groups will not fly patients or supplies when insurance or other funds can provide commercial transport via air ambulance, charter, or airline. ACA volunteers fly only when financial need or other special circumstances mean a compelling human need would go unfulfilled.

Contact: Air Care Alliance, 4620 Haygood Road Suite 8, Virginia Beach, VA 23455; {E-mail: aircare@aol.com}; {www.aircareall.org}.

Free Air Travel To Needed Medical Care

AirLifeLine is a national non-profit charitable organization of private pilots who donate their time, skills, aircraft and fuel to fly medical missions, provides an immediate solution during a time of crisis. AirLifeLine pilots assist ambulatory patients who must receive life-sustaining treatment at a medical facility far from home and cannot afford the cost of travel.

In addition to flights for patients to their medical treatment centers, AirLifeLine also provides flights for final wishes of terminally ill patients. To a limited degree, AirLifeLine also flies time-critical cargo such as blood and donor organs for transplants.

Contact: AirLifeLine National Office, 50 Fullerton Court, Suite 200, Sacramento, CA 95825; 800-446-1231; 916-641-7800; Fax: 916-641-0600; {E-mail: staff@ AirLifeLine.org}.

$ 1,500 In Travel Money To Receive Epilepsy Care

When people with seizures need specialized care, it may not be available in the local area. Travel expenses for individuals and families may sometimes be a barrier to such care, especially when other medical expenses mount up. The J. Kiffin Penry Travel Assistance Program of the Epilepsy Foundation offers a limited number of travel assistance grants, up to $1,500 each, for people who must travel for specialized epilepsy care or testing.

Contact: Epilepsy Foundation, 4351 Garden City Drive, Landover, MD 20785; 301-459-3700; 800-EFA-1000; Fax: 301-577-4941; {E-mail: webmaster@efa.org}; {www.efa.org/programs/ps_services.html}.

Coping With The High Cost of Health Insurance

3 Million Seniors & Disabled
Don't Apply for Their Free $1,000 For Health Care

Women Without Health Insurance

15% of all adult women have no insurance
500,000 pregnant women have no insurance

Source: Center for Policy Alternatives www.cfpa.org/publications/index.html

Each year over 3 million eligible seniors and people with disabilities fail to apply for a little-known program that will give them up to an extra $1,051 annually in their Social Security check. That's how much the government deducts from their Social Security to pay for their Medicare premiums. It amounts to $87.60 a month for couples and $43.80 for individuals. There are three basic programs:

1) *Pays for Medicare premiums, deductibles and co-payments under the Qualified Medicare Beneficiaries (QMBs) plan.*
2) *Pays for Medicare Part B premiums under the Specified Low-Income Medicare Beneficiaries (SLMBs) plan.*

3) Pays for Medicare Part B premiums under the Qualified Individuals Plan for people with incomes up to $14,892.

Studies show that only 5,000 of the 500,000 eligible apply for this program. With so few eligible people applying, it's understandable that many people don't know about this program.

Here's where to go. Contact your local Social Security Office. If they don't know, contact your state Office of Social Services listed in the Appendix. You can also contact the Medicare Hotline and request the publication, *Guide to Health Insurance for People With Medicare.* Contact Medicare Hotline at 800-638-6833; {www.medicare.gov}.

Working People With Disabilities Can Get Cheap Health Insurance

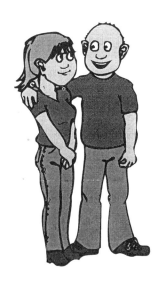

A change to the Balanced Budget Act of 1997 passed by Congress allows states to offer Medicaid to individuals who are working and who have a disability. Prior to this, states could only offer Medicaid to people with disabilities who were NOT working. The income limits goes up to $40,000 and the state can charge premiums on an income-related sliding scale.

Contact your state Department of Health listed in the Appendix to identify your Medicaid office or page 397 for your state contact. You can contact the local office of your congressman or senator for more information on the law. You can also check out the website of the Bazelon Center at {www.bazelon.org}.

Free Audio Tapes Describe Medicare Benefits To Disabled

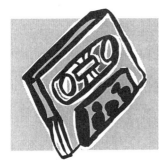

If you have use of a high speed cassette player (talking book reader), you can learn about Medicare benefits with free audio copies of:

1) Medicare Home Health
2) Medicare and Medicaid Guide To Choosing a Nursing Home
3) Medicare Hospice Benefits
4) Medicare Managed Care
5) Medicare Savings for Qualified Beneficiaries
6) Medicare & Other Health Benefits: Who Pays First?

Contact your local Medicare office, order from 800-318-2596, or order online at {www.medicare.gov}.

Free Health Insurance Counseling

Free one-on-one counseling is available to seniors and, in most areas, people with disabilities, to answer questions like:

★ How much insurance is too much?
★ If something sounds like fraud, where can I go for help?
★ What's the best Medigap insurance plan?
★ Do I qualify for government health benefits?
★ Should I buy long-term care insurance?

The program is called **Health Insurance Counseling and Advocacy Program (HICAP)** and is sponsored by the U.S. Health Care Financing Administration. In most states, it is usually run by the state Department on Aging or the State Insurance Commissioner's office. The office for each state is listed in the Appendix. If that fails, contact the Eldercare Locator hotline at 1-800-677-1116. They can give you the local number.

State Health Insurance Assistance Program

Alabama
800-243-5463
334-242-5743

Alaska
800-478-6065
907-269-3680

Arizona
800-432-4040
602-542-6595

Arkansas
800-224-6330
501-371-2782

California
800-434-0222
800-510-2020
916-323-7315

Colorado
800-544-9181
303-894-7499 ext. 356

Connecticut
800-994-9422
860-424-5245

Delaware
800-336-9500
302-739-6266

District of Columbia
202-676-3900

Florida
800-963-5337
850-414-2060

Georgia
800-669-8387
404-657-5334

Hawaii
808-586-7299

Idaho
800-247-4422
208-334-4350

Illinois
800-548-9034
217-785-9021

Indiana
800-452-4800
317-233-3475

Iowa
8000-351-4664
515-281-6867

Kansas
800-860-5260
316-337-7386

Kentucky
502-564-7372

Louisiana
800-259-5301
225-342-0825

Maine
800-750-5353
207-623-1797

Maryland
800-243-3425
410-767-1100

Massachusetts
800-882-2003
617-727-7750

Michigan
800-803-7174
517-373-8230

Minnesota
800-333-2433

Mississippi
800-948-3090
601-359-4929

Missouri
800-390-3330

Montana
800-332-2272
406-444-7781

Nebraska
800-234-7119
402-471-2201

Nevada
800-307-4444
702-486-3478

New Hampshire
800-852-3388
603-225-9000

New Jersey
800-792-8820
609-588-3139

New Mexico
800-432-2080
505-827-7640

New York
800-333-4114
212-869-3850

North Carolina
800-443-9354
919-733-0111

North Dakota
800-247-0560
701-328-2440

Ohio
800-686-1578
614-644-3458

Oklahoma
800-763-2828
405-521-6628

Oregon
800-722-4134
503-947-7984

Pennsylvania
800-783-7067

Rhode Island
800-322-2880
401-222-2880

South Carolina
800-868-9095
803-898-2850

South Dakota
800-822-8804
605-773-3656

Tennessee
800-525-2816
615-741-4955

Texas
800-252-9240

Utah
800-541-7735
801-538-3910

Vermont
800-642-5119
802-748-5182

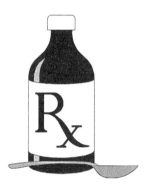

Virginia
800-552-3402
804-622-9333

Washington
800-397-4422
360-407-0383

West Virginia
877-987-4463
304-558-3317

Wisconsin
800-242-1060
608-266-2536

Wyoming
800-856-4398
307-856-6880

Solving Insurance and Money Problems For Cancer Patients

Cancer Care Inc. provides Free Patient and Family Education Program workshops, clinics, and seminars for people with cancer, their families, and caregivers on the following topics:

♦ *Medicare: How to Maximize Your Benefits*. This workshop discusses the basics of Medicare, Medicare HMOs and related health insurance, little known and hard-to-get benefits, appealing a denial of coverage, and programs for middle and low-income Medicare beneficiaries.

♦ *Maximizing Your Health Insurance Benefits.* This workshop can help you find your way through medical paperwork so that you or your doctor can receive the money you are entitled to after filing an insurance claim.

♦ *Getting to Know Your Entitlements.* This session discusses Medicaid and Medicare, the differences between Supplemental Security Income (SSI) and Social Security Disability (SSD), and how to access these and other benefits.

♦ *Managed Care: What You Need to Know.* This workshop will help you with information on getting your insurance to cover your treatment if you have cancer. Discussions include the basics of managed care, problems and solutions, and how to advocate for yourself.

♦ *Learn Your Right to Appeal a Denial or Discontinuance of Government Benefits.* In this workshop you will learn how to appeal a denial or discontinuance of SSD, SSI, Medicaid, food stamps, home care, or other government benefits.

♦ *Strategies and Solutions to Help Pay for a Serious Illness.* This workshop helps cancer patients and their families explore options to help pay for the high cost of cancer treatment.

♦ *Planning for Important Health Care Decisions: A Review of Advance Directives*. The presenter of this workshop will discuss and review important documents, including the Health Care Proxy and Living Will, which protect your right to receive the care you want in the event you lose the ability to make decisions yourself.

♦ *The Most Common Estate Planning Mistakes*. One of the concerns of many citizens today is how they can preserve their estates from the high cost of settling an estate. The presenters of this workshop will discuss why you should plan ahead to prevent problems that can cost your estate thousands of dollars. Topics to be addressed: joint ownership, federal and state taxes, gifts, liquidity, charitable trusts, selection of executor, disposition of assets and special needs trusts, and will documents.

♦ *A Financial Planning Seminar for Bereaved Spouses, Partners, and Adult Children*. This workshop helps people dealing with bereavement with their finances and answers financial planning questions.

♦ *All You Want to Know About Legal Issues and Cancer*. This is a free legal planning seminar to discuss estate planning, power-of-attorney, wills, living wills, and health care proxy.

A schedule of the workshops is available on the Cancer Care webpage. For more information, contact Cancer Care, Inc., 1180 Avenue of the Americas, 2nd Floor, New York,

NY 10036; 212-221-3300; 800-813-HOPE (800-813-4673); {www.cancercareinc.org}; {E-mail: info@cancercare.org}.

Medicare/Medicaid: Free Medical Care For Elderly, Disabled And Low Income

How do you know if you qualify for Medicare or Medicaid? The Medicare Program is a federal health insurance program for persons over 65 years of age and certain disabled persons. It is funded through Social Security contributions, premiums, and general revenue. The

LEARN HOW TO BE YOUR OWN HEALTH CARE ADVOCATE

"How to Be an Effective Advocate for Yourself or Others" is a free workshop offered by Cancer Care, Inc. that will help you identify and prioritize your health care needs, navigate the health care system, communicate your needs more effectively, and advocate individually locally and nationally. A schedule of the workshops is available on their webpage.

For more information contact: Cancer Care, Inc., 1180 Avenue of the Americas, 2nd Floor, New York, NY 10036; 212-221-3300; 800-813-HOPE (800-813-4673); {www.cancercareinc.org}; {E-mail: info@cancercare.org}.

Medicaid Program is a joint federal/state program that provides medical services to the needy and the medically needy. Eligibility and services for this program vary from state to state. To locate an office near you, look in the blue pages of your phone book under Human Services or:

Contact:
Medicare Hotline
Health Care Financing Administration
330 Independence Ave., SW
Washington, DC 20201
800-638-6833
800-492-6603
www.medicare.gov

This hotline can provide you with information regarding Medicare, Medicaid, and Medigap questions. They can refer you to the proper people to answer your questions, as well as provide you with publications on your topic of interest. This is also the number to call if you suspect Medicare or Medicaid fraud or abuse, as well as if you suspect improper sales practices of Medigap policies.

Medicaid

Medicaid is a federal/state assistance program that varies from state to state within federal guidelines. Medical bills are paid from federal, state and local tax funds. It serves low-income people of every age. Patients usually pay no part of costs for covered medical expenses although a small co-payment is sometimes required.

Benefits

No two states' Medicaid programs are alike, yet there are certain federally mandated standards common to all Medicaid programs across the nation. Within these broad federal guidelines, states determine the amount and duration of services offered under their Medicaid programs. In most states, recipients may seek medical services from any provider who accepts Medicaid patients.

Though coverage varies by state, Medicaid typically covers services from doctors, hospitals, outpatient care, prenatal services, family planning services, preventive health education, well-child checkups, dental care, eye care, psychiatric care, nursing 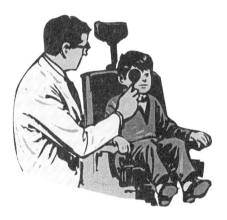 home care, health care clinics and centers, mental health services, home health care, case management services, hospice services, ambulance services, non-emergency transportation, prescription drugs, laboratory and x-ray services, renal dialysis, transplants, out-of-state services when necessary, and more. Note that there may be restrictions such as limits on the number of services you can receive and the length of time you may be eligible to receive services. Medicaid patients are sometimes asked to pay a small amount of the cost of services they receive. This is called a co-payment.

Eligibility and Applying

Each state determines their own eligibility intake processes and benefits. Eligibility guidelines are generally based on income and favor elderly and disabled people, families with dependent children, people in nursing homes who meet financial, resource and medical requirements, foster children, pregnant women and young children who meet financial requirements, people whose Social Security has stopped but federal law makes it possible for them to stay on Medicaid, and people on Medicare who meet financial and resource requirements.

Eligibility requirements are complex as there are many factors to be considered. For example, you may still be eligible for coverage even if your income exceeds the guidelines because of your situation (such as if you are pregnant). Some states provide partial coverage to higher income participants. The best way to determine your eligibility is to contact your state Medicaid official using the list below. You may also contact your local state welfare office, state public health department, or a state social service agency.

State Medicaid Officials
(source: {www.hcfa.gov/medicaid/scontact.htm})

Alabama
Mr. W. Dale Walley, Acting
Commissioner
Alabama Medicaid Agency
501 Dexter Avenue
P.O. Box 5624
Montgomery, AL 36103-5624
334-242-5010
800-362-1504
Fax: 334-242-5097
www.medicaid.state.al.us/

Alaska
Mr. Robert Labbe, Director
Division of Medical Assistance
Department of Health and
Social Services
P.O. Box 110660
Juneau, AK 99811-0660
907-465-3355
Fax: 907-465-2204
www.hss.state.ak.us/dma/
table.htm

American Samoa
Mr. Niuatoa A. Puletasi
State Medicaid Officer
Department of Health
LBJ Tropical Medical Center
Pago Pago, AS 96799
011-684-633-4590
Fax: 011-684-633-1869

Arizona
Ms. Phyllis Beidess, Director

Arizona Health Care Cost
Containment System
(AHCCCS)
801 East Jefferson Street
Phoenix, AZ 85034
602-417-4680
800-654-8713
TDD: 800-826-5140
Fax: 602-252-6536
www.ahcccs.state.az.us/

Arkansas
Mr. Ray Hanley, Director
Division of Medical Services
Department of Human
Services
P.O. Box 1437, Slot 1100
Little Rock, AR 72203-1437
501-682-8292
800-482-8988
TDD: 510-682-6789
Fax: 501-682-1197
www.state.ar.us/dhs

Mr. Mark Hemingway
Assistant Director
Office of Long-Term Care
Division of Medical Services
Department of Human
Services
P.O. Box 8059, Slot 400
Little Rock, AR 72203-8059
501-682-8487
Fax: 501-682-6955
www.state.ar.us/dhs

California

Mr. J. Douglas Porter, Deputy
Director
Medical Care Services
Department of Health Services
714 P. Street, Room 1253
Sacramento, CA 95814
916-654-0391
Fax: 916-657-1156
www.dhs.cahwnet.gov/

Colorado

Mr. Richard Allen, Executive
Director
Department of Health Care
Policy and Financing
1575 Sherman Street
Denver, CO 80203-1714
303-866-2993
800-221-3943
TDD 303-866-3883
Fax: 303-866-4411
www.state.co.us/gov_dir/
chcpf/index.html

Connecticut

Mr. David Parella, Deputy
Commissioner
Department of Social Services
25 Sigourney Street
Hartford, CT 06106-5116
860-424-5110
Fax: 860-424-5114
www.dss.state.ct.us/svcs/
medical.htm

Delaware

Mr. Philip Soulé, Sr., Director
Medical Assistance Program

Department of Health and
Social Services
P.O. Box 906
Lewis Building
1901 North DuPont Highway
New Castle, DE 19720
302-577-4901
800-372-2022
TDD: 800-924-3958
Fax: 302-577-4557
E-mail: PSoule@state.de.us
www.state.de.us/govern/
agencies/dhss/irm/dss/
dsshome.htm

District of Columbia

Mr. Paul Offner
Deputy Director
Medical Assistance
Administration
Department of Health
2100 ML King Jr. Avenue,
S.E., Suite 302
Washington, DC 20020
202-727-0735
Fax: 202-610-3209
www.dchealth.com/offices.htm

Florida

Mr. Gary Crayton
Director of Medicaid
Agency for Health Care
Administration
2727 Mahan Drive
Building 3
Tallahassee, FL 32308
850-922-6463
Fax: 850-488-3560
www.fdhc.state.fl.us/

Georgia

Gary B. Redding, Director
Department of Medical
Assistance
2 Peachtree Street, NW
Suite 4043
Atlanta, GA 30303-3159
404-656-4479
800-282-4536
Fax: 404-657-5238
www.state.ga.us/Departments/
DMA/

Guam

Ms. Ma Theresa Arcangel,
Acting Administrator
Bureau of Health Care
Financing
Department of Public Health
and Social Services
P.O. Box 2816
Agana, GU 96910
671-735-7269
Fax: 671-734-6860

Hawaii

Mr. Chuck C. Duarte,
Administrator
Med-Quest Division
Department of Human
Services
P.O. Box 399
Honolulu, HI 96809-0339
808-692-8056
587-3521 (Oahu)
933-4112 (Hawaii East)
329-3454 (Hawaii West)
243-5780 (Maui)
241-3575 (Kauai)

808-553-3295 (Molokai)
800-894-5755 (Lanai toll-free
calls to Maui)
Fax: 808-692-8173
www.state.hi.us/icsd/dhs/
dhs.html

Idaho

Mr. Joe Brunson,
Administrator
Division of Medicaid
Department of Health and
Welfare
Americana Building
P.O. Box 83720
Boise, ID 83720-0036
208-364-1802
Fax: 208-364-1811
www.state.id.us/dhw/
hwgd_www/home.html

Illinois

Mr. A. George Hovanec,
Administrator
Medical Operations
Department of Public Aid
201 South Grand Avenue, East
Third Floor
Springfield, IL 62763-0001
217-782-2570
Fax: 217-782-5672
www.state.il.us/dpa/

Indiana

Ms. Kathleen D. Gifford,
Assistant Secretary
Medicaid Policy and Planning
Family and Social Services
Administration

Room W382, 402 W.
Washington Street
Indianapolis, IN 46204-2739
317-233-4455
Fax: 317-232-7382
Email: KGifford@FSSA.
STATE.IN.US
www.ai.org/fssa/HTML/
PROGRAMS/2d.html

Iowa
Mr. Donald Herman, Director
Division of Medical Services
Department of Human
Services
Hoover State Office Building
Fifth Floor
Des Moines, IA 50319-0114
515-281-8621
Fax: 515-281-7791
www.dhs.state.ia.us/
HomePages/DHS/medical.htm

Kansas
Mr. Oliver Green,
Commissioner
Adult and Medical Services
Department of Social and
Rehabilitation Services
Docking State Office Building
Room 628 South
915 SW Harrison Street
Topeka, KS 66612
785-296-8904
800-792-4884
TDD: 800-792-4202
Fax: 785-296-4813
www.ink.org/public/srs/
srsservices.html

Kentucky
Mr. Dennis Boyd,
Commissioner
Department for Medicaid
Services
275 East Main Street
Third Floor
Frankfort, KY 40621
502-564-4321
Fax: 502-564-3866
http://cfc-chs.chr.state.ky.us/
medicaid/medimap.htm

Louisiana
Mr. Thomas D. Collins,
Director
Bureau of Health Services
Financing
Department of Health and
Hospitals
P.O. Box 91030
Baton Rouge, LA 70821-9030
504-342-3891
Fax: 504-342-9508
www.dhh.state.la.us/

Maine
Mr. Francis T. Finnegan, Jr.,
Director
Bureau of Medical Services
Department of Human
Services
State House Station 11
Augusta, ME 04333-0011
207-287-2674
Fax: 207-287-2675
www.state.me.us/bms/
bmshome.htm

Maryland

Debbie Chang
Deputy Secretary for Health
Care Financing
Department of Health and
Mental Hygiene
201 West Preston Street
Baltimore, MD 21201
410-767-4664
Fax: 410-333-5185
Email: dchang@dhmh.
md.state.us
www.dhmh.state.md.us/health
choice/

Massachusetts

Mr. Bruce M. Bullen
Commissioner
Division of Medical Assistance
600 Washington Street
Boston, MA 02111
617-210-5690
800-841-2900
Fax: 617-210-5697
www.state.ma.us/dma/

Michigan

Mr. Robert M. Smedes, Chief
Executive Officer
Medical Services
Administration
Dept. of Community Health
400 S. Pine St.
Lansing, MI 48909
517-335-5001
888-858-5929
Fax: 517-335-5007
www.mdch.state.mi.us/
mdch2/index_g.htm

Minnesota

Mary B. Kennedy
Medicaid Director
Assistant Commissioner
Health Care
Minnesota Department of
Human Services
444 Lafayette Road
St. Paul, MN 55155-3852
651-282-9921
800-657-3672
TTY: 800-366-8930
Fax: 651-215-9453
www.dhs.state.mn.us/

Mississippi

Ms. Helen Wetherbee
Executive Director
Division of Medicaid
Office of the Governor
Robert E. Lee Building
239 N. Lamar St., Suite 801
Jackson, MS 39201-1399
601-359-6050
Fax: 601-359-6048
www.dom.state.ms.us/

Missouri

Mr. Gregory A. Vadner
Division of Medical Services
Department of Social Services
615 Howerton Court
P.O. Box 6500
Jefferson City, MO 65102-
6500
573-751-6922
800-348-6627
Fax: 573-751-6564
www.dss.state.mo.us/

Montana

Ms. Nancy Ellery
Administrator
Division of Health Policy and
Services
Department of Public Health
and Human Services
1400 Broadway
Helena, MT 59601
406-444-4141
Fax: 406-444-1861
www.dphhs.mt.gov/

Nebraska

Cec Brady, Acting
Administrator
Medicaid Division
Nebraska Department of
Health and Human Services
301 Centennial Mall South
Fifth Floor
Lincoln, NE 68509-5026
402-471-9506
Fax: 402-471-9092
www.hhs.state.ne.us/med/
medindex.htm

Nevada

Ms. Myla Florence,
Administrator
Nevada State Welfare Division
2527 North Carson Street
Carson City, NV 89710
775-687-4128
Fax: 775-687-5080

Ms. Janice Wright, Acting
Administrator
Division of Health Care
Financing and Policy

1100 E. William St., Suite 119
Carson City, NV 89710
775-687-4176, ext. 251
Fax: 775-684-8792
www.state.nv.us/dhcfp

New Hampshire

Ms. Lee Bezanson
Medicaid Director
Medicaid Administration
Bureau
Department of Health and
Human Services
6 Hazen Drive
Concord, NH 03301-6521
603-271-4912
Fax: 603-271-4376
www.state.nh.us/dhhs/ohm/
ohm_ind.htm

New Jersey

Ms. Margaret A. Murray,
Director
Division of Medical Assistance
and Health Services
Dept. of Human Services
CN-712
7 Quakerbridge Plaza
Trenton, NJ 08625-0712
609-588-2600
800-356-1561
Fax: 609-588-3583
www.state.nj.us/
humanservices/dhshc1.html

New Mexico

Mr. Charles J. Milligan,
Director
Medical Assistance Division

New Mexico Human Services
Department
P.O. Box 2348
Santa Fe, NM 87504-2348
505-827-3100
888-997-2583
888-997-2583
TDD: 800-609-4833
Fax: 505-827-3185
www.state.nm.us/hsd/

New York
Ms. Kathryn Kuhmerker,
Deputy Commissioner
NYS Department of Health
Office of Medicaid
Management
Empire State Plaza
Room 1466, Corning Tower
Building
Albany, NY 12237
518-474-3018
Fax: 518-486-6608
www.health.state.ny.us/
index.htm

North Carolina
Mr. Paul R. Perruzzi, Director
Division of Medical Assistance
Department of Health and
Human Services
1985 Umstead Drive
P.O. Box 29529
Raleigh, NC 27626-0529
919-857-4011
Fax: 919-733-6608
www.state.nc.us/DHR/docs/
divinfo/dma.htm

North Dakota
Mr. David J. Zentner, Director
Division of Medical Assistance
Department of Human
Services
600 East Boulevard Avenue
Bismarck, ND 58505-0261
701-328-3194
800-755-2604
Fax: 701-328-3194
www.health.state.nd.us/
ndhd/default.asp

Northern Mariana Islands
Ms. Helen Sablan, Acting
Medicaid Administrator
Department of Public Health
and Environmental Services
Commonwealth of the
Northern Mariana Islands
P.O. Box 409 CK
Saipan, MP 96950
670-664-4880 or 4882
Fax: 670-234-8931

Ohio
Ms. Barbara Edwards, Deputy
Director
Office of Medicaid
Department of Human
Services
30 E. Broad St., 31st Floor
Columbus, OH 43266-0423
614-644-0140
800-324-8680
Fax: 614-752-3986
E-mail: Medicaid@
dsotol.psoto2
www.ohio.gov/odhs/R11.html

Oklahoma

Mr. Michael Fogarty
State Medicaid Director
Oklahoma Health Care
Authority
4545 North Lincoln
Boulevard, Suite 124
Oklahoma City, OK 73105
405-522-7439
800-522-0310
Fax: 405-530-3470
www.state.ok.us/~ohca/
index.htm

Oregon

Mr. Hersh Crawford,
Administrator
Senior and Disabled Services
Division
Department of Human
Resources
500 Summer Street, NE
2nd Floor
Human Resources Building
Third Floor
Salem, OR 97310-1015
503-945-5772
800-273-0557
Fax: 503-373-7823
www.omap.hr.state.or.us/

Pennsylvania

Ms. Christine M. Bowser
Acting Deputy Secretary
Medical Assistance Programs
Department of Public Welfare
Health and Welfare Building
Room 515
Harrisburg, PA 17120

717-787-1870
800-842-2020
Fax: 717-787-4639
E-mail: cbowser@dpw.
state.pa.us
www.state.pa.us/PA_Exec/
Public_Welfare/overview.html

Puerto Rico

Ms. Margarita Latorre
Medicaid Director
Office of Economic Assistance
to the Medically Indigent
Department of Health
G.P.O. Box 70184
San Juan, PR 00936
809-765-1230
800-981-2737
Fax: 809-250-0990

Rhode Island

Mr. John Young, Associate
Director
Division of Medical Services
Department of Human
Services
600 New London Avenue
Cranston, RI 02920
401-462-3113
800-346-1004
Fax: 401-464-6338
www.state.ri.us/

South Carolina

J. Samuel Griswold, Director
Department of Health and
Human Services
P.O. Box 8206
Columbia, SC 29202-8206

803-898-2500
Fax: 803-253-4137
www.dhhs.state.sc.us/

South Dakota
Mr. David M. Christensen
Program Administrator
Medical Services
Department of Social Services
Richard F. Kneip Building
700 Governors Drive
Pierre, SD 57501-2291
605-773-3495
800-452-7691
Fax: 605-773-4855
www.state.sd.us/state/
executive/social/medicaid/

Tennessee
Mr. Brian Lapps, Sr.
Director of Operations
Department of Finance and
Administration
729 Church Street
Nashville, TN 37247-6501
615-741-0213
Fax: 615-741-0882
www.state.tn.us/commerce/
tncardiv.html

Texas
Ms. Linda K. Wertz
State Medicaid Director
Health and Human Services
Commission
P.O. Box 13247
Austin, TX 78711
512-424-6549
Fax: 512-424-6547

www.hhsc.state.tx.us/
HP1.html

Utah
Mr. Michael Deily, Director
Department of Health
Division of Health Care
Financing
P.O. Box 143101
Salt Lake City, UT 84116-
3101
800-662-9651
Fax: 801-538-6099
http://hlunix.ex.state.ut.us/
medicaid/

Vermont
Mr. Paul Wallace-Brodeur,
Director
Office of Health Access
Department of Social Welfare
103 South Main Street
Waterbury, VT 05671-0201
802-241-3985
Fax: 802-241-2974
www.dsw.state.vt.us/

Virginia
Mr. Dennis G. Smith, Director
Department of Medical
Assistance Services
600 E. Broad St., Suite 1300
Richmond, VA 23219
804-786-8099
800-884-9730
Fax: 804-371-4981
E-mail: DSmith@dmas.
state.va.us
www.state.va.us/~dmas

Virgin Islands
Ms. Priscilla Berry-Quetel,
Director
Bureau of Health Insurance
and Medical Assistance
Department of Health
210-3A Altona
Suite 302 Frostco Center
Charlotte Amalie, VI 00802
809-774-4624
Fax: 809-774-4918

Washington
Mr. Tom Bedell, Acting
Assistant Secretary
Medical Assistance
Administration
P.O. Box 45080
Olympia, WA 98504-5080
360-664-0008
800-562-3022
Fax: 360-902-7855
www.wa.gov/dshs/

West Virginia
Ms. Elizabeth Lawton,
Commissioner
Bureau for Medical Services
Department of Health and
Human Resources
7011 MacCorkle Avenue, SE
Charleston, WV 25304

304-926-1703 (ask for Ms.
Lawton's Secty)
800-688-5810
Fax: 304-926-1818
E-mail: ELawton@
wvdhhr.org
www.wvdhhr.org/bms

Wisconsin
Ms. Peggy Bartels, Director
Division of Health
Department of Health and
Social Services
One West Wilson Street
Room 250
Madison, WI 53701
608-266-2522
Fax: 608-266-1096
www.dhfs.state.wi.us/

Wyoming
Mr. James Shepard,
Administrator
Division of Health Care
Financing
Department of Health
North Building, Room 259B
6101 Yellowstone Road
Cheyenne, WY 82002
307-777-7531
Fax: 307-777-6964
http://wdhfs.state.wy.us/
wdh/medicaid.htm

Dieting, Fitness and Nutrition

Is Your Food Safe?
E-coli, Salmonella, and Listeria Monocytogenes

Fungi, viruses, parasites, and bacteria in foods are
estimated to account for 6.5 to 33 million cases of human
illness and up to 9,000 deaths in the United States each
year.

Since 1992, when E coli contaminated hamburger in a fast-
food restaurant in Washington and made 500 people ill,
consumers seem to be more aware of the potential
problems with food safety. Now the Center for Disease
Control and Prevention estimates as many as 20,000 cases
of E coli infections happen every year. And many people

Free Nutrition Analysis Tool

Allows you to analyze the foods you eat for various
different nutrients. Developed by the Department of
Food Science and Human Nutrition, University of
Illinois, Urbana-Champaign at

{http://spectre.ag.uiuc.edu/~food-lab/nat/}.

even know that the nitrates in your water may cause "blue baby syndrome."

If you need the facts on food safety, contact the government's main information center on the topic: USDA/FDA Foodborne Illness Education Information Center, National Agricultural Library/ USDA, Beltsville, MD 20705; 301-504-5719; Fax: 301-504-6409; {foodborne@nal.usda.gov}.

FREE FOOD AT SCHOOL FOR YOUR KIDS

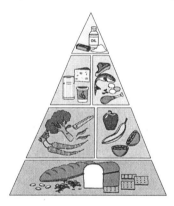

A 1998 Tufts University study states: "Children who participate in the U.S. Department of Agriculture's School Breakfast Program were shown to have significantly higher standardized achievement test scores than eligible non-participants. Children getting school breakfasts also had significantly reduced absence and tardiness rates."

Your child can get a free breakfast at one of the 70,000 participating schools at one income level ($21,385 for family of 4) and at a reduced fee at another level ($30,433 for family of 4). Families who pay full price still get a bargain. Over 6.9 million kids participate and 5.9 million get it for free or at a reduced rate.

Lunch is also available under the U.S. Department of Agriculture's National School Lunch program at 95,000 schools serving 26 million children. The same general requirements apply to both programs.

Ask your school if they participate, or contact your local School Food Service Authority in your school system. If all this fails, contact your state Department of Education listed in the Appendix.

Check out the Food and Nutrition Services web page at {www.fns.usda.gov}.

Rich Kids Pay 2 Cents For Half-Pint of Milk

Milk at this price is available to students, no matter what the family income, at over 8,000 schools, 1,400 summer camps, and 500 non-residential child care institutions. The program is called the U.S. Department of Agriculture's **Special Milk Program** and is available to institutions that do not use the School Breakfast Program or the National School Lunch program.

Ask your school if they participate, or contact your local School Food Service Authority in your school system. If all this fails, contact your state Department of Education listed in the Appendix. If you cannot get satisfaction from these offices, contact your local office of your state or federal elected official.

Work Out With Your Own Personal Trainer

You don't need to spend a fortune having someone coming to your house to motivate you to exercise. The President's Council on Physical Fitness and Sports has several free publications to spark your new exercise program.

Some titles include: Fitness *Fundamentals*, *Exercise and Weight Control*, and *Walking for Exercise and Pleasure*. Each of these titles provides technique guides, motivational tips, and more to get you up and moving.

For these publications and more information contact President's Council on Physical Fitness and Sports, HHH Bldg., Room 738H, 200 Independence Ave., SW, Washington, DC 20201; 202-690-9000; {www.indiana. edu/~preschal}.

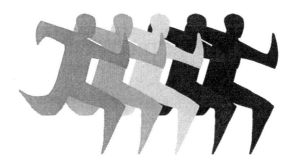

ASK A REGISTERED DIETITIAN!

You can call a Registered Dietitian for customized answers to your food and nutrition questions. Simply call the American Dietetic Association's (ADA). The cost of the call will be $1.95 for the first minute and $.95 for each additional minute.

Contact: American Dietetic Association, 216 West Jackson Boulevard, Chicago, IL 60606; 312-606-6995; 312-899-0040; 900-CALL-AN-RD (900-225-5267)- $1.95 for first minute; {E-mail: hotline@eatright.org}; {www.eatright.org}.

Find a Dietitian!

Nutrition is a key component of a healthy lifestyle. Call the American Dietetic Association's (ADA) award-winning Consumer Nutrition Hot Line for a referral to a Registered Dietitian (RD) in your area and to listen to food and nutrition messages recorded by a Registered Dietitian in English or Spanish from 9:00 a.m. to 4:00 p.m. Central Time, Monday through Friday. You can also e-mail your food and nutrition questions.

Contact: American Dietetic Association, 216 West Jackson Boulevard, Chicago, IL 60606; 312-606-6995; 312-899-0040; 800-366-1655; {E-mail: hotline@eatright.org}; {www.eatright.org}.

Free Women's Exercise Program

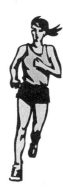

You don't have to join a gym or health club to fit a daily routine of physical activity into your life! The American Heart Association's "Choose To Move" campaign begins with only 10 minutes of moderate physical activity per day in the first two weeks, moves up to 20 minutes per day in the second two weeks, and tops off at 30 minutes per day in the final six weeks. The new 1999 program focuses on both physical activity and nutrition.

Contact: Women's Health Information, American Heart Association, National Center, 7272 Greenville Avenue, Dallas, TX 75231; 888-MY-HEART; {www.women.americanheart.org/}.

Free 10-Minutes-A-Day Fitness Book

The "Take Wellness To Heart" program at the American Heart Association will send you a fitness handbook written in collaboration with the highly respected Cooper Institute of Aerobics Research in Dallas. It contains health and fitness tips, and resource lists showing you how you can start a program with only 10 minutes a day.

Contact: American Heart Association, National Center, 7272 Greenville Avenue, Dallas, TX 75231; 888-MY-HEART; {www.americanheart.org}.

Free Fitness and Training Books From the Experts

The American College of Sports Medicine will send you the following free booklets:

1) *Stay Cool to Perform Your Best*

Addresses the importance of including fluids in your daily exercise routines. Based on ACSM's Position Stand "Exercise and Fluid Replacement," Stay Cool gives tips on the importance of drinking fluids before, during, and after exercise. Stay Cool also gives advice on exactly what fluids you should drink when exercising, focusing on those that include carbohydrates and electrolytes (sodium). Finally, this colorful brochure gives several tips to beat the heat such as exercising in the morning or evening to avoid high temperatures, wearing light-colored, absorbent clothing when exercising in the heat, and cutting back your exercise time period to allow for acclimatization. So, if you're going to do your part by exercising regularly, make sure to do it right by including fluids in your physical activity regimen!

2) *Fitting Fitness In, Even When You're Pressed for Time*

Offers advice on incorporating fitness into a busy day. ACSM guidelines recommend accumulating 30 minutes of physical activity most days of the week. Fitting Fitness In helps you schedule this time into your daily routine with helpful suggestions such as: taking the stairs instead of the elevator, parking farther away from a destination and walking, and eating lunch three or four blocks away versus just one.

3) *Eating Smart, Even When You're Pressed for Time*

Addresses important nutritional needs for the '90s person on the move. For full health benefits, people need to not just exercise, but eat well, too. Tips include: balancing your diet to include fruits and vegetables instead of cookies and candies for your afternoon snack, planning ahead to include valuable carbohydrates and proteins in your meals, and combining exercise and eating habits to establish a well-rounded approach to a healthy lifestyle.

Send a self-addressed stamped envelope to: American College of Sports Medicine, c/o Public Information, P.O. Box 1440, Indianapolis, IN 46206-1440; {www.acsm.org}.

Choosing a Safe and Successful Weight-Loss Program Very Low-Calorie Diets Weight Loss for Life.

Weight-Control Information Network, 1 Win Way, Bethesda, MD 20892; 301-984-7378; 800-WIN-8098; {www.niddk.nih.gov}.

Great Chefs Share Their Healthy Heart Recipes

The Heart Healthy Cooking recipes at the American Medical Association's (AMA) website {www.ama-assn.org} come from chefs in several restaurants of the Lettuce Entertain You Enterprises, Inc, group. These recipes meet the American Heart Association's (AHA) requirements for calories, cholesterol, fat, and sodium. New recipes are posted every 2 weeks. Previously posted recipes will be placed in an Archive file.

The Newstart® Recipes are from the Newstart® Lifestyle Cookbook, developed by the Weimar Institute. These recipes are plant-based, free of all animal products (vegan), and high in fiber, low in fat, and cholesterol-free.

The *Vibrant Life* recipes are taste-tempting vegetarian recipes. *Vibrant Life* is a magazine for healthy living. To find out what is known and what is not known about the connection between nutrition and breast cancer, and to find out how the interaction of diet and exercise in adults affects the risk of breast cancer, read the fact sheet provided by the American Dietetic Association's (ADA) at its website, as part of ADA's Nutrition & Health Campaign for Women.

Contact: American Dietetic Association, 216 West Jackson Boulevard, Chicago, IL 60606-6995; 312-899-0040; 800-366-1655; {www.eatright.org/women'shealth}.

OSTEOPOROSIS AND YOUR DIET

To find out what is known and what is not known about the connection between nutrition and osteoporosis and how nutrition education can be used more reliably in the treatment as well as prevention of osteoporosis, read the fact sheet provided by the American Dietetic Association's (ADA) at its web site, as part of ADA's Nutrition & Health Campaign for Women.

For further information and additional free resources contact the ADA. Contact: American Dietetic Association, 216 West Jackson Boulevard, Chicago, IL 60606-6995; 312-899-0040; {www.eatright.org/womenshealth/ osteoporosis.html}.

Free Nutritional Quiz

Take the online "Rate Your Plate" nutritional quiz from the American Dietetic Association and find out how you can make your diet a healthier one. Contact American Dietetic Association 216 W. Jackson Blvd., Chicago, IL 60606-6995; 312-899-0040; 800-366-1655; {E-mail: hotline@eatright. org}; {www.eatright.org/ nuresources.html} (Rate Your Plate).

Watching Your Weight Can Help Prevent Breast Cancer

To raise awareness of the link between weight and breast cancer, the National Alliance of Breast Cancer Organizations (NABCO) and Weight Watchers International teamed up and developed the educational brochure called, *Take Charge of Your Breast Health...Here's How.* Free copies are available from National Alliance of Breast Cancer Organizations (NABCO), 9 East 37th Street, 10th Floor, New York, NY 10016; 888-80-NABCO; {www.nabco.org}; {E-mail: NABCOinfo@aol.com}.

The Fountain of Food

One of the Food and Drug Administration's (FDA) missions is to protect the safety and wholesomeness of food. They regulate what's termed fresh, what's low fat, and more. They test samples of food to see if any substances, such as pesticide residues, are present in unacceptable amounts. If contaminants are identified, FDA takes corrective action. FDA also sets labeling standards to help consumers know what is in the foods they buy.

Information is available (for free) on a wide variety of topics including, but not limited to: calcium and other special needs of women, cellulite removal gimmicks, eating disorders, fad diets and diet books, fast food and nutrition, food preparation, nutrition labels, organic foods, saccharin, salt, vitamins. Contact: Information Office of Consumer Affairs, Food and Drug Administration, 5600 Fishers Lane, Rockville, MD 20857; 800-532-4440, 301-827-4420; or online at {http://www.fda.gov}.

The Road to Good Health

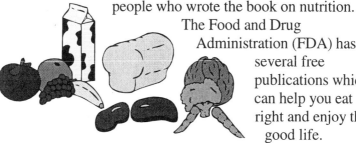

Starts with a good diet. One day you're told to eat carbohydrates, the next day it's fruit. Get the facts from the people who wrote the book on nutrition. The Food and Drug Administration (FDA) has several free publications which can help you eat right and enjoy the good life.

★ *Women and Nutrition: A Menu of Special Needs*
★ *A Consumer Guide to Fats*
★ *Fiber: Something Healthy To Chew On*
★ *Dietary Guidelines For Americans*
★ *Olestra and Other Food Substitutes*

For these and other publications on food, contact: Food and Drug Administration, Division of Consumer Affairs, HFE-88, 5600 Fishers Lane, Rockville, MD 20857; 800-532-4440, 301-827-4420; or online at {http://www.fda.gov}.

Free Mammograms, Cervical and Breast Cancer Treatment

An estimated 2 million American women have been diagnosed with breast or cervical cancer in the 1990s, and half a million will lose their lives from these diseases. Screening could have prevented up to 30% of these deaths for women over 40.

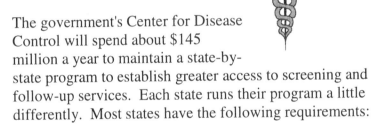

The government's Center for Disease Control will spend about $145 million a year to maintain a state-by-state program to establish greater access to screening and follow-up services. Each state runs their program a little differently. Most states have the following requirements:

→ women starting at 40 or 50 years old,
→ are underinsured or have no insurance
→ have income below a certain level (usually $32,000 or $40,000 for family of 4)

Some states can adjust eligibility requirements for special cases. States vary in the array of services covered but they normally include:

→ breast and cervical cancer screening
→ mammograms
→ treatment if diagnosed with cancer
→ breast reconstruction or prosthesis

States that don't have direct funds for treatment often make arrangements with other facilities to provide treatment for free. If your screening has been done elsewhere, you can still receive free treatment under this program. Men

Breast Cancer Facts

* In 1998, there were 178,00 new cases of breast cancer in women and 1,600 new cases in men.

* In 1998, 43,500 women died from breast cancer, and 400 men died of breast cancer. 97% of women diagnosed with cancer have survived 5 years, in 1940 it was only 72%.

* 67% of women diagnosed with breast cancer survive 10 years.

* 57% of women diagnosed with breast cancer survive 15 years.

* By age 40 one in 217 women are diagnosed with breast cancer.

* By age 70 one in 14 women are diagnosed with breast cancer.

Source: American Cancer Society {www.cancer.org},
U.S. Dept of Health and Human Services Press Office
{www.hhs.gov/news/1998pres/981125.html}.

diagnosed with breast cancer can also receive free
treatment.

Contact your county office of public health listed in your
telephone book or your state Department of Health listed in
the Appendix. You can also contact the main office of this
program at Division of Cancer Prevention and Control,
National Center for Chronic Disease Prevention and Health
Promotion, Center for Disease Control and Prevention,
4770 Buford Highway, NE, MS K-64, Atlanta, GA 30341,
770-488-4751; {www.cdc.gov/nccdphp/dcpc/nbccedp/
index.htm}; or see listing on page 431.

HOW NOT TO FORGET YOUR NEXT BREAST EXAM

Sign up online with the National
Alliance of Breast Cancer
Organizations' (NABCO) E-
mail Reminder, and in 10
months from your last clinical
breast exam or mammogram, they
will send you an e-mail reminder
to schedule your next exam.

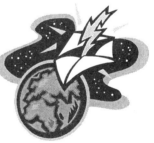

Contact: National Alliance of Breast Cancer Organizations
(NABCO), 9 East 37th Street, 10th floor, New York, NY
10016; 888-80-NABCO; {www.nabco.org}; {E-mail:
NABCOinfo@aol.com}.

Do You Have Your Own Breast Health Program?

No matter what your age, you need to have your breast health program of regular check-ups. A good program includes:

♦ Regular screening mammograms (breast x-rays) each year starting at age 40,

♦ Having your breasts checked by a doctor or nurse every year starting at age 20, and

♦ Checking your breasts yourself every month. Learn what feels normal for you, and if you feel a change, see a doctor or nurse.

Free information, assistance, and referral on your breast cancer questions are available at National Alliance of Breast Cancer Organizations (NABCO), 9 East 37th Street, 10th floor, New York, NY 10016; 888-80-NABCO; {www.nabco.org}; {E-mail: NABCOinfo@aol.com}.

Breast Cancer and Sexuality

A new pamphlet called *Breast Cancer and Sexuality* is now available free of charge from Cancer Care, Inc. The pamphlet covers information on a woman's normal sexual response, sex and menopause, how breast cancer treatment affects a woman's sexuality, ways to cope with difficulties in sexuality and intimacy, communicating with your partner, issues for single women and where to go for more help.

Contact: Cancer Care, Inc., 1180 Avenue of the Americas, 2nd Floor, New York, NY 10036; 212-221-3300; 800-813-HOPE (800-813-4673); {www.cancercareinc.org}; {E-mail: info@cancercare.org}.

Free Breast Prostheses, Bras, Wigs and Beauty Tips for Cancer Patients

Cancer Care, Inc offers free breast prostheses and/or bras available for women who have had a mastectomy. Also, assistance in selecting and fitting and practical tips on prosthesis care. Other services include:

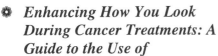

* ***Enhancing How You Look During Cancer Treatments: A Guide to the Use of Cosmetics***. A licensed cosmetician brings the newest make-up techniques and tips to help enhance your well-being.
* ***Facial on the Go***. A beauty consultant will provide glamour tips with highlights designed for maturing

skin, eyeglass wearers, women of color, day into evening looks and beauty techniques during cancer treatment.

⚫ *All You Want to Know About Wigs*. Free wig and fitting or help re-styling a wig you already have. A stylist will be on hand to assist.

For a location near you, contact: Cancer Care, Inc., 1180 Avenue of the Americas, 2nd Floor, New York, NY 10036; 212-221-3300; 800-813-HOPE (800-813-4673); {www.cancercareinc.org}; {E-mail: info@cancercare.org}.

HOW TO GET A LOW COST MAMMOGRAM

Excluding skin cancer, breast cancer is the most common cancer among American women. A mammogram, though not perfect, is the best way to detect breast cancer in its earliest, most treatable stage — an average of 1.7 years before the woman can feel the lump. Regular mammograms — not just one — find breast cancer at its earliest, most treatable stage and should be included among the healthy lifestyle choices of women in their forties or older.

A mammogram is an x-ray of the breast made with special equipment that can find a breast cancer even when it is too small to be felt. Using a low-radiation machine, the breast is gently squeezed between two plates to get a good picture.

This takes only a few seconds and should not cause pain. The resulting x-rays are examined by a radiologist who is trained to look for abnormalities in breast tissue.

A screening mammogram at most facilities costs between $50 and $150. However, most states now have laws requiring health insurance to cover all or part of the cost of screening mammograms. Medicare will pay for a mammogram every year. Since coverage varies by state, you are encouraged to call Medicare for details on coverage for mammograms at 800-638-6833.

Even if you do not have health insurance, you still have a lot of options for obtaining a low-cost mammogram. Many mammography facilities are willing to work out a lower fee or payment schedule that will make the test more affordable. Explain your financial situation and ask the facility if they are willing to discuss these options with you. Many mammography facilities offer special fees and extended hours in October in observance of National Breast Cancer Awareness Month. You are urged to call as early as

1 Out Of 4 Women Who Show Breast Cancer Don't Have It

A study published in the April 16, 1998 issue of The New England Journal of Medicine suggests that almost 25% of women will have a false-positive result at some point in 10 years of clinical breast exams.
{www.cancer.org/ bottomjoining.html}

September to reserve an appointment. There are many non-profit and public agencies that can assist you in locating a low-cost service provider. Please refer to the lists below.

Breast Cancer Resources

The following national organizations can refer you to a low-cost breast cancer screening service provider in your specific area. They can also answer your questions and offer information about all aspects of breast cancer.

✔ The **American Cancer Society** has chapters throughout the nation. They also host a comprehensive online information source called the Breast Cancer Network. For more information, contact your local American Cancer Society, (number and address in your phone book); or American Cancer Society, 1599 Clifton Rd., NE, Atlanta, GA 30329; 800-ACS-2345 (national); {www.cancer.org/}; {www2.cancer.org/bcn/index.html}.

✔ The **National Alliance of Breast Cancer Organizations**, (NABCO), provides information on all aspects of breast health. Their web site includes breast cancer news, information on clinical trails, a list of resources, a list of support groups, and more. For more information, contact National Alliance of Breast Cancer Organizations, 9 East 37th Street, 10th Floor, New York, NY 10016; 888-80NABCO (806-2226); {E-mail: NABCOinfo@aol.com}; {www.nabco.org/}

✔ The **US Government**: The FDA regulates the quality of all mammograms. A low-cost mammogram must meet the same requirements as any other mammogram. Order the free booklet *Things to Know About Quality Mammograms* in English or Spanish from the US Government's Agency for Health Care Policy and Research, P.O. Box 8547, Silver Spring, MD 20907; 800-358-9295; {www.ahcpr.gov).

✔ The **National Cancer Institute** (NCI) is the Federal Government's principal agency for cancer research and training. They can refer you to FDA-certified, accredited mammography facilities in your area as well as offer you the latest, most accurate cancer information. Through a network of 19 regional offices located throughout the country, the CIS serves the entire United States. For more information, contact Office of Communication, Public Inquiry Section, National Cancer Institute, Bldg. 31, Rm. 10A16, 9000 Rockville Pike, Bethesda, MD 20892; 800-4-CANCER (422-6237); {www.fda.gov/cdrh/faclist.html}; {www.nci.nih.gov/}.

• **Y-ME National Breast Cancer Organization** has a commitment to provide information and support to anyone who has been touched by breast cancer. Their services include a 24-hour national hotline, referrals, support meetings, public education seminars, wig and prosthesis bank and a teen program introducing high school senior girls to breast health awareness. Their web site includes breast health information, breast self-examination guidelines, a Kid's Corner, newsletters, ordering information for publications, "Ask Y- ME," a unique opportunity to have questions answered quickly and confidentially, and links to many other resources. Most of the information is also available in Spanish. For more information, contact Y-ME National Breast Cancer Organization, Inc., 212 W. Van Buren Street, Chicago, IL 60607-3908; 312-986-8338 (office); Fax: 312-294-8597; National Hotline: 800-221-2141; Spanish Hotline: 800-986-9505; {www.y-me.org/}

YWCA

The YWCA's ENCOREplus® is a community-based program that targets underserved women in need of early detection education and breast and cervical cancer screening and support services. It also provides women under treatment and recovering from breast cancer with a unique, combined peer group support and exercise program. Components of the program include community outreach and breast health education, referral to breast and cervical screening, and an on-going information resource service. This is a growing national program.

To find a participating YWCA facility near you, refer to the list below, call 1-800-95EPLUS, or your local YWCA. For more information, contact Myrna Candreia, Director, Office of Women's Health Initiatives, YWCA of the U.S.A., 624 Ninth Street, N.W. Third Floor, Washington, DC 20001-5303; 202-628-3636; 800-95EPLUS (953-7587); Fax: 202-783-7123; {E-mail: mcandreia@ ywca.org}; {www.ywca.org/mission/health_care.html}.

ONLINE RESOURCES

Avon's Breast Cancer Awareness Crusade is the largest corporate supporter of breast health programs in America. Its mission is to provide more women, through grants to qualified non-profit and university- based programs, direct access to breast cancer education and early

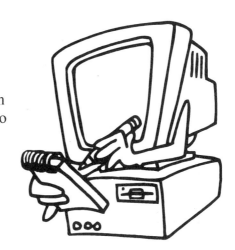

detection screening services, at little or no cost. Their web site includes a resource center with information about breast cancer, including a list of support groups by state, a glossary of breast cancer terms, the definition of a mammogram and guidelines for when and where to obtain one, and ten frequently asked questions about breast cancer. Contact Avon's Breast Cancer Awareness Crusade at {www.avoncrusade.com/}.

BreastCancer.Network is an online listing of current breast cancer Internet sites and breaking news and medical developments. Contact BreastCancer.Network at {www.breastcancer.net/ bcn.html}.

Breast Cancer Information Clearinghouse is a web server maintained by the New York State Education and Research Network. Its purpose is to provide information for breast cancer patients and their families. Contact Breast Cancer Information Clearinghouse at {www.acor.org/}.

The mission of the **National Action Plan on Breast Cancer** (NAPBC) is to speed progress toward eradicating breast cancer. A critical national health priority is to reduce suffering and death from breast cancer in the United States and internationally. Their website features up-to-date information about breast cancer, reports and recommendations, products you can use to educate yourself about breast cancer, links to dozens of breast cancer-related sites and organizations including listservs, late-breaking information regarding ongoing clinical trials for breast cancer, and a frequently asked question list about breast cancer. Contact National Action Plan on Breast Cancer at {www.napbc.org}.

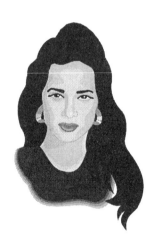

The **National Breast Cancer Coalition** (NBCC) is a grassroots advocacy organization dedicated to fighting breast cancer. NBCC was formed in 1991 with one mission: to eradicate breast cancer through action and advocacy. Their website has information on becoming an advocate for change, outreach and educational activities, legislative priorities, and how NBCC-trained advocates have helped change the world of breast cancer research. Contact National Breast Cancer Coalition at {www.natlbcc.org/}.

State and Regional Contacts for Low-Cost Mammograms

Alabama
Viki L. Brant, MPA
Director, Cancer Branch
Alabama Department of Public
Health
Bureau of Health Promotion
and Information
201 Monroe Street
Suite 900
P.O. Box 303017
Montgomery, AL 36130-3017
334-206-5535
Fax: 334-206-5534
www.alapubhealth.org/inform/
frames4.htm

Alaska
Jeanne Roche, RN, MPH, CTR
Program Director
Barbara Berner, ANP, EdD
Program Coordinator
Alaska Breast and Cervical
Cancer Program
Department of Health and
Social Services
Division of Public Health
Epidemiology Office
3601 C Street
Suite 540
P.O. Box 240249
Anchorage, AK 99524-0249
907-269-8000
Fax: 907-561-1896
www.epi.hss.state.ak.us/
programs/chronic/cancer.htm

YWCA of Anchorage
ENCOREplus Program
P.O. Box 102059
245 West 5th Avenue
Anchorage, AK 99510-2059
907-274-1572

American Samoa
Diana Tuimei
Program Director
Department of Health
American Samoa Government
Pago Pago, AS 96799
011-684-633-4606
Fax: 011-684-633-5379

Arizona
Joan Smith, BSN, MBA
Program Director
Adult Program Operations
Administrator
Arizona Department of Health
Services
1400 West Washington
Suite 330
Phoenix, AZ 85007
602-542-7534
Fax: 602-542-7520
www.hs.state.az.us/

YWCA of Tuscon
ENCOREplus Program
738 N. Fifth Ave., Suite 110
Tucson, AZ 85705-8400
520-884-7810

Arkansas
Lynda Lehing, BSN, MBA
Program Director
Breast and Cervical Cancer
Control Program
Arkansas Department of
Health
4815 West Markham Street
Slot #11
Little Rock, AR 72205
501-661-2231
Fax: 501-661-2009
http://health.state.ar.us/

YWCA of Greater Little Rock
ENCOREplus Program
1200 South Cleveland Street
Little Rock, AR 72204
501-663-8406

California
Jacquolyn Duerr
Program Director
Medical Advisor
California Chronic Disease and
Injury Control
Cancer Detection Services
601 North Seventh Street
MS-662
P.O. Box 942732
Sacramento, CA 94234-7320
916-323-4790
Fax: 916-445-1890
www.dhs.cahwnet.gov/org/ps/
cdic/cdicindex.htm

YWCA of Contra Costa
County
ENCOREplus Program

1320 Arnold Drive, Suite 170
Martinez, CA 94553-6537
925-372-4213

YWCA of Glendale
ENCOREplus Program
735 East Lexington Drive
Glendale, CA 91206-3797
818-242-4155

YWCA of the Harbor Area
ENCOREplus Program
437 West 9th Street
San Pedro, CA 90731-3281
310-547-0831

YWCA of Greater Los
Angeles
3345 Wilshire Boulevard
Suite 300
Los Angeles, CA 90010-0814
213-365-2991

YWCA of North Orange
County
ENCOREplus Program
1514 East Katella Avenue
Anaheim, CA 92805
714-935-9720

YWCA of Sacramento
ENCOREplus Program
1122 17th Street
Sacramento, CA 95814-4079
916-264-8080

Colorado
Sharon Michael, Director
Cancer Control Program

Colorado Department of Public
Health and Environment
Cancer Prevention
Building A, Fifth Floor
4300 Cherry Creek Dr., South
Denver, CO 80246-1530
303-692-2505
Fax: 303-782-0095
E-mail: smichael@smtpgate.
dphe.state.co.us
www.state.co.us/gov_dir/
cdphe_dir/pp/ccphom.html

Connecticut
Christine Parker, MPH
Program Director
Connecticut Department of
Public Health
Cancer Early Detection
Program
410 Capitol Avenue
MS# 11HLS
Hartford, CT 06134-0308
860-509-7804
Fax: 860-509-7854
www.state.ct.us/dph/

Delaware
Debra Lightsey, MSW
Director
Delaware Breast and Cervical
Cancer Early Detection Project
Delaware's Division of Public
Health
Delaware Department of
Health and Social Services
Blue Hen Corporate Center
655 Bay Road, Suite 4H
Dover, DE 19901

302-739-4651
Fax: 302-739-2352
www.state.de.us/govern/
agencies/dhss/irm/dph/
dphhome.htm

District of Columbia
Barbara Baldwin
Program Coordinator
Breast and Cervical Cancer
Prevention
PHSA/Department of Health
800 Ninth St., SW, Third Floor
Washington, DC 20024
202-645-5573
www.dchealth.com/

Florida
Margo C. Blake
Program Director
Florida Department of Health
HSFHG
1317 Winewood Boulevard
Building 5, Room 404
Tallahassee, FL 32399-0700
850-414-5638
Fax: 850-922-9321
www.doh.state.fl.us/

YWCA of Greater Miami &
Dade County
ENCOREplus Program
351 NW Fifth Street
Miami, FL 33128-1615
305-377-9922

Georgia
Carol B. Steiner, RN, MN
Program Director

24569128792030

Cancer Control Section
Division of Public Health
Georgia Department of Human
Resources
2 Peachtree Street, NE
Sixth Floor Annex
Atlanta, GA 30303
404-657-6606
Fax: 404-657-4338
E-mail: cbs0600@ph.dhr.
state.ga.us
www.ph.dhr.state.ga.us/
org/cancercontrolsection.
screening.htm

YWCA of Greater Atlanta
ENCOREplus Program
957 North Highland Avenue
Atlanta, GA 30309
404-892-3476

YWCA of Macon
ENCOREplus Program
775 Second Avenue
Macon, GA 31201-8392
912-743-5468

Hawaii
Doug Kreider
Hawaii Breast and Cervical
Cancer Control Program
Hawaii Department of Health
838 South Beretania Street
Room 205
Honolulu, HI 96813-2498
808-587-3900
Fax: 808-587-3911
www.hawaii.gov/doh/resource/
Cancer/index.html

Idaho
Minnie Inzer
Idaho's Women's Health Check
Breast and Cervical Cancer
Early Detection Program
Idaho Department of Public
Health
450 West State Street
First Floor, Suite 1
P.O. Box 83720
Boise, ID 83720-5450
208-332-7311
Fax: 208-334-6573
www.bhp-whc.state.id.us/

Illinois
Doris Garrett
Program Director
Office of Women's Health
Illinois Dept. of Public Health
535 West Jefferson Street
Springfield, IL 62761
217-524-3300
Fax: 217-782-1235
www.idph.state.il.us/about/
owhservices.htm

YWCA of Metropolitan
Chicago
ENCOREplus Program
320 West 202nd Street
Chicago Heights, IL 60411
708-754-0486

YWCA of Freeport
ENCOREplus Program
641 West Stephenson Street
Freeport, IL 61032-5093
815-235-9421

YWCA of Lake & McHenry
Counties
ENCOREplus Program
2133 Belvidere Road
Waukegan, IL 60085-6153
847-662-4247

YWCA of Peoria
ENCOREplus Program
301 NE Jefferson
Peoria, IL 61602-1293
309-674-1167

Indiana
Dena L. Watts
Program Director
Breast and Cervical Cancer
Early Detection Program
Indiana State Department of
Health
2 N. Meridian St., Sixth Floor
Indianapolis, IN 46204-1964
317-233-7901
Fax: 317-233-7127
E-mail: dwatts@gwnet.isd.
state.in.us
www.state.in.us/isdh/

YWCA of Greater Lafayette
ENCOREplus Program
605 North Sixth Street
Lafayette, IN 47901-1022
765-742-0075

Iowa
Gloria Vermie, RN
Program Coordinator
Division of Substance Abuse
and Health Promotion

Iowa Dept. of Public Health
Lucas State Office Building
321 East 12th Street
Des Moines, IA 50319-0075
515-281-4909
Fax: 515-242-6384
www.idph.state.ia.us/sa/
hprom/bcc.htm

Kansas
Julia Francisco, Director
Office of Chronic Disease and
Health Promotion
Department of Health and
Environment
Landon State Office Building
900 SW Jackson, Room 901N
Topeka, KS 66612-1290
913-296-8126
Fax: 913-296-8059
www.kdhe.state.ks.us/

Kentucky
Greg Lawther
Program Director
Paula Alexander, RN, MS
Program Coordinator
Nurse Consultant
Department for Public Health
Commonwealth of Kentucky
275 East Main Street
Frankfort, KY 40621-0001
502-564-7996
Fax: 502-564-4553
cfc-chs.chr.state.ky.us/ph.htm

Louisiana
Lynn Buggage
Program Director

Chronic Disease Control
Section
Office of Public Health
Louisiana Department of
Health and Hospitals
234 Loyola Avenue
P.O. Box 60630
New Orleans, LA 70112
504-599-1095
Fax: 504-599-1085
www.dhh.state.la.us./OPH/
chrondis/default.htm

YWCA of Northern Louisiana
ENCOREplus Program
710 Travis
Shreveport, LA 71101-2999
318-222-2116

YWCA of Greater Baton
Rouge
250 S. Foster Dr., 2nd Floor
Baton Rouge, LA 70806
225-926-3820

Maine
Barbara A. Leonard, MPH
Program Director
Maine Breast and Cervical
Health Program
Maine Department of Human
Services
11 State House Station
151 Capitol Street
Augusta, ME 04333-0011
207-287-5387
Fax: 207-287-8944
E-mail: barbara.a.leonard@
state.me.us

www.state.me.us/dhs/hpe/bcp/
homepage.htm

Maryland
Donna Gugel
Program Manager
Division of Cancer Control
Office of Chronic Disease
Prevention
Maryland Department of
Health and Mental Hygiene
Maryland Breast and Cervical
Cancer Program
Community and Public Health
Administration
201 West Preston Street
Room 304, Third Floor
Baltimore, MD 21201
410-767-5281
Fax: 410-333-7279
mdpublichealth.org/ocd/cctrl/
html/b_csprog.html

Massachusetts
Dorothy Tucker, Director
Women's Health Unit
Massachusetts Department of
Public Health
Women's Health, Fourth Floor
250 Washington Street
Boston, MA 02108-4619
617-624-5454
Fax: 617-624-5075
www.state.ma.us/dph/
bccan.htm

YWCA of Boston
ENCOREplus Program
140 Clarendon Street

Boston MA 02116-5193
617-351-7600

YWCA of Central
Massachusetts
ENCOREplus Program
1 Salem Square
Worcester, MA 01608-2090
508-791-3181

YWCA of Greater Lawrence
ENCOREplus Program
38 Lawrence Street
Lawrence, MA 01840-1493
978-687-0331

YWCA of Maiden
ENCOREplus Program
54 Washington Street
Maiden, MA 02148-8298
781-322-3760

YWCA of Newburyport
ENCOREplus Program
13 Market Street
Newburyport, MA 01950-2584
978-465-0981

YWCA of Southern
Massachusetts
ENCOREplus Program
20 South Sixth Street
New Bedford, MA 02740-
5912
508-990-3010

Michigan
Carol Callaghan, MPH
Program Director

Chief, Cancer Section
CHP/CDP
Michigan Department of
Community Health
Community Public Health
Agency
3423 North Logan/Martin
Luther King, Jr. Boulevard
Lansing, MI 48909
517-335-8379
Fax: 517-335-9397
E-mail: callaghanc@
state.mi.us
www.mdmh.state.mi.us/

YWCA of Grand Rapids
ENCOREplus Program
25 Sheldon Boulevard, SE
Grand Rapids, MI 49503-4295
616-459-4681

YWCA of Western Wayne
County
ENCOREplus Program
26279 Michigan Avenue
Inkster, MI 48141-2480
313-561-4110

Minnesota
Shelly D. Heck
Program Coordinator
Assistant Chief
Cancer Control Section
Minnesota Department of
Health
717 Delaware Street, SE
Minneapolis, MN 55440-9441
612-623-5500
Fax: 612-623-5520

www.health.state.mn.us/
divs/dpc/dpc.html

YWCA of Duluth
ENCOREplus Program
202 West Second Street
Duluth, MN 55802-1918
218-722-7425

YWCA of Minneapolis
ENCOREplus Program
1130 Nicollet Mall
Minneapolis, MN 55403-2475
612-332-0501

Mississippi
Alan Penman
Program Coordinator
Women's Health
Mississippi State Department
of Health
2423 North State Street
Jackson, MS 39215-1700
601-960-7725
Fax: 601-354-6061
www.msdh.state.ms.us/
OSHO/GENERAL/
Msdhorg.htm#ochs

Missouri
Marianne Ronan, MPA
Program Director
Chief, Missouri Breast and
Cervical Cancer Control
Program
Bureau of Cancer Control
Division of Chronic Disease
Prevention and Health
Promotion

Missouri Department of Health
101 Park Deville Dr., Suite A
Columbia, MO 65203
573-876-3233
Fax: 573-446-8777
www.health.state.mo.us/
StatePrograms/SP_BCa.html

YWCA of St. Joseph
ENCOREplus Program
304 North Eighth Street
St. Joseph, MO 64501-1988
816-232-4481

Montana
Richard Paulsen
Program Director
Cancer Control Program
Health Policy and Services
Division
Montana Department of Public
Health and Human Services
Cogswell Building
1400 Broadway
Helena, MT 59620
406-444-3624
Fax: 406-444-1861
www.dphhs.state.mt.us/hpsd/

Nebraska
Debra T. Hartmann
Program Manager
Chronic Disease Division
Nebraska Department of
Health
301 Centennial Mall South
Third Floor
Lincoln, NE 68509-5007
402-471-0370

Fax: 402-471-6446
E-mail: dhoffma@hhs.
state.ne.us
www.hhs.state.ne.us/hew/
ewm.htm

YWCA of Adams County
ENCOREplus Program
604 North St. Joseph
Hastings, NE 68901-7500
402-462-8080

Nevada
Pamela S. Graham, BS, RN
Nevada Department of Human
Resources
Breast and Cervical Cancer
Control and Prevention
Program
Capitol Complex
410 East John Street, No. 3
Carson City, NV 89710-4761
702-687-4800
Fax: 702-687-1688
www.state.nv.us/health/
bdcis/bdcis.htm

YWCA of Reno-Sparks
ENCOREplus Program
1301 Valley Road
Reno, NV 89512-2296
702-322-4531

New Hampshire
Margaret Murphy
Program Director and Program
Coordinator
Office of Chronic Disease and
Health Data

Breast and Cervical Cancer
Early Detection Program
New Hampshire Division of
Public Health Services
6 Hazen Drive
Concord, NH 03301-6527
603-271-4886
Fax: 603-271-3745
www.dhhs.state.nh.us/

New Jersey
Doreleena Sammons-Posey
Program Coordinator
Breast and Cervical Cancer
Control Initiative
Division of Family Health
Services
New Jersey State Department
of Health and Senior Services
50 East State Street
Sixth Floor, Capital Plaza
P.O. Box 364
Trenton, NJ 08625-0364
609-292-8540
Fax: 609-292-3580
www.state.nj.us/health/fhs/
broch4.htm

YWCA of Bergen County
ENCOREplus Program
75 Essex Street
Hackensack, NJ 07601
201-487-2224

YWCA of Camden & Vicinity
ENCOREplus Program
565 Stevens Street
Camden, NJ 08103
609-963-7614

YWCA of Montclair-North
Essex
ENCOREplus Program
159 Glenridge Avenue
Montclair, NJ 07402-3692
973-746-5400

New Mexico
Barbara Hickok
Project Director
New Mexico Dept. of Health
Public Health Division
2329 Wisconsin St., NE
Suite A
Albuquerque, NM 87110
505-827-2380
Fax: 505-841-8333
www.health.state.nm.us/

YWCA of Albuquerque
ENCOREplus Program
7201 Paseo del Norte, NE
Albuquerque, NM 87113-1750
505-822-9922

New York
David C. Momrow, Director
Bureau of Chronic Disease
Prevention and Adult Health
Corning Tower, Room 584
New York State Department of
Health
Empire State Plaza
Albany, NY 12237-0620
518-474-0512
Fax: 518-473-0642
www.health.state.ny.us/
nysdoh/consumer/cancer/
about.htm

YWCA of Binghamton &
Broome County
ENCOREplus Program
80 Hawley Street
Binghamton, NY 13901-3805
607-772-0340

YWCA of Brooklyn
ENCOREplus Program
30 Third Avenue, 11th Floor
Brooklyn, NY 11217-1897
718-875-1601

YWCA of Elmira and the
Twin Tiers
ENCOREplus Program
211 Lake Street
Elmira, NY 14901-3193
607-733-5575

YWCA of Mowhawk Valley
ENCOREplus Program
1000 Cornelia Street
Utica, NY 13502-4684
315-732-2159

YWCA of Orange County
ENCOREplus Program
565 Union Avenue
New Windsor, NY 12553-
6140
914-561-8050

YWCA of Schenectady
ENCOREplus Program
44 Washington Avenue
Schenectady, NY 12305-1799
518-374-3394

YWCA of Western New York
ENCOREplus Program
190 Franklin Street
Buffalo, NY 14202-2462
716-852-6120

YWCA of White Plains &
Central Westchester
ENCOREplus Program
515 North Street
White Plains, NY 10605-3096
914-949-6227

North Carolina
Larry K. Jenkins, MPH
Acting Program Director
Breast and Cervical Cancer
Control Program
Division of Community Health
P.O. Box 29605
Raleigh, NC 27626-0605
919-715-0123
Fax: 919-733-0488
www.dhhs.state.nc.us/docs/
divinfo/dch.htm

YWCA of Asheville
ENCOREplus Program
185 South French Broad
Avenue
Asheville, NC 28801-3954
828-254-7206

YWCA of High Point
ENCOREplus Program
112 Gatewood Avenue
High Point, NC 27260
336-882-4126

YWCA of Wake County
ENCOREplus Program
554 East Hargett Street
Raleigh, NC 27601
919-834-7386

North Dakota
Danielle Kenneweg
Program Director
Cancer Prevention and Control
North Dakota Department of
Health
600 East Boulevard Avenue
Bismarck, ND 58505-0200
701-328-4514
Fax: 701-328-1412
E-mail: dkennewe@pioneer.
state.nd.us
www.health.state.nd.us/ndhd/

Northern Mariana Islands
Dr. Isamu J. Abraham
Secretary of Health
Commonwealth Health Center
Department of Public Health
Service
P.O. Box 409 CK
Saipan, MP 96950
670-234-8950
Fax: 670-234-8930
www.mtccnmi.com/
community/CHCSaipan/
index.htm

Ohio
Lois Hall, MS
Program Coordinator
Bureau of Health Promotion
and Risk Reduction

Ohio Department of Health
246 North High Street
Columbus, OH 43266-0588
614-752-2464
Fax: 614-644-7740
www.odh.state.oh.us/

YWCA of Cincinnati
ENCOREplus Program
898 Walnut Street
Cincinnati, OH 45202-2088
513-241-7090

YWCA of Cleveland
ENCOREplus Program
3101 Euclid Avenue, Suite 711
Cleveland, OH 44115-2573
216-881-6878

YWCA of Columbus
ENCOREplus Program
65 South Fourth Street
Columbus, OH 43215-4383
614-224-9121

YWCA of Lorain
ENCOREplus Program
200 Ninth Street
Lorain, OH 44052-1997
440-244-1919

YWCA of Summit County
ENCOREplus Program
670 West Exchange Street
Akron, OH 44302
330-253-6131

YWCA of Toledo
ENCOREplus Program

1018 Jefferson Avenue
Toledo, OH 43624-1924
419-241-3235

YWCA of Youngstown
ENCOREplus Program
25 West Rayen Avenue
Youngstown, OH 44503-1091
330-746-6361

Oklahoma
Adeline Yerkes, RN, MPH
Program Director
Chief, Chronic Disease Service
Oklahoma Dept. of Health
1000 Northeast Tenth Street
Oklahoma City, OK 73117-
1299
405-271-4072, ext. 57123
Fax: 405-271-5181
www.health.state.ok.us/
PROGRAM/cds/charge.html

Oregon
Jane Moore, PhD, RD
Project Director
Health Promotion and Chronic
Disease Prevention
Oregon Health Division
800 NE Oregon St., No. 730
Portland, OR 97232
503-731-4025
Fax: 503-731-4082
www.ohd.hr.state.or.us/cdpe/
hpcdp/docs/bcc.htm

YWCA of Greater Portland
ENCOREplus Program
1111 SW 10th Avenue

Portland, OR 97205-2496
503-294-7400

YWCA of Salem
ENCOREplus Program
768 State Street
Salem, OR 97301-3884
503-581-9922

Palau, Republic of
Yorah Demei
Ministry of Health
Republic of Palau
P.O. Box 6027
Koror, PW 96940
011-680-488-2552
Fax: 011-680-488-1211

Pennsylvania
Diane Hergenrather
Program Director
Pennsylvania Healthy Women
50+
Pennsylvania Dept. of Health
Cancer Control Program
Health and Welfare Building
Commonwealth and Forster
Street, Room 1011
Harrisburg, PA 17120
717-787-5251
Fax: 717-772-0608
www.health.state.pa.us/PHP/
HW/default.htm

YWCA of Carlisle
ENCOREplus Program
301 G Street
Carlisle, PA 17013-1389
717-243-3818

YWCA of McKeesport
ENCOREplus Program
410 Ninth Avenue
McKeesport, PA 15132-4001
412-664-7146

YWCA of Greater Pittsburgh
ENCOREplus Program
305 Wood Street
Pittsburgh, PA 15222-1982
412-365-1915

Puerto Rico
Mariwilda Padilla Diaz
Program Administrator
Cancer Prevention and
Detection Program
Commonwealth of Puerto Rico
Department of Health
P.O. Box 9342
San Juan, PR 00908
787-274-7860
Fax: 787-274-7863

Rhode Island
Mary Ann Miller, MS, RN
Program Director
Rhode Island Women's Cancer
Program
Rhode Island Dept. of Health
Cannon Building, Room 103
Three Capitol Hill
Providence, RI 02828
401-222-1171, ext.135
Fax: 401-222-4415
www.health.state.ri.us/

YWCA of Greater Rhode
Island

ENCOREplus Program
1035 Branch Avenue
Providence, RI 02904
401-831-9922

YWCA of Northern Rhode
Island
ENCOREplus Program
514 Blackstone Street
Woonsocket, RI 02895-1891
401-769-7450

South Carolina
Brenda C. Nickerson, RN,
MSN, Director
Division of Cancer Prevention
and Control
South Carolina Department of
Health and Environmental
Control
Center for Health Promotion
Mills Jarrett Building
2600 Bull Street
Columbia, SC 29201
803-737-3934
Fax: 803-253-4001
E-mail: nickerbc@columb61.
dhec.state.sc.us
www.state.sc.us/dhec/

YWCA of Greenville
ENCOREplus Program
700 Augusta Street
Greenville, SC 29605-3899
864-467-3700

South Dakota
Norma Schmidt, MA
Program Director

Breast and Cervical Cancer
Program
Division of Health, Medical,
and Laboratory Services
445 East Capitol Avenue
Pierre, SD 57501-3185
605-773-5728
Fax: 605-773-5509
www.state.sd.us/doh/
Disease2/cancer.htm

Tennessee
Barbara Lynn, RN
Program Director
Breast and Cervical Cancer
Prevention and Control
Community Health Services
Section
Tennessee Department of
Health
Cordell Hull Building
426 Fifth Avenue, North
Sixth Floor
Nashville, TN 37247-5210
615-532-8480
Fax: 615-532-8478
www.state.tn.us/health/
links.html

YWCA of Memphis
ENCOREplus Program
7553 Old Poplar Pike
Germantown, TN 38138
901-754-4356

Texas
Margaret C. Mendez, MPA
Director, Breast and Cervical
Cancer Control Program

Texas Department of Health
Bureau of Chronic Disease
Prevention and Control
1100 West 49th Street
General Building, Room G407
Austin, TX 78756-3199
512-458-7644
Fax: 512-458-7650
E-mail: margaret.mendez@
tdh.state.tx.us
www.tdh.state.tx.us/bcccp/

YWCA of Abilene
ENCOREplus Program
1350 North Tenth Street
Abilene, TX 79601-4195
915-677-5321

YWCA of Metropolitan Dallas
ENCOREplus Program
4621 Ross Avenue
Dallas, TX 75204-4997
214-821-9595

YWCA of Houston
ENCOREplus Program
3621 Willia
Houston, TX 77007-7427
713-868-9922

YWCA of Lubbock
ENCOREplus Program
3101 35th Street
Lubbock, TX 79413-2399
806-792-2723

YWCA of San Antonio &
Bexar County
ENCOREplus Program

405 N. Saint Mary's Street
Suite 500
San Antonio, TX 78205
210-228-9922

Utah
Catherine Hoelscher
Program Coordinator
Breast Cancer Awareness
Utah Cancer Control Program
Utah Department of Health
P.O. Box 142868
Salt Lake City, UT 84114-2868
800-717-1811
801-538-7049
Fax: 801-538-9495
http://hlunix.hl.state.ut.us/cfhs/
chronic/cancer/index.html

Vermont
Jean Ewing, MS
Program Director
Cancer Control Chief
Vermont Department of
Health, Epidemiology
Third Floor, 108 Cherry Street
P.O. Box 70-05402
Burlington, VT 05401
802-863-7331
Fax: 802-865-7701
www.state.vt.us/health/
hvcancer.htm

Virginia
Elizabeth McGarvey, EdD
Program Director
Breast and Cervical Cancer
Early Detection Program

Division of Women's and
Infant's Health
Virginia Department of Health
1500 East Main Street
Suite 106
P.O. Box 2448
Richmond, VA 23218
804-924-1868
Fax: 804-371-6032
www.vdh.state.va.us/fhs/
women/breast/breast.htm

Virgin Islands
Darlene Carty Petty, Director
Breast and Cervical Cancer
Early Detection Program
Knud Hansen Health Complex
Old Municipal Hospital
Building F
St. Thomas, VI 00802
340-774-9000, ext. 4643
Fax: 340-776-720

Washington
Veronica Foster
Program Manager
Breast and Cervical Health
Program
Washington State Department
of Health
New Market Industrial
Campus, Building 10
P.O. Box 47835
Olympia, WA 98504-7835
360-236-3695
Fax: 360-664-2619
E-mail: vif1303@doh.wa.gov
www.fhcrc.org/cipr/bchp/

YWCA of Seattle, King, &
Snohomish Counties
ENCOREplus Program
1118 Fifth Avenue
Seattle, WA 98101-3012
206-461-4888

YWCA of Spokane
ENCOREplus Program
829 West Broadway Avenue
Spokane, WA 99201
509-248-7796

YWCA of Yakima
ENCOREplus Program
15 North Naches Avenue
Yakima, WA 98901-2795
509-248-7796

West Virginia
Nancye Bazzle, MPH
Program Director
Office of Maternal and Child
Health
Breast and Cervical Cancer
Screening Program
West Virginia Department of
Health and Human Resources
1411 Virginia Street
East Charleston, WV 25301-
3013
304-558-5388
Fax: 304-558-2183
www.hsc.wvu.edu/radrx/
bccsp.htm

YWCA of Charleston
ENCOREplus Program
1114 Quarrier Street

Charleston, WV 25301-2495
304-340-3550

YWCA of Wheeling
ENCOREplus Program
1100 Chapline Street
Wheeling, WV 26003-2999
304-232-0511

Wisconsin
Gale D. Johnson
Program Manager
Bureau of Public Health
Wisconsin Department of
Health and Social Services
1414 East Washington
Avenue, Room 96
Madison, WI 53703-3044
608-261-6872
Fax: 608-266-8925
www.dhfs.state.wi.us/

YWCA of Green Bay-DePere
ENCOREplus Program
230 South Madison Street

Green Bay, WI 54301-4592
920-432-5581

YWCA of Waukesha
ENCOREplus Program
306 North West Avenue
Waukesha, WI 53186-4534
414-547-1872

Wyoming
Judith Kluever
Program Manager
Breast and Cervical Cancer
Program
Division of Preventive
Medicine
Wyoming Dept. of Health
Hathaway Building, Room 482
Cheyenne, WY 82002
307-777-6006
Fax: 307-777-5402
E-mail: jkluev@missc.
state.wy.us
http://wdhfs.state.wy.us/
WDH/Programs.htm

Special Help For Cancer Patients

Editor's Note: Information on and resources for cancers of women's reproductive organs are found in the chapter on mammograms.

The National Cancer Institute

Many people view the government's ability to address real

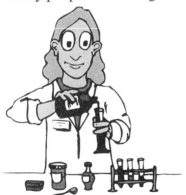

people's real problems with a great deal of skepticism, but when it comes to cancer, the National Cancer Institute (NCI) is the center of the hub for cancer research and information.

The NCI coordinates the government's cancer research program. It is the largest of the 17 biomedical research institutes and centers at the National Institutes of Health. In addition to the institute's research activities, the NCI provides vast amounts of easily accessible, up-to-date information on cancer for patients and their caregivers.

The NCI offers several means of accessing their vast informational resources. For persons with access to the

Internet, the "Information for People with Cancer" site is the most direct. (Go to {www.nci.nih.gov}, select "Information for Patients, the Public and the Mass Media," then click on "Patients.") Follow the links in the following categories to pull up specific information:

❑ **Cancer Sites and Types** connects you to comprehensive information about your specific cancer diagnosis and treatment options.

❑ **Challenges During Treatment** provides you with information about challenges faced when undergoing treatment, including tips and resources for managing side effects and eating well during treatment.

❑ **Clinical Trials** is your comprehensive resource center for clinical trials information.

❑ **Living with Cancer** includes information on the challenges of living with cancer, as well as resources for cancer survivors. Find useful materials and information for managing emotional and practical aspects of cancer.

❑ **Science Behind the News** is a series of self-teaching modules, consisting of text and graphics, designed to explain the complex scientific concepts involved in cancer research and seen in today's news.

❑ **History Behind the Research** includes information on the history of NCI and of cancer research.

❑ **Cancer Information Service** provides information about the Cancer Information Service, the NCI's nationwide information and education service.

❑ **Publication Index** has full-text illustrated publications for patients, the public and health professionals.

❑ **Cancer Facts Index** includes fact sheets on cancer-related topics, cross-listed by subject.

❑ **Communication Internships** provides information about six-month paid internships available to graduate students in the areas of health communications and science writing.

❑ **Glossary** provides a comprehensive list of definitions of cancer-related terms.

The NCI's CancerNet site {http://cancernet.nic.nih.gov} links to the same information.

800-4-CANCER

If you prefer to do your research by phone, you can call the NCI's toll-free hotline 800-4-CANCER (800-422-6237), where an information specialist will answer questions about prevention, treatment, symptoms and risks, diagnosis and research studies, as well as provide NCI materials and referrals to cancer-related services such as treatment centers, pain clinics, mammography facilities, or other cancer organizations.

NCI Public Inquiries Office
Building 31, Room 10A03
31 Center Drive, MSC 2580
Bethesda, MD 20892-2580
301-435-3848
Cancer Information Service: 800-4-CANCER
(800-422-6237); {www.nci.nih.gov}
CancerNet: {http://cancernet.nci.nih.gov}

FREE COUNSELING AND EMOTIONAL SUPPORT WHEN YOU HAVE CANCER

Cancer Care has more than 45 professional oncology social workers on staff, who can speak to you in a private consultation, work with you in a support group, or talk with you over the phone. They can provide emotional support, assist you in coping with treatment and treatment side effects, help you understand and talk to your doctor, nurse or other health care provider, and guide you to resources that can make you better able to focus on your health. All the services of Cancer Care Inc. are free of charge to the public.

Contact: Cancer Care, Inc, 1180 Avenue of the Americas, 2nd Floor, New York, NY 10036; 212-221-3300; 800-813-HOPE, (800-813-4673) - Cancer Care Support Line; {E-mail: info@cancercare.org}; {www.cancercareinc.org}.

FREE CANCER CARE TELEPHONE Educational Program

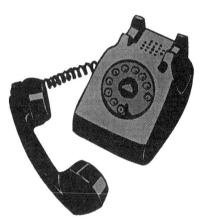

Are you unable to visit a Cancer Care office, but would like to take part in Cancer Care's educational programs? Throughout the year, Cancer Care offers a number of telephone educational programs (or 'teleconferences', as they are called) for people with cancer, their families and their friends. These teleconference seminars are completely free (you will not be charged for the call).

A Sample Teleconference Seminar Topic is Relaxation Techniques and Visualization Exercises to Cope with the Stress of Cancer. You will learn relaxation techniques to counter the discomforts of cancer. Exercises led by a leading expert include focused breathing, muscle relaxation, and visualization. All the services of Cancer Care Inc. are free of charge to the public.

Contact Cancer Care, Inc., 1180 Avenue of the Americas, 2nd Floor, New York, NY 10036; 212-221-3300; Cancer Care Counseling Line 800-813-HOPE (800-813-4673); {E-mail: info@cancercare.org}; {www.cancercareinc.org}.

Free Hotels For Cancer Patients

For patients who must travel far from home to receive cancer treatment, lodging assistance is sometimes available. In some areas, patients may stay at a Hope Lodge, the American Cancer Society's home away from home for patients and an accompanying family member. The American Cancer Society offers patients, their families, their caregivers, and the community the full range of emotional and practical help from the time of diagnosis throughout one's life to life's end. In 1996, almost one million cancer patients were helped through the programs of the American Cancer Society.

How To Prevent, Stop and Treat Melanoma

Although melanoma accounts for only about 5 percent of all skin cancer cases, it is the leading cause of all skin cancer-related deaths. A free booklet describes how to reduce your risk, how to spot melanoma, and options for treatment.

Contact: The Cancer Research Institute, 681 Fifth Avenue, New York, NY 10022, 800-99 CANCER; 800-992-2623; {www.cancerresearch.org}; {E-mail: cancerres@ aol.com}.

Contact: American Cancer Society, 1599 Clifton Rd., NE, Atlanta, GA 30329; 800-ACS-2345; {www.cancer.org}.

Man to Man:
Prostate Cancer Support Group

Man to Man is a group program offered by the American Cancer Society that provides information about prostate cancer and related issues to men and their partners in a supportive atmosphere. Some areas offer a group program for the partners of men with prostate cancer and a visitation program in which a trained prostate cancer survivor provides support to a man newly diagnosed with prostate cancer. Contact: American Cancer Society, 1599 Clifton Rd., NE, Atlanta, GA 30329; 800-ACS-2345; {www.cancer.org}.

Control Your Pain So It
Doesn't Control You

The fear of becoming addicted to pain medication is just one of many 'myths' explained in a new free booklet from Cancer Care, *Control Your Pain So It Doesn't Control You.* It provides a general explanation of pain medication categories, general tips on controlling side effects of pain medication, suggestions for reducing pain without the use of drugs, and a detailed explanation of the issues of addiction.

Contact: Cancer Care, Inc., 1180 Avenue of the Americas, 2nd Floor, New York, NY 10036; 212-221-3300; 800-813-

HOPE (800-813-4673); {www. cancercareinc.org};
{E-mail: info@cancercare.org}.

One-On-One Support For Melanoma Patients

Malignant melanoma accounts for only 5 percent of
reported skin cancer cases, but it causes over 75 percent of
skin cancer-related deaths. Over the past two decades, the
incidence of malignant melanoma in Caucasians increased
at a faster rate than that of any other cancer, with the
number of cases doubling.

Crossing Bridges is a program that provides patients with
support, help to better communicate with caregivers, and
skills to handle side effects more effectively. You get a
buddy, a coach, a newsletter, and a
one-on-one counselor to help
you through the therapy
process.

Crossing Bridges

Contact the Crossing Bridges
Hotline at 888-77BRIDGE (772-7434). The program is run
by Cancer Care, Inc., 1180 Avenue of the Americas, 2nd
Floor, New York, NY 10036; 212-221-3300; 800-813-
HOPE (800-813-4673); {www.cancercareinc.org}; {E-
mail: info@cancercare.org}.

One Page Briefs On Lung Cancer

The topic titles are:

- ♦ What is Lung Cancer?
- ♦ What Are the Symptoms of Lung Cancer and How Is It Diagnosed?
- ♦ What are the Different "Stages" of Lung Cancer and What is the Recommended Treatment?
- ♦ Your Lung Cancer Health Team: Your Doctor Is Only the Beginning
- ♦ "Doctor, Can We Talk?" Tips for Communicating With Your Doctor, Nurse of Health Care Team If You Have Lung Cancer
- ♦ Lung Cancer and Clinical Trials: How Do I Decide if a Clinical Trial Is Right for Me?

The Briefs are available free from: Cancer Care, Inc., 1180 Avenue of the Americas, 2nd Floor, New York, NY 10036; 212-221-3300; 800-813-HOPE (800-813-4673); {www.cancercareinc.org}; {E-mail: info@cancercare.org}.

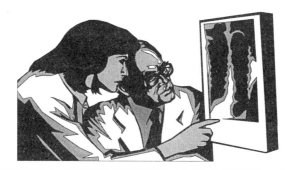

Free Resource Directory for Cancer Patients

A Helping Hand: The Resource Directory for People with Cancer. Recently updated by Cancer Care, this 144-page book, which comes to you free of charge, is the first nation-wide directory of free services and resources for people with cancer and their families. All of the major listings in the book have 'icons' that tell the reader at a glance the type of services each provides. In addition, all listings are indexed alphabetically, by service, by cancer site, and by e-mail and "800" number.

Contact: Cancer Care, Inc., 1180 Avenue of the Americas, 2nd Floor, New York, NY 10036; 212-221-3300; 800-813-HOPE (800-813-4673); {www.cancercareinc.org}; {E-mail: info@cancercare.org}.

Learning About Pancreatic Cancer

A new booklet for people with pancreatic cancer is now available free of charge from Cancer Care, Inc. Called *Learning About Pancreatic Cancer: It Helps to Understand*, this 60-page publication has extensive information on pancreatic cancer symptoms, stages, recommended treatments and treatment side effects, tips on managing cancer pain, how to assess clinical trials, how to eat well during treatment, and how to get help and support.

Contact Cancer Care, Inc., 1180 Avenue of the Americas, 2nd Floor, New York, NY 10036; 212-221-3300; 800-813-HOPE (800-813-4673); {www.cancercareinc.org}; {E-mail: info@cancercare.org}.

Free Workshops On Cancer Diagnosis & Treatments

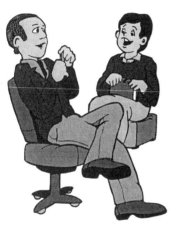

Cancer Care Inc. provides Free Patient and Family Education Program workshops, clinics, and seminars for people with cancer, their families, and caregivers on the following topics:

- ***It Doesn't Have to Hurt: Coping with the Discomforts of Cancer***. In this workshop experts will discuss the major causes of pain, myths about pain medication, and practical strategies to get pain relief.

- ***Understanding Your Treatment***. This workshop offers to help people with cancer, their families, and friends understand state-of-the-art treatment, scheduling, and dosing for chemotherapy and radiation. Information about managing the side effects of treatment will also be discussed.

- *What's New in Oncology Treatment*. In this workshop you will get the most up-to-date information on new cancer treatments for a variety of types of cancers.

- *What You Can Do About Fatigue and Treatment Side Effects*. This workshop focuses on fatigue as a side effect of chemotherapy and radiation treatments, and offers suggestions for you and your doctor and/or health care team, as well as caregivers, on how to lessen its effect.

- *Mouth Care During Cancer and Cancer Treatment: Maintaining Optimum Oral Hygiene*. Your expert presenter in this workshop will provide state-of-the-art information on how to care for and prevent oral health problems during cancer treatment.

- *Acupuncture for Pain Control*. No cancer patient should have to deal with overwhelming pain. In this workshop acupuncture will be demonstrated and explained as an effective pain control technique.

- *"Can We Talk?": Communicating with Your Health Care Team*. In this workshop experts will discuss with you what questions to ask, the importance of advocating for yourself, and practical tips for successful communication with your health care team.

- *Research, Because Lives Depend on It: Clinical Trials Could Improve the Quality of Care You Receive*. In this workshop experts will define clinical trials and research studies, review issues to consider in thinking about clinical trials, and discuss how to get information about them.

- *Coping with Grief: A Journey in Time* is a free workshop offered by Cancer Care, Inc., providing people who are living with loss information and practical tips helpful in coping with bereavement.

A schedule of the workshops is available on their webpage. For more information, contact Cancer Care, Inc., 1180 Avenue of the Americas, 2nd Floor, New York, NY 10036; 212-221-3300; 800-813-HOPE (800-813-4673); {www.cancercareinc.org}; {E-mail: info@cancercare.org}.

HOW TO COPE WITH CANCER IN THE WORKPLACE

Cancer Care offers the following free workshops:

★ *The Challenge of Cancer in the Workplace: How to Communicate with Your Employer*. The presenter of this workshop discusses the Americans with Disabilities Act (ADA), and the Family and Medical Leave Act; "reasonable accommodation" in the workplace; talking with your employer; and the Employee Retirement Income Security Act (ERISA).

★ *Your First Impression: Putting Your Best Foot Forward*. A business fashion designer and consultant will show you how to enhance your physical

appearance for work following cancer treatment or
illness.

A schedule of the workshops is available on their webpage.
For more information, contact: Cancer Care, Inc., 1180
Avenue of the Americas, 2nd Floor, New York, NY
10036; 212-221-3300; 800-813-HOPE (800-813-4673);
{www.cancercareinc.org}; {E-mail: info@cancercare.org}.

How To Use the Internet To Find Resources and Treatment Information for Cancer

This Cancer Care workshop
introduces cancer patients
to the Internet and the
World Wide Web and
shows you how to find
the information you
need, use medical and
health libraries, send
e-mail, and locate newsgroups.
No Internet experience necessary. A schedule of the
workshops is available on their webpage.

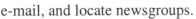
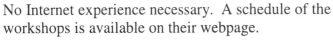

For more information, contact: Cancer Care, Inc., 1180
Avenue of the Americas, 2nd Floor, New York, NY
10036; 212-221-3300; 800-813-HOPE (800-813-4673);
{www.cancercareinc.org}; {E-mail: info@cancercare.org}.

How To Take Care of Yourself With Cancer

Cancer Care offers the following free workshops:

✦ *All You Want to Know About Nutrition*. This workshop discusses eating difficulties during or after cancer treatment and offers suggestions to help you eat well.

✦ *Healthy Eating for Cancer Patients and Family Members*. Learn the latest nutritional information to help enhance the quality of one's life before, during, and after a diagnosis of cancer. This workshop will offer a general overview of a nutritious diet for cancer recovery and prevention, as well as dietary approaches to coping with side effects from treatment.

✦ *How to Stay Safe in the Sun While Enjoying the Outdoors*. This workshop reviews myths and facts about sun exposure and teach techniques for protection when outdoors.

✦ *Breast Health Awareness*. These sessions are designed to educate women about breast cancer and the importance of early detection and treatment.

✦ *Helping Men Become Active Participants in Their Own Health Care.* This workshop explores how gender roles affect men's approach to physical and mental health, and assists men in communicating with their doctors and health care team. (Men and women welcome.)

✦ ***Men's Health Issues: What You Need to Know About Prostate Cancer.*** This workshop will focus on the importance of annual exams and explains new therapies that can effectively treat and often cure this disease.

✦ ***Using Relaxation Techniques to Cope with the Stress of Cancer.*** In this workshop you will learn relaxation techniques to counter the discomforts of cancer and demonstrates exercises including focused breathing, muscle relaxation, and visualization.

✦ ***Healing Circle.*** The presenter in this workshop will conduct a Healing Circle incorporating meditation, sharing, support, and energy healing. This session is designed for people who have cancer and, if space permits, their family members.

✦ ***A Helping Hand, A Healing Word: Drawing on the Resources of Judaism to Cope with Cancer.*** At this workshop patients and families will learn how they can find comfort and strength in the prayers, beliefs, and practices of Judaism. The session is open to people of all backgrounds.

✦ ***Story Telling Through Photography.*** This workshop will help you focus on: 1) how to look at a photograph and how a photograph tells a story, and 2) the art of photography in coping with cancer. Practical tips on taking photos will be reviewed, including an introduction to the various techniques of photography. Participants are encouraged to bring in photos to discuss with the group.

✦ *A Retreat on Humor Therapy: For People Living with Cancer and Their Caregivers*. (In Recognition of National Humor Month). The retreat leaders will show you how to relieve stress, develop a humor perspective, exercise through humorobics, and enhance your health. If you are feeling burned out, in need of a good laugh, and want to increase your energy, this retreat is for you.

✦ *A Laugh a Day Keeps the Stress Away*. This workshop will help people learn to use humor as a stress reducer and health enhancer.

✦ *Fitness Exercises for People Living with Cancer and Their Caregivers*. This workshop will help you decipher your roadblocks to fitness, find fitness incentives and set a plan that works for you. There will be demonstrations of basic exercise tips, including aerobics, strength training, and stretching. Participants will be invited to take part in a mini exercise session. Comfortable clothing is suggested.

✦ *Healthy All Over*. Exercise is not only healthy but it is also psychologically therapeutic. Women with breast cancer still have the ability to exercise. In this workshop a fitness trainer, will demonstrate simple exercises for breast cancer patients. Dress comfortably.

✦ *"Let's Talk About It": Helping Children Cope When a Parent Has Cancer* is a free workshop for parents with cancer, their partners, and their children (ages 6-12). Provided by Cancer Care, Inc., this workshop helps families learn to cope with and communicate more effectively about cancer. Discussions include children's need for information and emotional support. Parents and children meet together and separately.

A schedule of the workshops is available on their webpage. For more information, contact: Cancer Care, Inc., 1180 Avenue of the Americas, 2nd Floor, New York, NY 10036; 212-221-3300; 800-813-HOPE (800-813-4673); {www.cancercareinc.org}; {E-mail: info@cancercare.org}.

Learn About the Genetics of Cancer and Genetic Testing!

"Genetics and Cancer" is a free workshop offered by Cancer Care, Inc., which discusses the concept of the genetics of cancer, heritable and non-heritable genetic aspects of cancer, the characteristics of a heritable cancer, and genetic testing. A schedule of the workshops is available on their webpage.

For more information, contact: Cancer Care, Inc., 1180 Avenue of the Americas, 2nd Floor, New York, NY 10036; 212-221-3300; 800-813-HOPE (800-813-4673); {www.cancercareinc.org}; {E-mail: info@cancercare.org}.

FREE BABY SITTING AND TRANSPORTATION FOR FAMILIES WITH CANCER

The Candlelighters Childhood Cancer Foundation is an international, nonprofit organization. CCCF provides free babysitting and transportation services to and from treatments.

For free information and support for families of children with cancer, contact The Candlelighters Childhood Cancer Foundation, 7910 Woodmount Ave, Suite 460, Bethesda, MD 20814-3015; 800-366-2232; 301-657-8401; Fax: 301-718-2686; {www.candlelighters.org}.

How to Help the Underserved With Health Care

This book has listed thousands of resources and services to try to offer something for everyone. But we want to make sure we have covered all the bases. Here in this chapter are the main offices for many different government programs, which all provide services across the country. You can contact these offices to find resources near you. We have also 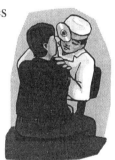 included the headquarters for the three major social service organizations. You are never alone in your battle, but it may take a little digging to find the help you need.

Government Resources
Bureau of Primary Health Care

Over 43 million people in the United States lack access to primary health care. The Bureau of Primary Health Care (BPHC) assures that underserved and vulnerable people get the health care they need.

BPHC is one of four Bureaus of the Health Resources and Services Administration (HRSA), an agency in the

Department of Health and Human Services. Working in partnership with the states, the BPHC funds community health centers that provide free or low-cost quality care for seven different categories of underserved populations. These include: those who have economic, geographic, or cultural barriers which limit their access to primary health care; migrant workers; homeless persons; homeless children: public housing residents; those who suffer from black lung disease; and at-risk school-aged children. Each is described in more detail below.

To receive an updated list of BPHC-supported health care centers in your vicinity, you can write directly to the BPHC, but calls are not recommended. You can also access a searchable online database of Bureau supported programs through their website. Contact Bureau of Primary Health Care, Division of Community and Migrant Health, 4350 East-West Highway, 7th Floor, Bethesda, MD 20814; 301-594-4300; Fax: 301-594-4497; {www.bphc.hrsa.gov}.

Bureau of Primary Health Care Programs and Services

Community Health Center Program
The Community Health Centers (CHCs) provide family-oriented primary and preventive health care services for people living in rural and urban medically underserved communities. CHCs exist in areas where economic, geographic, or cultural barriers limit access to primary health care for a substantial portion of the population; and

they tailor services to the needs of the community. Their
services include providing: primary and preventive care,
outreach, and dental care; links to welfare, Medicaid,
substance abuse treatment, WIC, and related services; other
essential ancillary services such as laboratory tests, X-ray,
environmental health, and pharmacy services as well as
related services such as health education, transportation,
translation, and prenatal services. For more information,
contact Division of Community and Migrant Health,
Bureau of Primary Health Care, 4350 East-West Highway,
7th Floor, Bethesda, MD 20814; 301-594-4300; Fax: 301-
594-4497; {www.bphc.hrsa.gov}.

Migrant Health Center Program
Migrant Health Centers (MHC) and Migrant Health
Program (MHP) provide migrant and seasonal
farmworkers and their families access to comprehensive
medical care services with a culturally sensitive focus.
Migrant farmworkers have some of this nation's most
severe health and social problems and are at greater risk
than the general population because of poverty,
malnutrition, infectious diseases, exposure to pesticides,
and poor housing. MHC and MHP services may include
primary care, preventive health care, transportation,
outreach, dental, pharmaceutical, and environmental health.
These programs use lay outreach workers, bilingual,
bicultural health personnel, and culturally appropriate
protocols often developed by the Migrant Clinicians
Network. They also provide prevention-oriented and
pediatric at MHCs, such as immunizations, well baby care,
and developmental screenings. For more information,

contact Migrant Health Program, Division of Community and Migrant Health, Bureau of Primary Health Care, 4350 East-West Highway, 7th Floor, Bethesda, MD 20814; 301-594-4303; Fax: 301-594-4997; {www.bphc.hrsa.gov}.

Health Care for the Homeless Program

The program emphasizes a multi-disciplinary approach to delivering care to homeless persons, combining aggressive street outreach with integrated systems of primary care, mental health and substance abuse services, case management, and client advocacy. Particular emphasis is placed on coordinating efforts with other community health providers and social service agencies. Grantees recognize the complex needs of homeless people and strive to provide a coordinated, comprehensive approach to the care they provide their homeless clients, and in such a way that welcomes them as patients. Specifically, programs provide primary care and substance abuse services at locations accessible to homeless people; provide around-the-clock access to emergency health services; refer homeless persons for necessary hospital services; refer homeless persons for needed mental health services unless these services are provided directly; provide outreach services to inform homeless individuals of the availability of services; and aid homeless individuals in establishing eligibility for housing assistance and services under entitlement programs. For additional information, contact Health Care for the Homeless Program, Division of Programs for Special Populations, Bureau of Primary Health Care, 4350 East-West Highway, 9th Floor, Bethesda, MD 20814; 301-594-4430; Fax: 301-594-2470; {www.bphc.hrsa.gov}.

Outreach And Primary Health Services For Homeless Children

The Homeless Children's Program supports innovative programs for the delivery of outreach, health services, and referral for homeless children and children at imminent risk of homelessness. The needs of homeless children and at-risk children are addressed through prevention, assessment of primary care needs, and provision of comprehensive primary care services. The Homeless Children's Program serves homeless children and their families by providing, or arranging for, services to address their health and social service needs. Programs must provide the following services, either directly or through contract: conduct outreach activities to identify homeless children and children at risk of homelessness and inform parents and guardians of the availability of health care and other support services; provide comprehensive primary health care services, (including diagnostic laboratory and radiology, as well as preventive health, dental and pharmaceuticals) in a variety of settings, including clinics and mobile medical units; establish referrals to organizations which provide other health, social, and educational services, such as hospitals, community and migrant health centers, Head Start and other educational programs, and programs that prevent and treat child abuse. For additional information, contact Homeless Children Program Coordinator, Health Care for the Homeless Branch, Division of Programs for Special Populations, Bureau of Primary Health Care, 4350 East-West Highway, 9th Floor, Bethesda, MD 20814; 301-594-4430; Fax: 301-594-2470; {www.bphc.hrsa.gov}.

Public Housing Primary Care Program

The mission of the Public Housing Primary Care (PHPC) Program is to provide residents of public housing with increased access to comprehensive primary health care services through the direct provision of health promotion and disease prevention activities and primary health care services. Services are provided on the premises of public housing developments, or at least other locations immediately accessible to residents of public housing. To improve the health status of public housing residents, the PHPC Program supports health centers and other health delivery systems in providing services in the partnership with other community-based providers. PHPC grantees carry out the following major activities: provide primary health care services, including health screening, health counseling, health education, preventive dental, prenatal and perinatal, preventive health, diagnostic and laboratory, patient case management services, and immunizations against disease; aid residents to establish eligibility for assistance under entitlement programs and to obtain government support for health, mental health, or social services; refer residents, as appropriate, to qualified facilities and practitioners for other necessary services, including substance abuse and mental health services train and employ residents of public housing to provide health screenings and health education services; conduct outreach services to inform residents about health services availability; emphasize HIV services for pregnant women and their infants, and violence prevention services. For additional information, contact Public Housing Primary Care Program, Division of Programs for Special Populations, Bureau of Primary Health Care, 4350 East-West Highway, 9th Floor, Bethesda, MD 20814; 301-594-4430; Fax: 301-594-2470; {www.bphc.hrsa.gov}.

Black Lung Clinics Program

The Black Lung Clinics Program provides funding to 36 clinics, which provide diagnosis, treatment, and rehabilitation of active and retired coal miners with respiratory and pulmonary impairments. These clinics also provide educational programs to help respiratory disease patients and their families cope with their disease, improve their breathing and endurance, and improve the quality of their life. In addition to treatment of Black Lung disease and directly related conditions,

Black Lung Clinics

coverage includes prescription drugs, office visits, hospitalizations, and with specific approval, durable medical equipment, outpatient pulmonary rehabilitation therapy, and home nursing visits. For further information, contact Black Lung Clinics Program, Division of Programs for Special Populations, Bureau of Primary Health Care, 4350 East-West Highway, 9th Floor, Bethesda, MD 20814; 301-594-4461; Fax: 301-594-2470; {www.bphc.hrsa.gov}.

Healthy Schools, Healthy Communities Program
The Healthy Schools, Healthy Communities Program provides comprehensive primary care and preventive health care services including ancillary and enabling services. These services are culturally sensitive, appropriate, family-oriented and tailored to meet the specific needs of the community and youth served. For more information contact School Health Services, Division of Programs for Special Populations, Bureau of Primary Health Care, 4350 East-West Highway, 9th Floor, Bethesda, MD 20814; 301-594-4450; Fax: 301-594-2470; {www.bphc.hrsa.gov}.

Locate Outstanding Health Care Programs

The Models That Work Campaign (MTW) is a public-private partnership led by the Health Resources and Services Administration (HRSA) whose mission is to increase access to primary health care, especially for more than 40 million Americans without health insurance, and millions of other underserved Americans.

While their primary function lies in working with community health care systems, you, the consumer, can benefit from their online database. Each year they host a competition honoring health care programs that demonstrate innovation, quality and outcomes in primary health care. All of the programs that apply are included in a database that lists detailed information about their programs. You can do a search using key words such as "maternal" or "mental health." This is a great place to get a listing of successful health programs providing services for vulnerable populations.

Contact: Models That Work, 4350 East-West Highway, Bethesda, MD 20814; 800-859-2386, 301-594-4312; Fax: 703-852-2901; E-mail: {models@hrsa.gov}; {www.bphc.hrsa.dhhs.gov/mtw/mtw.htm}.

Service Organizations

Need help with child care, elderly services, substance abuse treatment? What about youth programs or disaster assistance? Many large service organizations have local offices that provide all this and more. Services vary depending upon the needs of the community, but before you fight your battles alone, contact these main offices to find out about local programs:

✦ *Catholic Charities USA*, 1731 King St., #200, Alexandria, VA 23314; 703-549-1390; {www.catholiccharitiesusa.org}.

✦ *Salvation Army*, 615 Slaters Lane, P.O. Box 2696, Alexandria, VA 22313; 703-684-5500; 800-SAL-ARMY; {www.salvationarmyusa.org}.

✦ *United Way of America*, 701 N. Fairfax St., Alexandria, VA 22314; 800-411-UWAY; {www.unitedway.org}.

How To Fight Your Doctor, Hospital, Or Insurance Company — Call The Marines

Well, not the actual Marines from the Department of Defense, dressed in fatigues and armed with high tech weapons. But you can call other government offices and advocacy groups that will do your fighting for you or give you the needed weapons to do your own fighting. Before you call a lawyer, call these free offices first:

◆ *State Insurance Commissioner*: will help you learn your legal rights regarding insurance, as well as your HMO.

◆ *State Medical Boards*: will review your complaint (including billing issues) and help resolve disputes.

◆ *The Center for Patient Advocacy*, 1350 Beverly Road, Suite 108, McLean, VA 22101; 800-846-7444; {www.patientadvocacy.org}: provides free advice and publications on how to fight the system,

also does advocacy work for patients rights on
Capitol Hill)

♦ *Center for Medicare Advocacy, Inc*, P.O. Box 350,
Willimantic, CT 06226; 860-456-7790;
{www.medicareadvocacy.org}. Attorneys,
paralegals, and technical assistants provide legal
help for elderly and disabled who are unfairly
denied Medicare coverage in the states of
Connecticut and New York. They will send
materials to people in other states to learn how to
fight for themselves.

♦ *American Self Help Clearinghouse*, Northwest
Covenant Medical Center, 25 Pocono Rd., Denville,
NJ 07834; 973-625-9565; Fax: 973-635-8848; TTD
973-625-9053; {www.cmhc.com/selfhelp}: makes
referrals to self-help organizations world wide and
helps people interested in starting their own self
help group.

♦ *National Self-Help Clearinghouse*, c/o CUNY,
Graduate School and University Center, 25 West
43rd St., Room 620, New York, NY 10036; 212-
354-8525; Fax: 212-642-1956; {www.selfhelpweb.
org}: makes referrals to self-help groups
nationwide.

♦ *National Commission for Quality Assurance*, 2000
L St., NW, Suite 500, Washington, DC 20036; 202-
955-3500; 888-275-7585 (accreditation status);
{www.ncqa.org}: this organization accredits

managed care organizations and you can contact them to see if an HMO passed inspection. They also accept complaints, although they do not act upon them. They use the complaints as the key when the HMO comes up for re-accreditation. NCQA carefully looks at how your complaint was handled.

♦ *Medicare HMOs*, Medicare Hotline, Health Care Financing Administration, 330 Independence Ave., SW, Washington, DC 20201; 800-638-6833; {www.medicare.gov}: every Medicare HMO is required to tell you how to appeal their decisions, and that needs to be your first course of action. If you are not getting satisfaction, contact the Medicare Hotline and they can direct you to the proper channel for complaints.

♦ *Medicaid HMOs*, Center for Medicaid and State Operations, Health Care Financing Administration, 7500 Security Blvd., Baltimore, MD 21244;

FIGHT BACK — What to Do When Your HMO Says No

This booklet is free from The Center for Patient Advocacy, 1350 Beverly Road, Suite 108, McLean, VA 22101; 800-846-7444; {www.patientadvocacy.org}.

{www.hcfa.gov/medicaid/medicaid.htm}: if you have a complaint regarding your Medicaid HMO, you must first go through the HMO appeal process which the HMO is required to explain to you. If you are not getting satisfaction, contact your local Medicaid office or the state Medicaid office listed in the Health Insurance chapter (see page 384). Information on who to contact can also be found on the website listed above.

State Insurance Commissioners

Alabama
Insurance Commissioner
201 Monroe St., Suite 1700
Montgomery, AL 36104
334-269-3550
800-243-5463

Alaska
Director of Insurance
P.O. Box 110805
Juneau, AK 99811-0805
907-465-2515
http://www.commerce.state.
ak.us/insurance

Arizona
Director of Insurance
2910 N. 44th St.
Suite 210
Phoenix, AZ 85018
602-912-8400
800-325-2548
http://www.state.az.us/id/

Arkansas
Insurance Commissioner
1200 W. 3rd St.
Little Rock, AR 72201
501-371-2600
800-852-5494

California
Commissioner of Insurance
300 S. Spring St., 13th Floor
Los Angeles, CA 90013
916-492-3500 (Sacramento)
213-346-6400 (Los Angeles)
800-927-HELP (complaints)
http://www.insurance.ca.gov/
docs/index.html

Colorado
Commissioner of Insurance
1560 Broadway, Suite 850
Denver, CO 80202
303-894-7499
800-544-9181

http://www.state.co.us/gov_dir/
regulatory_dir/insurance_reg.
html

Connecticut
Insurance Commissioner
P.O. Box 816
Hartford, CT 06142-0816
860-297-3802
800-203-3447
http://www.state.ct.us/cid/

Delaware
Insurance Commissioner
841 Silver Lake Blvd.
Rodney Bldg.
Dover, DE 19903
302-739-4251
800-282-8611
http://www.state.de.us/govern/
elecoffl/ inscom.htm

District of Columbia
Commissioner of Insurance
441 4th St., NW
8th Floor N.
Washington, DC 20001
202-727-8000

Florida
Insurance Commissioner
200 E. Gaines St.
Tallahassee, FL 32399-0300
850-922-3100
800-342-2762
http://www.doi.state.fl.us/

Georgia
Insurance Commissioner

7th Floor, West Tower
Floyd Bldg.
2 Martin Luther King, Jr. Dr.
Atlanta, GA 30334
404-656-2070
800-656-2298
http://www2.state.ga.us/
gains.commission/

Hawaii
Insurance Commissioner
250 S. King Street, 5th Floor
Honolulu, HI 96813
808-586-2790
http://www.state.hi.us/insurance

Idaho
Director of Insurance
P.O. Box 83720
Boise, ID 83720-0043
208-334-2250
http://www.doi.state.id.us/

Illinois
Director of Insurance
320 W. Washington St.
4th Floor
Springfield, IL 62767-0001
217-782-4515
800-548-9034
http://www.state.il.us/ins/

Indiana
Commissioner of Insurance
311 W. Washington St.
Suite 300
Indianapolis, IN 46204-2787
317-232-2385
800-622-4461

http://www.ai.org/idoi/
index.html

Iowa
Insurance Commissioner
330 E. Maple St.
Des Moines, IA 50319
515-281-5705
800-351-4664
http://www.state.ia.us/
government/com/ ins/ins.htm

Kansas
Commissioner of Insurance
420 SW 9th St.
Topeka, KS 66612-1678
785-296-3071
800-432-2484
http://www.ink.org/public/kid/

Kentucky
Insurance Commissioner
215 W. Main St.
P.O. Box 517
Frankfort, KY 40602
502-564-3630
800-595-6053
http://www.state.ky.us/agencies/
insur/default.htm

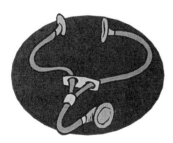

Louisiana
Commissioner of Insurance
P.O. Box 94214
Baton Rouge, LA 70804-9214
504-342-5900
800-259-5300
http://wwwldi.ldi.state.la.us/

Maine
Superintendent of Insurance
34 State House Station
Augusta, ME 04333
207-624-8475
800-750-5353
http://www.state.me.us/pfr/ins/
inshome2.htm

Maryland
Insurance Commissioner
525 St. Paul Place
Baltimore, MD 21202
410-486-2090
800-492-6116
http://www.gacc.com/mia/

Massachusetts
Commissioner of Insurance
470 Atlantic Ave., 6th Floor
Boston, MA 02210-2223
617-521-7794
800-882-2003

Michigan
Commissioner of Insurance
Insurance Bureau
P.O. Box 30220
Lansing, MI 48909-7720
517-373-9273
800-803-7174

http://www.commerce.state.
mi.us/ins/

Minnesota
Commissioner of Commerce
133 E. 7th St.
St. Paul, MN 55101-2362
612-297-7161
800-657-3602
800-657-3978
http://www.commerce.state.mn.
us/mainin.htm

Mississippi
Commissioner of Insurance
1804 Walter Sillers Bldg.
P.O. Box 79
Jackson, MS 39205
601-359-3569
800-562-2957
http://www.doi.state.ms.us

Missouri
Director of Insurance
301 W. High St.
Room 630
P.O. Box 690
Jefferson City, MO 65102-0690
573-751-4126
800-726-7390
http://services.state.mo.us/
insurance/ mohmepg.htm

Montana
Commissioner of Insurance
P.O. Box 4009
Helena, MT 59604-4009
406-444-2040
800-332-6148

Nebraska
Director of Insurance
941 O St., Suite 400
Lincoln, NE 68508-3690
402-471-2201
800-833-0920
http://www.nol.org/home/ndoi/

Nevada
Commissioner of Insurance
1665 Hot Springs Rd.
Capitol Complex 152
Carson City, NV 89706-0646
702-687-4270
800-992-0900
http://www.state.nv.us/b&i/id/

New Hampshire
Insurance Commissioner
169 Manchester St.
Concord, NH 03301-5151
603-271-2261
800-852-3416
http://www.state.nh.us/
insurance/

New Jersey
Commissioner
Department of Insurance
20 W. State St.
P.O. Box 325
Trenton, NJ 08625-0325
609-292-5316
800-792-8820
http://www.naic.org/nj/
div_ins.htm

New Mexico
Superintendent of Insurance

P.O. Drawer 1269
Santa Fe, NM 87504-1269
505-827-4601
800-947-4722

New York
Superintendent of Insurance
25 Beaver St.
New York, NY 10004
212-480-6400
800-342-3736 (in NY)
http://www.ins.state.ny.us

North Carolina
Commissioner of Insurance
Dobbs Bldg.
P.O. Box 26387
Raleigh, NC 27611
919-733-7349
800-662-7777 (in NC)
http://www.doi.state.nc.us/

North Dakota
Commissioner of Insurance
Capitol Bldg., 5th Floor
600 E. Boulevard Ave.
Bismarck, ND 58505-0320
701-328-2440
800-247-0560 (in ND)

Ohio
Director of Insurance
2100 Stella Court
Columbus, OH 43215-1067
614-644-2651
800-686-1526 (consumer)
800-686-1527 (fraud)
800-686-1578 (senior health)
http://www.state.oh.us/ins/

Oklahoma
Insurance Commissioner
P.O. Box 53408
Oklahoma City, OK 73152-3408
405-521-2828
800-522-0071
http://www.oid.state.ok.us

Oregon
Insurance Commissioner
440 Labor and Industries
Building
330 Winter St., NE
Salem, OR 97310
503-378-4271
800-722-4134
http://www.state.or.us/agencies.
ns/44000/ 00070/index.html

Pennsylvania
Insurance Commissioner
1326 Strawberry Square
Harrisburg, PA 17120
717-787-2317
800-783-7067
http://www.state.pa.us/pa_exec/
insurance/ overview.html

Rhode Island
Insurance Commissioner
233 Richmond St., Suite 233
Providence, RI 02903
401-277-2223
800-322-2880

South Carolina
Chief Insurance Commissioner
P.O. Box 100105

Columbia, SC 29202-3105
803-737-6150
800-768-3467
http://www.state.sc.us/doi/

South Dakota
Director of Insurance
Insurance Bldg.
118 W. Capitol St.
Pierre, SD 57501
605-773-3563
800-822-8804
http://www.state.sd.us/
insurance/

Tennessee
Commissioner of Insurance
500 James Robertson Parkway
Nashville, TN 37243-0565
615-741-2241
800-342-4029
http://www.state.tn.us/
commerce

Texas
Director, Claims and
Compliance Division
State Board of Insurance
P.O. Box 149104
Austin, TX 78714-9104
512-463-6464
800-252-3439
http://www.tdi.state.tx.us

Utah
Commissioner of Insurance
3110 State Office Bldg.
Salt Lake City, UT 84114
801-538-3805

800-439-3805
http://www.ins-dept.state.ut.us/

Vermont
Commissioner of Banking and
Insurance
89 Main St.
Drawer 20
Montpelier, VT 05620-3101
802-828-3301
800-642-5119
http://www.state.vt.us/bis/

Virginia
Commissioner of Insurance
1300 E. Main St.
P.O. Box 1157
Richmond, VA 23218
804-371-9741
800-552-7945
http://dit1.state.va.us/scc/
division/ boi/index.htm

Washington
Insurance Commissioner
Insurance Bldg. AQ21
P.O. Box 40255
Olympia, WA 98504-0255
360-753-7301
800-562-6900
http://www.wa.gov/ins/

West Virginia
Insurance Commissioner
2019 Washington St., E.
P.O. Box 50540
Charleston, WV 25305-0540
304-558-3394
800-642-9004

Wisconsin
Commissioner of Insurance
P.O. Box 7873
Madison, WI 53707-7873
608-266-3585
800-236-8517
http://badger.state.wi.us/
agencies/oci/oci_home.htm

Wyoming
Commissioner of Insurance
Herschler Bldg. 3 East
122 W. 25th St.
Cheyenne, WY 82002
307-777-7401
800-438-5768

State Medical Boards

Alabama
Alabama State Board of
Medical Examiners
P.O. Box 946
Montgomery, AL 36101
334-242-4116
800-227-2606
http://bmedixon.home.
mindspring.com

Alaska
Alaska State Medical Board
3601 C St.
Suite 722
Anchorage, AK 99503
907-269-8160

Arizona
Arizona Board of Medical
Examiners
1651 E. Morten Ave.
Suite 210
Phoenix, AZ 85020
602-255-3751
877-255-2212 (toll-free in AZ)
www.docboard.org/bomex/
index.htm

Arizona Board of Osteopathic
Examiners in Medicine and
Surgery
9535 E. Doubletree Ranch Rd.
Scottsdale, AZ 85258
602-657-7703

Arkansas
Arkansas State Medical Board
2100 Riverfront Dr., Suite 200
Little Rock, AR 72202
501-296-1802

California
Medical Board of California
1426 Howe Ave., Suite 54
Sacramento, CA 95825
916-263-2466
800-633-2322
www.medbd.ca.gov

Osteopathic Medical Board of
California
2720 Gateway Oaks Dr.
Suite 350
Sacramento, CA 95833
916-263-3100

Colorado
Colorado Board of Medical
Examiners
1560 Broadway, Suite 1300
Denver, CA 80202
303-894-7690
www.dora.state.co.us/medical

Connecticut
Connecticut Medical
Examining Board
410 Capitol Ave., MS12APP
P.O. Box 340308
Hartford, CT 06134
860-509-7563
www.ct-clic.com

District of Columbia
District of Columbia Board of
Medicine
614 H St., NW, Room 108
Washington, DC 20001
202-727-4087

Florida
Florida Board of Medicine
Northwood Centre
1940 N. Monroe St.
Tallahassee, FL 32399
850-488-0595
www.doh.state.fl.us/mqa

Florida Board of Osteopathic
Medicine
Northwood Centre
1940 N. Monroe St.
Tallahassee, FL 32399
850-488-0595
www.doh.state.fl.us/mqa

Georgia
Georgia Composite State
Board of Medical Examiners
166 Pryor St., SW
Atlanta, GA 30303
404-656-3913
www.state.ga.us/gch

Hawaii
Hawaii Board of Medical
Examiners
Department of Commerce and
Consumer Affairs
P.O. Box 3469
Honolulu, HI 96801
808-586-2699

Idaho
Idaho State Board of Medicine
P.O. Box 83720
Statehouse Mail
Boise, ID 83720
208-334-2822

Illinois
Illinois Department of
Professional Regulation
R. James Thompson Center
100 W. Randolph St., 9-300
Chicago, IL 60601
312-814-4500
www.state.il.us/dpr

Indiana
Indiana Health Professions
Bureau
402 W. Washington St.
Room 041
Indianapolis, IN 46204

317-232-2960
www.ai.org/hpb

Iowa
Iowa State Board of Medical
Examiners
Executive Hills West
400 SW 8th St., Suite C
Des Moines, IA 50319
515-281-5171
www.docboard.org

Kansas
Kansas Board of Healing Arts
235 SW Topeka Blvd.
Topeka, KS 66603
785-296-7413
www.ink.org/public/boha

Kentucky
Kentucky Board of Medical
Licensure
Hurstbourne Office Park
310 Whittington Parkway
 Suite 1B
Louisville, KY 40222
502-429-8046
www.state.ky.us/agencies/
kbml

Louisiana
Louisiana State Board of
Medical Examiners
P.O. Box 30250
New Orleans, LA 70190
504-524-6763
www.dhh.state.la.us/
boards.HTM

Maine
Maine Board of Licensure in
Medicine
137 State House Station
Two Bangor St.
Augusta, ME 04333
207-287-3605
www.docboard.org/me/
me_home.htm

Maine Board of Osteopathic
Licensure
142 State House Station
Augusta, ME 04333
207-287-2480
www.docboard.org

Maryland
Maryland Board of Physician
Quality Assurance
P.O. Box 2571
Baltimore, MD 21215
410-764-4777
800-492-6836
www.docboard.org

Massachusetts
Massachusetts Board of
Registration in Medicine
10 West St., 3rd. Floor
Boston, MA 02111
617-727-3086
800-377-0550
www.massmedboard.org

Michigan
Michigan Board of Medicine
P.O. Box 30670

Lansing, MI 48909
517-335-0918

Michigan Board of
Osteopathic Medicine and
Surgery
P.O. Box 30670
Lansing, MI 48909
517-335-0918

Minnesota
Minnesota Board of Medical
Practice
University Park Plaza
2829 University Ave., SW
Suite 400
Minneapolis, MN 55414
612-617-2130
800-657-3709
www.bmp.state.mn.us

Mississippi
Mississippi State Board of
Medical Licensure
2600 Insurance Center Dr.
Suite 200-B
Jackson, MS 39216
601-987-3079
www.msbml.state.ms.us

Missouri
Missouri State Board of
Registration for the Healing
Arts
P.O. Box 4
Jefferson City, MO 65102
573-751-0098
www.ecodev.state.mo.us/
pr/healarts/

Montana
Montana Board of Medical
Examiners
P.O. Box 200513
Helena, MT 59620
406-444-4284
http://commerce.mt.gov/
license/POL/pol_boards/
med_board/board_page.htm

Nebraska
Nebraska Health and Human
Services System
P.O. Box 95007
Lincoln, NE 68509
402-471-2133
www.hhs.state.ne.us

Nevada
Nevada State Board of
Medical Examiners
P.O. Box 7238
Reno, NV 89510
775-688-2321
www.state.nv.us/medical

Nevada State Board of
Osteopathic Medicine
2950 E. Flamingo Rd.
Suite E-3
Las Vegas, NV 89121
702-732-2147

New Hampshire
New Hampshire Board of
Medicine
2 Industrial Park Dr., Suite 8
Concord, NH 03301
603-271-1203

800-780-4757
www.state.nj.us/lps/ca/
boards.htm

New Jersey
New Jersey State Board of
Medical Examiners
140 E. Front St., 2nd Floor
Trenton, NJ 08608
609-826-7100

New Mexico
New Mexico State Board of
Medical Examiners
Lamy Bldg., 2nd Floor
491 Old Santa Fe Trail
Santa FE, NM 87501
505-827-5022
800-945-5845

New Mexico Board of
Osteopathic Medical
Examiners
P.O. Box 25101
Santa Fe, NM 87504
505-476-7120

New York
New York State Board of
Medicine
Cultural Education Center,
Room 3023
Empire State Plaza
Albany, NY 12230
518-474-3841
www.nysed.gov/prof/

New York State Board for
Professional Medical Conduct

NY State Dept. of Health
Office of Professional Medical
Conduct
433 River St., Suite 303
Troy, NY 12180
518-402-0855
www.health.state.ny.us

North Carolina
North Carolina Medical Board
P.O. Box 20007
Raleigh, NC 27619
919-828-1100
800-253-9653 (in NC)
www.docboard.org/nc/

North Dakota
North Dakota State Board of
Medical Examiners
City Center Plaza
418 E. Broadway, Suite 12
Bismarck, ND 58501
701-328-6500

Ohio
State Medical Board of Ohio
77 S. High St., 17th Floor
Columbus, OH 43266
614-466-3934
800-554-7717
www.state.oh.us/med

Oklahoma
Oklahoma State Board of
Medical Licensure and
Supervision
P.O. Box 18256
Oklahoma City, OK 73154
405-848-6841

800-381-4519
www.osbmls.state.ok.us

Oklahoma State Board of
Osteopathic Examiners
4848 N. Lincoln Blvd.
Suite 100
Oklahoma City, OK 73105
405-528-8625
www.docboard.org/ok/ok.htm

Oregon
Oregon Board of Medical
Examiners
620 Crown Plaza
1500 SW First Ave.
Portland, OR 97201
503-229-5770
877-254-6263 (toll-free in OR)
www.bme.state.or.us

Pennsylvania
Pennsylvania State Board of
Medicine
P.O. Box 2649
Harrisburg, PA 17105
717-783-1400
www.dos.state.pa.us

Pennsylvania State Board of
Osteopathic Medicine
P.O. Box 2649
Harrisburg, PA 17105
717-783-4858
www.dos.state.pa.us

Rhode Island
RI Board of Medical Licensure
and Discipline

Department of Health
Cannon Building, Room 205
Three Capitol Hill
Providence, RI 02908
401-222-3855
www.docboard.org/ri/
main.htm

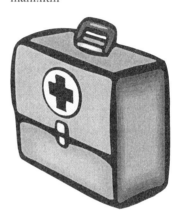

South Carolina
South Carolina Department of
Labor, Licensing and
Regulation
Board of Medical Examiners
P.O. Box 11289
Columbia, SC 29211
803-896-4500
www.llr.state.sc.us/me.htm

South Dakota
South Dakota State Board of
Medical and Osteopathic
Examiners
1323 S. Minnesota Ave.
Sioux Falls, SD 57105
605-334-8343

Tennessee
Tennessee Board of Medical
Examiners
425 5th Ave., North
1st Floor, Cordell Hull Bldg.
Nashville, TN 37247
615-532-5081
888-310-4650
www.state.tn.us/health/
links.html

Texas
Texas State Board of Medical
Examiners
P.O. Box 2018
Austin, TX 78768
512-305-7010
800-201-9353
www.tsbme.state.tx.us

Utah
Utah Dept. of Commerce
Division of Occupational and
Professional Licensure
P.O. Box 146741
Salt Lake City, UT 84114
801-530-6628

Vermont
Vermont Board of Medical
Practice
109 State St.
Montpelier, VT 05609
802-828-2673
www.docboard.org/vt/
vermont.htm

Vermont Board of Osteopathic
Physicians and Surgeons

109 State St.
Montpelier, VT 05609
802-828-2373
800-439-8683
www.sec.state.vt.us

Virginia
Virginia Board of Medicine
6606 W. Broad St., 4th Floor
Richmond, VA 23230
804-662-9908
800-533-1560 (VA only)
www.dhp.state.va.us

Washington
Washington Medical Quality
Assurance Commission
P.O. Box 47866
Olympia, WA 98504
360-664-8480
www.doh.wa.gov

Washington State Board of
Osteopathic Medicine and
Surgery
P.O. Box 47870
Olympia, WA 98504
360-664-8480
www.doh.wa.gov

West Virginia
West Virginia Board of
Medicine
101 Dee Dr.
Charleston, WV 25311
304-558-2921

West Virginia Board of
Osteopathy

334 Penco Rd.
Weirton, WV 26062
304-723-4638

Wisconsin
Wisconsin Medical Examining
Board
Department of Regulation and
Licensing
P.O. Box 8935
Madison, WI 53709

608-266-1188
http://badger.state.wi.us/
agencies/drl

Wyoming
Wyoming Board of Medicine
211 W. 19th St.
Colony Bldg., 2nd Floor
Cheyenne, WY 82002
307-778-7053

Your Very Own Strong Arm

You don't need to put up with cold food or rough care. Just make a call to your state's Nursing Home Ombudsman, and there will be another person on your side.

Ombudsmen are there to help people who are denied admission to nursing homes, improve the quality of the food, and even help report stolen property. The Ombudsman Program is designed to investigate and resolve complaints made by or on behalf of residents of long-term care facilities. They also make sure these places are running properly and up to code.

Ombudsman act as mediators, but they are not enforcement agencies. They cannot force a nursing home to change or correct their practices. But it is in the best interest of the nursing home to work with you, before you refer your complaint elsewhere. To locate the Nursing Home Ombudsman in your state, check the listings below.

Long-Term Care Ombudsman

Alabama
Marie Tomlin
State Long-Term Care
Ombudsman
Commission On Aging
RSA Plaza, Suite 470
770 Washington Avenue
Montgomery, AL 36130
334-242-5743
Fax: 334-242-5594
E-mail: mtomlin@
coa.state.al.us

Alaska
Suzann Armstrong
Acting State Long-Term Care
Ombudsman
Older Alaskans Commission
3601 C Street, Suite 260
Anchorage, AK 99503-5209
907-563-6393
Fax: 907-561-3862

Arizona
State Long-Term Care
Ombudsman
Aging And Adult
Administration
Department of Economic
Security

1789 West Jefferson, 950A
Phoenix, AZ 85007
602-542-4446
Fax: 602-542-6575

Arkansas
Alice Ahart
State Long-Term Care
Ombudsman
Arkansas Division Of Aging &
Adult Services
P.O. Box 1437
Slot 1412
Little Rock, AR 72201-1437
501-682-2441
Fax: 501-682-8155
E-mail: alice.ahart@
mail.state.ar.us

California
Phyllis Heath
State Long-Term Care
Ombudsman
Department Of Aging
1600 K Street
Sacramento, CA 95814
916-323-6681
Fax: 916-323-7299
E-mail: cda.pheath@
hw1.cahwnet.gov

Colorado
Jan Meyers & Virginia Fraser
State Long-Term Care
Ombudsman
The Legal Center
455 Sherman Street, Suite 130
Denver, CO 80203
303-722-0300
Fax: 303-722-0720
E-mail: CHGin28@aol.com

Connecticut
Teresa Cusano
Acting State Long-Term Care
Ombudsman
Department on Aging
25 Sigourney St., 10th Floor
Hartford, CT 06106-5033
860-424-5200, ext. 5221
Fax: 860-424-4966
E-mail: ltcop@po.state.ct.us

Delaware
Karen Michel
Acting State Long-Term Care
Ombudsman
Delaware Services for Aging-
Disabled
Health & Social Services
Oxford Building, Suite 200
256 Chapman Road
Newark, DE 19702
302-453-3820, ext. 46
Fax: 302-453-3836

District of Columbia
Deidre Rye & Anne Hart
State Long-Term Care
Ombudsman

AARP- Legal Counsel for the
Elderly
601 E Street, NW
4th Floor, Building A
Washington, DC 20049
202-434-2140

Florida
Steve Rachin Esquire
State Long-Term Care
Ombudsman
Florida State LTC
Ombudsman Council
Holland Building, Room 270
600 South Calhoun Street
Tallahassee, FL 32301
850-488-6190
Fax: 850-488-5657
E-mail: FLOmbuds@juno.com

Georgia
Becky Kurtz
State Long-Term Care
Ombudsman
Division of Aging Services
2 Peachtree Street, NW
36th Floor, Suite 36-385
Atlanta, GA 30303-3176
404-657-5319
Fax: 404-657-5285
E-mail: bkurtz@mail.doas.
state.ga.us

Hawaii
John McDermott
State LTC Care Ombudsman
Executive Office On Aging
Office of the Governor
250 South Hotel St., Suite 107

Honolulu, HI 96813-2831
808-586-0100
Fax: 808-586-0185
E-mail: jgmcderm@
mail.health.state.hi.us

Idaho
Cathy Hart
State Long-Term Care
Ombudsman
Office On Aging
P.O. Box 83720
700 West Jefferson, Room 108
Boise, ID 83720-0007
208-334-3833
Fax: 208-334-3033
E-mail: chart@icoa.state.id.us

Illinois
Beverly Rowley
State Long-Term Care
Ombudsman
Illinois Department On Aging
421 E. Capitol Ave., Suite 100
Springfield, IL 62701-1789
217-785-3143
Fax: 217-524-4477
E-mail: browley@age084rl.
state.il.us

Indiana
Arlene Franklin
State Long-Term Care
Ombudsman
Indiana Division of Aging &
Rehabilitation Services
P.O. Box 7083-W454
402 W. Washington Street
Indianapolis, IN 46207-7083

317-232-1750
Fax: 317-232-7867
E-mail: afranklin@
fssa.state.in.us

Iowa
Debi Meyers
Interim State LTC
Ombudsman
Iowa Department of Elder
Affairs
Clemens Building
200 10th Street, 3rd Floor
Des Moines, IA 50309-3609
515-281-8643
Fax: 515-281-4036
E-mail: debi.meyers@
dea.state.ia.us

Kansas
Matthew Hickam
State LTC Ombudsman
Office of the State Long-Term
Care Ombudsman
610 SW 10th Street, 2nd Floor
Topeka, KS 66612-1616
785-296-3017
Fax: 785-296-3916

Kentucky
Brenda Rice
State LTC Ombudsman
Division of Family/Children
Services
275 E Main St.
5th Floor West
Frankfort, KY 40621
502-564-6930
Fax: 502-564-4595

Louisiana
Linda Sadden
State LTC Ombudsman
Governor's Office of Elderly
Affairs
412 North 4th Street- 3rd Floor
P.O. Box 80374
Baton Rouge, LA 70802
225-342-7100
Fax: 225-342-7144
E-mail: Hchiang@aol.com

Maine
Brenda Gallant
State Long-Term Care
Ombudsman
Maine State Long Term Care
Ombudsman Program
1 Weston Court
P.O. Box 126
Augusta, ME 04332
207-621-1079
Fax: 207-621-0509
E-mail: BGallant@
maineombudsman.org

Maryland
Patricia Bayliss
State Long-Term Care
Ombudsman
Office On Aging
State Office Building
Room 1007
301 West Preston Street
Baltimore, MD 21201
410-767-1074
Fax: 410-333-7943
E-mail: plb@mail.ooa.
state.md.us

Massachusetts
Mary McKenna
State Long-Term Care
Ombudsman
Exec Office Of Elder Affairs
1 Ashburton Place, 5th Floor
Boston, MA 02108-1518
617-727-7750
Fax: 617-727-9368
E-mail: mary.e.mckenna@
state.ma.us

Michigan
Hollis Turnham Esquire
State Long-Term Care
Ombudsman
Citizens for Better Care
6105 West St. Joseph
Highway, Suite 211
Lansing, MI 48917-3981
517-886-6797
Fax: 517-886-6349
E-mail: Hturnham@aol.com

Minnesota
Sharon Zoesch
State Long-Term Care
Ombudsman
Office of Ombudsman For
Older Minnesotans
85 East Seventh Pl., Suite 280
St. Paul, MN 55155-3843
651-296-0382
Fax: 651-297-5654
E-mail: sharon.zoesch@
state.mn.us

Mississippi
Anniece McLemore

State Long-Term Care
Ombudsman
Division of Aging & Adult
Services
750 North State Street
Jackson, MS 39202
601-359-4929
Fax: 601-359-4970

Missouri
Carol Scott
State Long-Term Care
Ombudsman
Division On Aging
Department of Social Services
P.O. Box 1337
615 Howerton Court
Jefferson City, MO 65102-1337
573-526-0727
Fax: 573-751-8687
E-mail: cscott@mail.
state.mo.us

Montana
Robert Bartholomew
State Long-Term Care
Ombudsman
Office On Aging
Department of Health and
Human Services
Senior LTC Division
P.O. Box 4210
111 Sanders
Helena, MT 59604-4210
406-444-4077
Fax: 406-444-7743
E-mail: bbartholomew@
mt.gov

Nebraska
Cindy Kadavy
State Long-Term Care
Ombudsman
Department On Aging
P.O. Box 95044
301 Centennial Mall-South
Lincoln, NE 68509-5044
402-471-2306
Fax: 402-471-4619
E-mail: ckadavy@age1.
ndoa.state.ne.us

Nevada
Bruce McAnnany
State Long-Term Care
Ombudsman
Division For Aging Services
Department of Human
Resources
340 N. 11th St., Suite 203
Las Vegas, NV 89101
702-486-3545
Fax: 702-486-3572
E-mail: dasvegas@govmail.
state.nv.us

New Hampshire
Judith Griffin
State Long-Term Care
Ombudsman
Division of Elderly & Adult
Services
129 Pleasant Street
Concord, NH 03301-3857
603-271-4375
Fax: 603-271-4771
E-mail: Jgriffin@dhhs.
state.nh.us

New Jersey
Bernadette T. Kelly
State Long-Term Care
Ombudsman for
Institutionalized Elderly
P.O. Box 807
Trenton, NH 08625-0807
609-588-3614
Fax: 609-588-3365

New Mexico
Agapito Silva
State Agency On Aging
228 East Palace Avenue
Santa Fe, MN 87501
505-827-7640
Fax: 505-827-7649
E-mail: ajsilva@nm-us.
campus.mci.net

New York
Faith E. Fish
State Long-Term Care
Ombudsman
Office For The Aging
2 Empire State Plaza
Agency Building #2
Albany, NY 12223-0001
518-474-7329
Fax: 518-474-7761
E-mail: faith.fish@ofa.
state.ny.us

North Carolina
Wendy Sause
State Long-Term Care
Ombudsman
Division Of Aging
693 Palmer Drive

Caller Box #29531
Raleigh, NC 27626-0531
919-733-8395
Fax: 919-733-0443
E-mail: wendy.sause@
ncmail.net

North Dakota
Helen Funk
State Long-Term Care
Ombudsman
Aging Services Division
DHHS
600 South 2nd Street, Suite 1C
Bismarck, ND 58504
701-328-8910
Fax: 701-328-8989
E-mail: 88funh@state.nd.us

Ohio
Beverley Laubert
State Long-Term Care
Ombudsman
Department Of Aging
50 W. Broad St., 9th Floor
Columbus, ON 43215-5928
614-644-7922
Fax: 614-466-5741
E-mail: M_blaubert@msn.com

Oklahoma
Esther Houser
State Long-Term Care
Ombudsman
Aging Services Division, Dhs
312 NE 28th Street, Suite 109
Oklahoma City, OK 73105
405-521-6734
Fax: 405-521-2086

E-mail: eehouser@
hotmail.com

Oregon
Meredith A. Cote
State Long-Term Care
Ombudsman
Office of the Long Term Care
Ombudsman
3855 Wolverine NE, Suite 6
Salem, OR 97310
503-378-6533
Fax: 503-373-0852
E-mail: ombud@teleport.com

Pennsylvania
Joyce O'Brien
State Long-Term Care
Ombudsman
Department Of Aging
555 Walnut Street
5th Floor
P.(). Box 1089
Harrisburg, PA 17101
717-783-7247
Fax: 717-783-3382
E-mail: jobrien@
aging.state.pa.us

Puerto Rico
Norma Venegas
State Long-Term Care
Ombudsman
Governor's Office For Elder
Affairs
Call Box 50063
Old San Juan Station
San Juan, Puerto Rico 00902
787-725-1515

Fax: 787-721-6510
E-mail: nvenegas@
ogave.prstar.net

Rhode Island
Roberta Hawkins
Alliance For Better Long-Term
Care
422 Post Road, Suite 204
Warwick, RI 02888
401-785-3340
Fax: 401-785-3391
E-mail: nancy4cats@
earthlink.net

South Carolina
John Cook, SLTCO
State Long-Term Care
Ombudsman
Division on Aging
1801 Main Street
P.O. Box 8206
Columbia, SC 29202-8206
803-253-6177
Fax: 803-253-4173
E-mail: cook@dhhs.state.sc.us

South Dakota
Jeff Askew
State Long-Term Care
Ombudsman
Office Of Adult Services &
Aging
700 Governors Drive
Pierre, SD 57501-2291
605-773-3656
Fax: 605-773-6834
E-mail: jeffa@dss.state.sd.us

Tennessee
Adrian D. Wheeler
State Long-Term Care
Ombudsman
Commission On Aging
Andrew Jackson Bldg.
9th Floor
500 Deaderick Street
Nashville, TN 37243-0860
615-741-2056
Fax: 675-741-3309
E-mail: awheeler@
mail.state.tn.us

Texas
John Willis
State Long-Term Care
Ombudsman
Department On Aging
4900 North Lamar Boulevard
4th Floor
P.O. Box 12786
Austin, TX 78751-2316
512-424-6840
Fax: 512-424-6890
E-mail: john@tdoa.state.tx.us

Utah
Carol Bloswick
State Long-Term Care
Ombudsman
Division Of Aging & Adult
Services
Department of Social Services
120 North 200 West
Room 401
Salt Lake City, UT 84103
801-538-3910
Fax: 801-538-4395

E-mail: hsadm2.cbloswic@
email.state.ut.us

Vermont
Jacqueline Majoros Esquire
State Long-Term Care
Ombudsman
Vermont Legal Aid, Inc.
P.O. Box 1367
Burlington, VT 05402
802-863-5620
Fax: 802-863-7152
E-mail: jmajoros@
vtlegalaid.org

Virginia
Mark Miller
State Long-Term Care
Ombudsman
Virginia Association of Area
Agencies on Aging
530 E. Main St., Suite 428
Richmond, VA 23219
804-644-2923
Fax: 804-644-5640
E-mail: vaombudsman@
juno.com

Washington
Kary Hyre
State Long-Term Care
Ombudsman
South King County Multi-
Services Center
1200 South 336th Street
P.O. Box 23699
Federal Way, WA 98093
253-838-6810
Fax: 253-874-7831

West Virginia
Larry Medley
State Long-Term Care
Ombudsman
Commission On Aging
1900 Kanawha Blvd., East
Charleston, WV 25305-0160
304-558-3317
Fax: 304-558-0004

Wisconsin
George Potaracke
State Long-Term Care
Ombudsman
Board On Aging And Long
Term Care
214 North Hamilton Street

Madison, WI 53703-2118
608-266-8945, ext. DIR
Fax: 608-261-6570
E-mail: george.potaracke@
ltc.state.wi.us

Wyoming
Deborah Alden
State Long-Term Care
Ombudsman
Wyoming Senior Citizens, Inc.
756 Gilchrist
P.O. Box 94
Wheatland, WY 82201
307-322-5553
Fax: 307-322-3283

Free Expert Health Advice Online

The Internet can put you just a click and an instant away from free "expert" medical advice. The sites listed below all feature opportunities for you to pose your health questions to someone other than your own doctor. The advice you get could help save your life, but on the other hand, it could just as easily confuse you, misinform you, or even lead you to make a fatal mistake.

For instance, pediatric specialists at the Ohio State University College of Medicine and Public Health looked at web sites created by established, major medical institutions to see if the advice they provided on treating childhood diarrhea—a common problem most parents will have to deal with—matched the current guidelines established by the American Academy of Pediatrics. An astounding 80 percent of the institutions gave inaccurate advice that did not conform to current recommendations. (*Pediatrics*, Vol.101, No. 6, June 1998, a journal of the American Academy of Pediatrics.)

As you'll see from the list of "ask an expert" web sites below, you can find some one to consult everywhere from the massive Johns Hopkins Medical Institutions and small private practices to companies selling products with a doctor's advice column attached. And, as with any other Internet site, make sure you know what you're getting into before you reveal any information about yourself; you may well find yourself on a mailing list for products, services or solicitations you neither want nor need. Some sites bear the logos of organizations such as Medinex (www. medinx.com/code-ethics.html) or the Health On the Net (HON) Honor Code (www.hon.ch/HONcode/Conduct. html). Both these organizations offer guidelines that make a good baseline from which to evaluate a site before you send a message through the Internet.

Medical advice should only be provided by qualified medical or health professionals unless a statement clearly indicates the publisher is not appropriately qualified. The information contained in the site should support and encourage the relationship between the site visitor and his or her current physician. Web site owners should honor or exceed the legal requirements of medical/health information privacy laws that apply in the country and state where the web site originates. Web site publishers should protect the identity and confidentiality of the individuals visiting the site. Clear references to the sources of information, including HTML links, should be revealed whenever possible. Sponsors of the site should be identified and advertisements that fund the site should be clearly identified as such.

Finally, if you have a health problem, a timely call to your doctor is still the best way to take care of your health.

The "ask an expert" sites are listed below, with the large institutional sites covering many topics listed first, followed by specialties such as knee surgery, asthma, and diabetes.

General Sites With Multiple Health Topics

Medical Questions from A to Z:
Ask the Johns Hopkins Medical Institutions
www.intelihealth.com/IH/

This huge site run by the Johns Hopkins Medical Institutions includes an extensive section called "Ask the Doc," which you can access by clicking the button on the homepage. A Johns Hopkins physician will respond to questions from any of the following categories: AIDS/HIV/STDs, allergy, alternative/integrative medicine, arthritis/rheumatology, asthma, blood conditions, bone, muscles and joints, cancer, diabetes, digestive disorders, ears, nose and throat, eating disorders, eyes/vision, fitness/sports medicine, headaches/migraine, heart and circulatory conditions, infectious diseases, kidney, bladder and urinary tract, medical tests and procedures, medications, men's health, mental health, nervous system and stroke, nutrition, oral health, pain, pediatrics, pregnancy, seniors, sexuality, skin and hair, sleep, substance abuse, thyroid/other endocrine disorders, women's health, other diseases and conditions, and weight management. You can also check the archives for answers to previous questions on any of these topics. Responses include the name and professional profile of the doctor answering the question.

Ask the Doctors at Beth Israel in New York
www.bethisraelny.org/interactive/askdoctor.htm
The Beth Israel Medical Center in New York City hosts this site, which features extensive information and the opportunity to question physicians or other health professionals about specific problems. The question and answer sections also provide information about the physician who wrote the response. Topics covered include: allergies, asthma, back pain/spine, cancer, cardiology, diabetes, drug and alcohol abuse, ear and eye problems, gastroenterology/stomach, general medicine, men's health, neurology, orthopedics, pain medicine and palliative care, pediatrics, plastic surgery, and women's health.

Ask a Doctor
www.abilene.com/armc
You can ask the obstetrician/gynecologists and pediatricians at the Abilene Regional Medical Center and receive an e-mail reply within 10 days. You'll also find a list of frequently asked questions and responses on women and children's health issues, along with information on cardiology and family medicine.

Ask Colorado HealthNet
www.coloradohealthnet.org
Colorado HealthNet is a Colorado nonprofit corporation formed in 1995 to provide electronic access to factual and statistical information, support services, medical resources, and related health care information for persons with chronic medical conditions and for other users. Physicians with a

wide range of specialties have volunteered to field your questions, and you can check the archives for past questions and responses. QualMed, a health maintenance organization, is one of the site's sponsors.

Ask a Nurse: Nurse Healthline at Mercy Health System
www.mercyhealthsystem.org/ASKNURSE/askartcl.htm

The Mercy Health System, a network of 30 facilities in northern Illinois and southern Wisconsin, offers this opportunity to have your health questions answered by a nurse. The web site also links to articles by the nursing staff; topics range from new treatments for prostrate cancer, getting and staying fit, and preventing carpal tunnel syndrome, to name a few. The site does not provide any information concerning confidentiality, so be sure to ask before you send any e-mail that could make you feel uncomfortable. No answers to specific questions are posted on the web site.

Non-Emergencies: Ask a Nurse
www.harthosp.org/questions

Unless you ask something very complicated, you will get a reply from a registered nurse employed by the Hartford Hospital (Connecticut) within 24 hours. The site also has more general information on a range of health topics.

Aneurysms

Aneurysm Advice
www.westga.edu/~wmaples/aneurysm.html
www.westga.edu/~wmaples/doc.html
These web sites, hosted by the State University of West
Georgia, offer links to information about aneurysms,
including treatment and support for patients. You can also
ask a panel of specialists from around the world to field
your questions.

Allergies And Asthma

National Pollen Network: Ask an Allergist
www.allernet.com
E-mail: questions@allernet.com
The National Pollen Network can confirm what your nose
is telling you by providing daily maps of the national
allergy forecast for tree, grass, and weed pollen and mold
spores. The site offers lots of other allergy and asthma
information, including the opportunity to ask Dr. Steve
Kagan, an allergy specialist in Wisconsin and director of
the National Pollen Network, specific questions. You can
send your questions via e-mail or check out Dr. Kagan's
responses to previous queries at {www.allernet.com/
questions/default.asp}.

Ask the Asthma Experts
www.asthmacentre.com/index.html
You will receive an answer to your questions about asthma
within 14 days from the physicians and staff at the Asthma

Center at the Toronto Hospital. Before you send your
query, though, be sure to check out the extensive
information on the web site, including the Asthma
Education Handbook. Topics include managing asthma,
inhalers and other devices, allergies and their triggers, and
medications and their side effects.

Back And Spine

Back Problems: Ask the New York Spine Team
www.orthospine.com
Your questions will be answered by a team of New York
City doctors who diagnose and treat conditions affecting
the spinal column: spinal deformities, herniated discs,
spinal stenosis, spondylolisthesis, endoscopic surgery and
lower back pain. Answers to individuals' questions are not
posted on the site; however, you can link to a list of
frequently asked questions about specific spinal problems.
This site subscribes to the Health On the Net Code of
Conduct for medical and health web sites (see above).
Click on "Ask the Doctor" to e-mail your question.

Cancer

Ask the Cancer Specialists
www.cancerhope.com/ask_a_doctor/question.html
This site does not offer a lot of general information on
cancer, but you can ask a specific question via e-mail to the
physicians at the Cancerhope Foundation in Tallahassee,
Florida.

See Women's Health and Plastic Surgery

CPR

Refresh Your CPR Memory
www.learncpr.org/index.html
If it's been a while since your were last CPR (cardio-pulmonary resuscitation) certified, or you're heading out with the scout troop for a weekend camp out, this could be just the last-minute refresher you need. Along with lots of CPR information and a pocket-sized guide for you to print out, you can e-mail specific CPR-related questions to {gingy@learncpr.org}.

Death And Dying

Ask the Experts on Death and Dying
www.death-dying.com/experts/index.html
The "Death & Dying" web site is designed to provide comfort, support, and education about issues surrounding death at a time when people are confused, apprehensive, and dealing with shock and sorrow. This is a big site with lots of features to browse, but it also hosts a large panel of experts ready to field your questions on subjects such as grief in the workplace, loss of a loved one, loss of a pet, spirituality and sexuality, children and teen issues, funeral planning, legal questions, neonatal loss, and the physical process of dying itself. Each of the experts has provided his or her "introduction," so that you will have some idea of

who you are talking to before you send your message off into the Internet.

Dentistry And Orthodontia

Ask a Dentist
www.the-toothfairy.com

Dr. Marianne W. Schaeffer, a dentist in Chicago, includes a correspondence section in her office web site. She welcomes e-mail on the topics of cosmetic dentistry (including bleaching), alternative materials to replace silver amalgam, dental consumerism (how to choose a new doctor), crowns and bridges, root canal and associated materials, dental health care issues for women and children, forensic dentistry, and "terror teeth"—artificial false teeth intended to give friends a fright. Dr. Schaeffer is working toward board certification in forensic odontology and her web site provides extensive information on how dentistry can help solve crimes.

Ask an Orthodontist
www.bracesrus.com

Dr. Randall Ogata, an orthodontist practicing in Seattle, Washington, will respond to your questions about orthodontia and braces. You can also check out a very general question and answer page about braces.

Dermatology

Acne Anguish: Ask a Dermatologist
www.facefacts.com

Roche Pharmaceuticals hosts this site, which focuses on teenaged acne. When you click on the "e-mail a doctor" button you'll find a list of frequently asked questions and responses, and you can contact Dr. Michael S. Kaminer, M.D., if you need more information.

Diabetes

Children with Diabetes: Ask the Diabetes Team
www.childrenwithdiabetes.com/dteam/d_0d_000.htm

This extensive web site addresses many aspects of living with childhood diabetes. A team of diabetes health care professionals, including pediatric, adolescent, and adult endocrinologists, specialists in managing diabetes during pregnancy, diabetes nurse specialists, dietitians, exercise physiologists, researchers and counselors, will answer your questions. But first, check out the extensive archive of previous questions and answers. This site subscribes to the Health on the Net (HON) Code of Conduct for medical and health web sites. (See the introduction to this section.)

Eyes

Ask an Optometrist
www.visioncare.com

You can e-mail your vision care questions to optometrist Craig S. Steinberg, O.D. at City Eyes Optometry Center in

Los Angeles. You can also purchase sunglasses and contact lens (with a valid prescription) from the site.

Ask an Eye Doctor
www.magrudereye.com

The doctors at the Magruder Eye Institute in central Florida can field your questions on glaucoma treatment, pediatric eye care, diabetic and other eye diseases, cataract and corneal surgery, and surgery to correct nearsightedness or misalignment. They have posted lots of information for you to access, and you can also consult them by e-mail. This site is accessible in both English and Spanish.

Joint Pain And Arthritis

Back or Joint Paint: Ask Dr. Puentes
www.openmri-southtexas.com/askthe.html

Dr. Jairo A. Puentes, a board certified physician in the fields of physical medicine and rehabilitation and electrodiagnostic medicine and pain management, will respond to questions concerning low back pain, cervical spine pain, carpal tunnel syndrome, nerve injuries, muscle and ligament injuries and join pain. The site, which links to the Saratoga Medical Center in Corpus Christi, Texas, also contains a set of frequently asked questions on these topics.

Arthritis Expertise: Ask the Arthritis Foundation

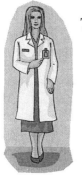

www.arthritis.org/forms/ask_help.asp
The national offices of the Arthritis Foundation in Atlanta offer a wealth of information about arthritis. Check their extensive archives at www.arthritis.org/resource or e-mail your question to their medical staff at the address above. You will receive a response within 24 to 48 hours, or, for a written response (perhaps for a friend or relative without computer access), you can e-mail a postal address.

Ask Dr. Bones: Information on Arthritis, Joint Pain and Sports Injuries

http://bunny.lek.net/~fed/

Dr. Bones identifies himself only as a rheumatologist who specializes in the diagnosis and treatment of arthritis and related diseases. His site includes information on various conditions and treatments. You can also send him an e-mail requesting information about your specific problem.

Knee Problems: Ask an Orthopedic Surgeon

www.knees.com

Dr. Jack Kriegsman, M.D., a board certified orthopedic surgeon, responds on how he would treat a specific knee problem. You can also visit an archive of previous questions and Dr. Kriegsman's answers. The site is hosted by the Center for Arthroscopic Surgery of Southern California and Sports Medicine. Dr. Krigsman has performed more than 6,500 arthroscopic surgical procedures since 1974.

Men's Health

Guy Stuff: Ask the Urologist
www.methodisthealth.com/Urology/ask.htm

A team of more than 20 physicians at the Urology Institute at the Methodist Hospital in Houston are standing by to respond to your plumbing questions. You can e-mail a specific question, or check the site's frequently answered questions section to see if it's already been addressed. Appropriate topics include: low sperm counts, cancer, medications, and sexual functions.

Mental Health

Ask a Mental Health Expert
www.mhsource.com/expert.html

Dr. Ron Pies, M.D., a clinical professor of psychiatry at Tufts University and columnist for Psychiatric Times, fields questions on a huge range of topics, including Attention Deficit Disorder, Alzheimer's Disease, caregiving issues, medications, schizophrenia, sexual issues, sleep disorders, bipolar mood disorder (manic-depressive illness), stress, substance abuse, and depression, to name just a few. You can e-mail your questions directly to him on the link provided; if your question is selected, in three weeks or less a response will be posted on this site. Your name and e-mail address will not appear. You may not need to wait so long, however; since answers to all previously posted questions are accessible by linking to the online archive at {www.mhsource.com/expert/consumer.html}. Chances are you'll find your question has been addressed already. The Psychiatric Times home page, "Mental Health Infosource," also provides an on-line locator service to identify a mental health practitioner near you.

Wisdom of the Ages: Ask Great-Granny
www.mbnet.mb.ca/crm/granny/granny.html#loc

Great-Granny, a.k.a. Rosaleen Dickson of Ottawa, Canada, may not have a M.D. after her name, but she does have a degree in psychology, six children, 14 grandchildren and four great grandsons. She dispenses practical thoughts on coping with problems arising from the increasing differences in attitudes and life styles between the generations. You can e-mail her directly, or check her archives for topics such as parents, young children, older children, children's boy or girl friends, grandparents, grandchildren, in-laws, siblings, husbands, sexual orientation and other topics.

Attention Deficit Disorder: Ask a Psychologist
www.erols.com/drleeb

Dr. Jack Leeb, a board certified psychologist as well as a board certified forensic examiner in independent practice in Silver Spring, Maryland, offers general information on attention deficit disorder and links to other related sites, along with an e-mail link if you want to ask a specific question. Although you can access various articles, there is no questions and answers document on the site.

Muscular Dystropy

Muscular Dystrophy Association: Ask the Experts
www.mdausa.org/experts
This extensive site provides information on 40 neuro-muscular diseases (click on "Diseases") and read responses to other site visitors' questions. You can query MDA-supported scientists and physicians on a broad range of topics.

Neurology

Ask a Neurosurgery Nurse
www.surgery.missouri.edu/ns/Services/nurse.html
You can question advanced practice nurses with specialized training and experience in neurosurgery on topics such as back pain, neck pain, surgery of the brain and nervous system in children and adults, vascular problems in the brain, neurological problems in children, and general neurosurgery. Clicking the "home" button will take you to the University of Missouri-Columbia neurosurgery home page, which has a link to the "Hyperbook of Neurosurgery" {www.neuroworld.com/hyperbook.index.html}, a series of articles on neurosurgery topics.

Ask a Neurosurgeon
www.dr-neurosurg.com/index.html
David F. Dean, M.D., a neurosurgeon practicing in San Antonio, Texas, will respond to questions related to neurosurgery. Unlike some other sites, Dr. Dean does not offer a lot of easily accessible general information—the

patient advice and care section dumps you into a neurology search engine. If Dr. Dean cannot answer your question, he will refer you to a doctor who can, and he will also try to recommend a specialist in your area if you tell him where you live.

Ask a Neurologist at Harvard
www.bih.harvard.edu/neurology/docbag.htm
This page is meant to provide a bulletin-board type forum for readers to ask questions of the experts at Harvard Medical School Department of Neurology. You can e-mail your queries if they are sufficiently general that posting both the question and the answer will be of interest to readers. Messages will be treated with complete confidentiality. If your question is very specific, or it involves details of your medical history, you should identify a specific staff member via the Department Staff listing, and click on the link to that doctor's e-mail. This page will also allow you to read the archives of past questions and answers.

Pain

Ask the Pain Doctor
www.pain.com/drfiles/default.cfm
This extensive site, which is hosted by the Dannemiller Memorial Education Foundation in San Antonio, Texas, covers many aspects of pain and pain management, from heel spurs to palliative care for cancer patients. You can ask physicians from various fields your question, or search the extensive archives for questions and answers from other pain sufferers.

Pediatrics

Baby Care: Ask Dr. Plain Talk
www.drplaintalk.org
Dr. Rob Payne, medical director of the
neonatal intensive care unit at Children's
Hospitals and Clinics in Minneapolis, edits
this site, which features medical answers in
parent-friendly language. You can e-mail
the doctor a children's health question, or search
the archives for information on topics previously covered.

Ask a Pediatrician
www.drs4kids.com/index.html
You can correspond with Dr. Frederic Suser, a pediatrician
practicing on Long Island, New York, on various child-
related topics, as well as read his answers to previous
queries. This site also markets childcare products under the
brand name Drs4Kids; it is not clear what connection, if
any, Dr. Suser has to the sale of these products.

Pediatrics: Electronic Consultations from the Children's Medical Center of the University of Virginia
www.med.virginia.edu/cmc/emailsrv.html
Doctors on the staff of the University of Virginia's
Children's Medical Center will take your e-mail questions
on pediatric gastroenterology and nutrition, pediatric
hematology and oncology, pediatric immunology, pediatric
infectious diseases, genetics and metabolism, and pediatric
organ transplantation.

See Diabetes

Plastic Surgery

"E-sthetics": Ask a Plastic Surgeon
www.phudson.com/WELCOME/form.html
Dr. Patrick Hudson, a board certified plastic surgeon practicing in Albuquerque, New Mexico, authors this extensive site, which features information about various cosmetic plastic surgery techniques, such as facial sculpturing, body sculpturing and scar revision, face lifting, liposuction, breast enlargement and reduction and tummy tucks. You can e-mail the doctor directly, but first check out the information on specific procedures he provides.

Plastic Surgery, Skin Cancer and Melanoma
www.ariyan.com/index.html
Dr. Stephan Ariyan is a plastic surgeon specializing in reconstructive and cosmetic surgery of the head, neck and breast and malignant melanoma who practices in New Haven, Connecticut. His site contains brief bits of information about a variety of procedures, but you can send him an e-mail with specific questions.

Radiology

Radiology: Get a Second Opinion
http://telescan.nki.nl/SecondOpinion/index.html
The radiology faculty of the Virchow Klinikum at Humbolt University in Berlin will provide a free second opinion on mammograms, CT scans and MRIs. You will need to send these images as attached files; be sure to check with your

radiologist to see whether they will scan with sufficient clarity before you make the effort to send them through cyberspace.

Veterinary

Ask a Veterinarian
www.prah.com/ask.htm
This quirky, entertaining site features a team of veterinarians at the Preston Road Animal Hospital in Dallas, Texas, who can field your questions on pet care. It may take several weeks for them to get back to you, and, due to the number of questions they receive, you may not receive an individualized response. However, the site also lists previous questions and the doctors' responses, as well as links to specific information on health issues for dogs, cats, birds and small mammals, so you may well find what you are looking for. Go to www.prah.com/Reference+ Library.htm for general information on specific topics. You'll also find a set of New Year's resolutions for dogs and samples of sayings you'll only hear in the South.

Good Dogs: Ask the K-9 Shrink
www.k9shrink.com/html/askdoc.html
Gail Clark, Ph.D., a.k.a. the K-9 Shrink, is a canine psychologist, dog behavior specialist, trainer and obedience and breed exhibitor. She has worked with more than 8,000 dogs of all sizes, breeds, and temperaments. You can e-mail her about your pet's peeves and, once a month; she will post the answer to one of the questions she receives.

Women's Health

A Forum for Women's Health: Ask Karen Sarpolis, M.D.
www.estronaut.com/n/ask.htm

This web site contains information on a large number of topics ranging from athletic issues, sexual function, nutrition and eating disorders, cancer, aging, osteoporosis, and more. You can e-mail your question directly to Dr. Sarpolis on the link provided. Like other services, your question may not be answered, but you are likely to find the information you seek in the archives, which are linked to the site. Dr. Sarpolis is the medical director of GenneX Healthcare Technologies, the sponsor of the site.

a Doctor: Cancers in Women's Reproductive Organs
www.143.111.212.41/cancerinfoask_doc.htm

This service is part of a much larger site for the M.D. Anderson Cancer Center in Houston, Texas, which, along with the Sloan Kettering Institute, is the largest cancer facility in the country. Physicians who are board certified in obstetrics, gynecology, and oncology will field your questions on cancers of the ovaries, fallopian tubes, uterus, cervix, vagina and vulva, and gestational trophoblastic disease. You will also find extensive information on these diseases by clicking "Women's Cancer Information Net."

Free Hotlines, Publications and Expertise on Any Health Topic

Don't know where to go or who to call? We have compiled a listing of resources you can call to receive information, support, assistance, and sometimes even treatment for a specific condition or disease! The following government and non-profit organizations are experts in their specific areas and will help you online or on the telephone with free expertise, publications, and referrals. You are not alone. Help is just a phone call or a click away.

General Health

National Women's Health Information
    Center
U.S. Public Health Service
Office on Women's Health
1600 Clifton Road, NE
Atlanta, GA 30333
800-944-WOMEN
www.4women.gov
National centers

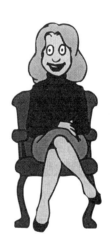

Some publications available include:
- ★ *Cancer Statistics*
- ★ *Pills, Patches and Shots: Can Hormones Prevent Aging?*
- ★ *Breast Cancer: a Report on the Fight to Prevent, Treat, and Cure the Disease*

★ *Women of Color Health Data Book*
★ and many more.

National Health Information Center
P.O. Box 1133
Washington, DC 20013
800-336-4797
301-565-4167
Fax: 301-984-4256
http://nhic-nt.health.org
Excellent phone referral service
Some publications available include:
★ *Toll-Free Numbers for Health Information*
★ *Federal Health Information Centers and Clearinghouses*
★ and many more

Adoption

National Adoption Information Clearinghouse
330 C Street, NW
Washington, DC 20447
703-352-3488
Fax: 703-385-3206
www.calib.com/naic
Some publications available include:
★ *State Adoption Statute Summaries*
★ *Adoption: Where Do I Start*
★ *After Adoption: The Need for Services*
★ *Foster Parents Adoption: What Parents Should Know*
★ and many more.

National Adoption Center
1500 Walnut Street, #701
Philadelphia, PA 19108
800-TO-ADOPT
215-735-9988
Fax: 215-735-9410
www.adopt.org
Some publications available include:

★ *When Adoption is the Answer: A Guidebook for Parents*
★ *Special Needs Adoption*
★ *Single Parent Adoption*
★ *Open Adoption*
★ and many more.

Aging

National Aging Information Center
U.S. Administration on Aging
330 Independence Avenue, NW
Room 4656
Washington, DC 20211
202-619-7501
Fax: 202-401-7620
www.aoa.dhhs.gov/naic/
Some publications available
include:

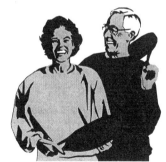

★ *Older Persons with Mobility and Self-Care Limitations*
★ *Elder Abuse Prevention*
★ *Housing Options for Older Americans*

★ *Protecting the Rights of Older Americans*
★ and many more.

National Institute on Aging Information Center
P.O. Box 8057
Gaithersburg, MD 20898
800-222-2225
301-587-2528
TDD: 800-222-4225
Fax: 301-589-3041
www.nih.gov/nia
Some publications available include:
★ *Accidental Hypothermia: Cold Weather Can be Trouble*
★ *Urinary Incontinence*
★ *Aging and Your Eyes*
★ *Don't Take it Easy — Exercise!*
★ *Age Pages*
★ *Menopause*
★ *Talking With Your Doctor*
★ and many more.

American Association of Retired Persons (AARP)
601 E Street, NW
Washington, DC 20049
800-424-3410
www.aarp.org
State Offices and Information Centers
Some publications available include:
★ *Home Improvement Fraud*
★ *Chronic Disease Management*

★ *Nursing Home Admission Contract*
★ *QMB: Dollars To Help Pay For Medicare*
★ and many more.

AIDS

CDC National Prevention Information Network
P.O. Box 6003
Rockville, MD 20849
800-458-5231
Fax: 301-738-6616
TDD: 800-243-7012
AIDS Clinical Trials: 800-874-2572
Fax-Back Service: 800-458-5231
HIV/AIDS Treatment: 800-448-0440; 301-519-0459
www.cdcnpin.org
Some publications available include:

★ *A Guide to AIDS in the Workplace Resources*
★ *Because You Love Them: A Parents Planning Guide Child Welfare League of America*
★ *Caring for Someone With AIDS at Home: A Guide*
★ *Does Sex Education Work?*
★ *AIDS Prevention Guide*
★ *Living with HIV/AIDS*
★ and many more

Alcoholism

National Clearinghouse for Alcohol and Drug Information
P.O. Box 2345
Rockville, MD 20847
800-729-6686

www.health.org
Some publications available include:
- ★ *Alcoholism: Getting the Facts*
- ★ *Growing Up Drug Free: A Parent's Guide to Prevention*
- ★ *Marijuana: Facts Parents Should Know*

Allergies

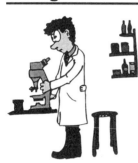

National Institute of Allergy and
Infectious Diseases
Office of Communications
Building 31, Room 7A50
900 Rockville Pike
Bethesda, MD 20892
301-496-5717
www.niaid.nih.gov
Some publications available include:
- ★ *Allergies: Living With Allergies*
- ★ *How to Create a Dust-Free Bedroom*
- ★ *Living With Food Allergies*
- ★ *Resources to Fight Indoor Pollution*
- ★ and many more.

Alternative Medicine

National Center for Complementary and Alternative
Medicine Clearinghouse
P.O. Box 8218
Silver Spring, MD 20907
888-644-6226 (toll-free)
800-531-7194 (Fax-back)
http://altmed.od.nih.gov/ncccam/clearinghouse/

Some publications available include:

★ *General Information*

★ *Frequently Asked Questions*

★ *Classification of Complementary and Alternative Health Care Practices*

★ *Alternative Medicine Research Using MEDLINE*

★ and many more.

Alzheimer's Disease

Alzheimer's Disease Education and Referral Center
National Institute on Aging
P.O. Box 8250
Silver Spring, MD 20907
800-438-4380
www.alzheimers.org
Centers in many states
Some publications available include:

★ *Alzheimer's Disease Genetics Fact Sheet*

★ *Estrogen and Alzheimer's Disease*

★ *Talking with Your Doctor: A Guide for Older People*

★ *Alzheimer's Disease: A Caregiver and Patient Resource List*

★ and many more.

Alzheimer's Association
919 North Michigan Avenue
Suite 1000
Chicago, IL 60611
800-272-3900
www.alz.org

Local chapters

Some publications available include:

★ *Information For Newly Diagnosed Individuals And Their Families*

★ *Caregiver Tips*

★ *Information for those who suspect*

★ *General Information about Alzheimer's*

★ and many more.

Arthritis

National Arthritis and Musculoskeletal and Skin Diseases
    Information Clearinghouse

1 AMS Circle

Bethesda, MD 20892

301-495-4484

301-881-2731 (Fax-back service)

www.nih.gov/niams

Some publications available include:

★ *Q&A Arthritis and Exercise*

★ *Q&A Arthritis Pain*

★ *Q&A Arthritis and Rheumatic Disease*

★ *Q&A Juvenile Rheumatoid Arthritis*

★ and many more.

Arthritis Foundation

1330 West Peachtree Street

Atlanta, GA 30309

404-872-7100, ext. 6350

800-238-7800

www.arthritis.org

Local chapters

Some publications available include:
- ★ *Exercise and Your Arthritis*
- ★ *Can You Prevent It?*
- ★ *Is It Arthritis?*
- ★ *What Treatments Work*
- ★ and many more.

Asthma

Allergy and Asthma Network/Mothers
   of Asthmatics
2751 Prosperity Avenue
Suite 150
Fairfax, VA 22031
703-641-9595
800-878-4403
Fax: 703-573-7794
www.aanma.org

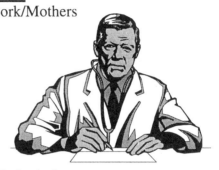

Some publications available include:
- ★ *When to See an Asthma Specialist*
- ★ *Asthma in Infants*
- ★ *Clearing The Air on Asthma and Allergy Medications*
- ★ *Your Health Insurance Plan, Questions You Should Ask*
- ★ and many more.

Asthma and Allergy Foundation of America
1125 Fifteenth Street, NW, Suite 502
Washington, DC 20005
202-466-7643
Fax: 202-466-8940

www.aafa.org
Local chapters
Some publications available include:
* ★ *You Can Control Asthma*
* ★ *Answers*
* ★ *What People With Asthma Should Know About Leukotrienes*
* ★ *AAFA Newsletters*
* ★ and much more.

National Asthma Education and Prevention Program
National Heart Lung, and Blood Institute Information
    Center
P.O. Box 30105
Bethesda, MD 20824
301-529-8573
www.nhlbi.nih.gov/nhlbi/nhlbi.htm
Some publications available include:
* ★ *Asthma and Physical Activity In The School*
* ★ *Your Asthma Can Be Controlled: Expect Nothing Less*

Bacterial Disease

National Center for Infectious Disease
1600 Clifton Road, NE
Atlanta, GA 30333
404-639-1338
888-4HEP-CDC
www.cdc.gov/ncidod/op/index.htm
Some publications available include:
* ★ *Emerging Infectious Disease Threats*

★ *Cholera Prevention*
★ *Bacterial and Mycotic Diseases*
★ *Group B Streptococcal Infections*
★ and many more.

Behavior Disorders

The Federation of Families for Children's Mental Health
1021 Prince Street
Alexandria, VA 22314-2971
703-684-7710
Fax: 703-836-1040
www.ffcmh.org
Local chapters and affiliates
Some publications available include:
★ *Fact Sheets on Childhood Disorders*
★ *Finding Help, Finding Hope*
★ *Principles on Family Support*
★ *Why Children Are Not Little Adults*
★ and many more.

American Academy of Child and Adolescent Psychiatry
3615 Wisconsin Avenue, NW
Washington, DC 20016-3007
202-966-7300
Fax: 202-966-2891
www.aacap.org
Some publications available include:
★ *The Autistic Child*
★ *Children and Grief*
★ *Children's Major Psychiatric Disorders*
★ *Know When to Seek Help for Your Child*

Bicycle Safety

Bicycle Helmet Safety Institute
4611 Seventh Street South
Arlington, VA 22204-1419
703-486-0100
703-486-0579
Fax: 703-486-0576
www.bhsi.org
Some publications available include:
- ★ *A Consumer's Guide to Bicycle Helmets*
- ★ *Must I Buy a Bicycle Helmet for My Child?*
- ★ *Teaching Your Child to Ride a Bicycle*
- ★ *Helmet Statistics*
- ★ and many more.

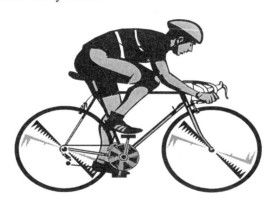

Think First Foundation
22 South Washington Street
Park Ridge, IL 60068
847-692-2740
800-THINK56
Fax: 847-692-2394

www.thinkfirst.org
Some publications available include:
* ★ *Bike Safety*
* ★ *Prevention Pages*
* ★ *Helmet Use*
* ★ *Bicycle Safety Rules*
* ★ and many more.

Birth Defects

March of Dimes Birth Defects Foundation
1275 Mamaroneck Avenue
White Plains, NY 10605
888-MODIMES
914-428-7100
www.modimes.org
Local chapters
Some publications available include:
* ★ *Think Ahead*
* ★ *Deliver The Best*
* ★ *Leading Categories of Birth Defects*
* ★ *Genetic Series*
* ★ and many more

Association of Birth Defect Children, Inc.
827 Irma Avenue
Orlando, FL 32803
800-313-ABDC
407-245-7035
Fax: 407-245-7087
www.birthdefects.org/
Parent matching
Some publications available include:

★ *How to Get Services for Your Child*
★ *How to Make Health Insurance Work for You*
★ *Limb Reduction Defects*
★ *Heart Defects*
★ and many more.

Brain Tumors

American Brain Tumor Association
2720 River Road
Des Plaines, IL 60018
847-827-9910
Patient Line: 800-886-2282
Fax: 847-827-9918
www.abta.org
Some publications available include:
★ *Radiation Therapy of Brain Tumors: A Basic Guide*
★ *Dictionary for Brain Tumor Patients*
★ *When Your Child is Ready to Return to School*
★ *Coping With a Brain Tumor Part I: From Diagnosis to Treatment*
★ and many more.

Burns

Shriners Hospital for Children
International Shrine Headquarters
2900 Rocky Point Drive
Tampa, FL 33607-1435
813-281-0300
800-237-5055
Canada: 800-361-7256
www.shrinershq.org/

Some publications available include:
- ★ *How Safe Is Your Kitchen?*
- ★ *Microwave Burn Prevention*
- ★ *Emergency Treatment Of Burns*
- ★ *How Safe Is Your Tent?*
- ★ and many more.

Phoenix Society for Burn Survivors, Inc.
2153 Wealthy Street, SE, #215
East Grand Rapids, MI 49506
616-458-2773
800-888-BURN (2876)
Fax: 616-458-2831
www.phoenix-society.org/
Local chapters
Some publications available include:
- ★ *Hidden Burns*
- ★ *Itching, What Helps*
- ★ *Burn Scars*
- ★ *Humor and the Burn Patient*
- ★ and many more.

Cancer

Cancer Information
   Service
National Cancer Institute
31 Center Drive
MSC2580
Building 31, Room 10A07
Bethesda, MD 20892-2580
800-4-CANCER
http://cis.nci.nih.gov

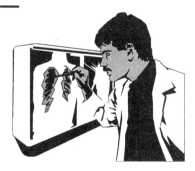

National and regional partners
Some publications available include:
★ *What You Need To Know About TM Cancer — An Overview*
★ *Moles and Dysplastic Nevi*
★ *Non-Hodgkins Lymphomas*
★ *Ovarian Cancer*
★ *Stomach Cancer*
★ and many more

The Candlelighters Childhood Cancer Foundation
7910 Woodmont Avenue, Suite 460
Bethesda, MD 20814-3015
800-366-2223
301-657-8401
Fax: 301-718-2686
www.candlelighters.org
Local chapters
Some publications available include:
★ *Educating the Child with Cancer*
★ *The Candlelighters Guide to Bone Marrow Transplants in Children*
★ *Know Before You Go: The Childhood Cancer Journey*
★ *CCCF Youth Newsletter*
★ and many more.

Cerebral Palsy

United Cerebral Palsy Associations
1660 L Street, NW, Suite 700
Washington, DC 20036
202-842-1266

Voice/TDD: 202-973-7197
Fax: 202-776-0414
202-776-0416
www.ucpa.org/html/
UCP affiliate partners in 43 states
Some publications available include:

★ *Parents Rights: How to be a Good Parent of a Child with Cerebral Palsy*
★ *Advocacy — Taking Charge: How To Do It: A Primer for Parents*
★ *Fast Facts on Individual Education Plans*
★ *VCP Research Fact Sheets*
★ and many more.

Child Abuse

National Clearinghouse on Child Abuse
   and Neglect Information
330 C Street, SW
Washington, DC 20447
800-FYI-3366
703-385-7565
www.calib.com/nccanch
Some publications available include:

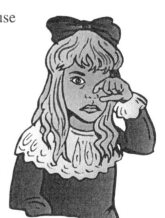

★ *Child Neglect: A Guide for Intervention*
★ *What is Child Maltreatment?*
★ *Resources for Prevention Activities*
★ *In Fact...Answers to Frequently Asked Questions on Child Abuse and Neglect*
★ and many more

National Committee to Prevent Child Abuse
200 South Michigan Ave., 17th Floor
Chicago, IL 60604-4357
800-55-NCPCA
312-663-3520
Fax: 312-939-8912
State chapters
Some publications available include:
- ★ *Child Abuse Hotline Numbers*
- ★ *When Parents Drink Too Much*
- ★ *Twelve Alternatives to Lashing Out at Your Child*
- ★ *Start Using Words That Help*
- ★ and many more.

Child Care

National Child Care Information Center
Administration For Children and Families
243 Church Street, NW, 2nd Floor
Vienna, VA 22180
800-616-2242
http://nccic.org
Linkages with national organizations and clearinghouses
Some publications available include:
- ★ *Baby Safety Shower*
- ★ *Care Around the Clock: Developing Child Care Resources Before 9 and After 5*
- ★ *Child Care and Early Program Participation of Infants, Toddlers, and Preschoolers*
- ★ *Child Care and Medicaid: Partners for Healthy Children*
- ★ and many more.

Child Health

National Institute on Child Health and
    Human Development
National Institutes of Health
31 Center Drive
MSC2425, Room 2A32
Bethesda, MD 20897
301-496-5133
www.nih.gov/nichd
Some publications available include:

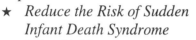

- ★ *Reduce the Risk of Sudden
  Infant Death Syndrome*
- ★ *Why Children Succeed or Fail at Reading*
- ★ *Children and Adolescent Nutrition: Why Milk
  Matters*
- ★ *NICHD Study of Early Child Care*
- ★ and many more.

American Academy of Family Physicians
Manager Information Services Department
11400 Tomahawk Creek Pkwy.
Leawood, KS 66211
913-906-6000
800-274-2237
Fax: 913-906-6095
www.aafp.org
Publications can be viewed online at {http://family
doctor.org}.

National Institute Of Child Health and Human
    Development
P.O. Box 3006

Rockville, MD 20847
800-370-2943
www.nih.gov/nichd
Some publications available include:
- ★ *Pituitary Tumors In Children*
- ★ *Why Children Succeed Or Fail At Reading*
- ★ *Uterine Fibroids*

Child Safety

National SAFE KIDS Campaign
1301 Pennsylvania Avenue, NW, Suite 1000
Washington, DC 20004-1707
202-662-0600
Fax: 202-393-2072
www.safekids.org
Local chapters
Some publications available include:
- ★ *Falls Brochure*
- ★ *Pedestrian Safety*
- ★ *Water Safety*
- ★ *Safe Kids Buckle Up*
- ★ and many more.

Cholesterol

National Cholesterol Education Program
National Heart Lung, and Blood Institute Information
    Center
P.O. Box 30105
Bethesda, MD 20824
301-529-8573
www.nhlbi.nih.gov/

Some publications available include:
- ★ *So You Have High Blood Cholesterol*
- ★ *Step By Step: Eating To Lower Your High Blood Cholesterol*

Craniofacial Deformities

Children's Craniofacial Association
9441 LBJ Freeway, Suite 115, LB 46
Dallas, TX 75243
972-994-9902
800-535-3643
Fax: 972-240-7607
www.masterlink.com/children/

Cleft Palate Foundation
104 South Estes Drive, Suite 204
Chapel Hill, NC 27514
919-933-9044
800-24-CLEFT
Fax: 919-933-9604
www.cleft.com/cpf.htm
Connects callers with parent-patient support groups in their area
Some publications available include:
- ★ *Information about Choosing a Cleft Palate or Craniofacial Team*
- ★ *Feeding an Infant with Cleft*
- ★ *Cleft Lip and Plate: The First Four Years*
- ★ *Genetics of Cleft Lip and Palate: Information for Families*
- ★ and many more.

Deafness

National Institute on Deafness and Other Communications
  Disorders Information Clearinghouse
1 Communication Avenue
Bethesda, MD 20892
800-241-1044
TTY: 800-241-1055
www.nih.gov/nidcd
Some publications available include:

  ★ *Early Identification of Hearing Impairment in
     Infants and Young Children*
  ★ *How Loud Is Too Loud?*
  ★ *Ten Best Ways To Recognize Hearing Loss*
  ★ *Cochlear Implants in Adults and Children*
  ★ and many more.

Alexander Graham Bell Association for the Deaf
3417 Volta Place, NW
Washington, DC 20007-2778
Voice-TTY: 202-337-5220
Fax: 202-337-8314
www.agbell.org
Local chapters in many states
Some publications available include:

  ★ *Oral Interpreters: Facts For Consumers*
  ★ *Speech and Hearing Checklist*
  ★ *Communicating With People Who Have a Hearing
     Loss*
  ★ *Speechreading for Better Communication*
  ★ and many more.

Depression

National Mental Health
   Association
Public Information
1021 Prince Street
Alexandria, VA 22314
703-684-7722
800-969-6642
www.nmha.org
Nationwide affiliates
Some publications available
include:

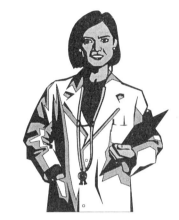

- ★ *Depression in Children*
- ★ *Controlling Your Anger*
- ★ *Coping With Loss: Bereavement and Grief*
- ★ *Mental Illness in the Family: Recognizing Warning Signs and How to Cope*
- ★ and many more

National Institute of Mental Health
National Institutes of Health
9000 Rockville Pike, MSC 80-30
Bethesda, MD 20892
301-443-4513
800-421-4211
800-64-PANIC (panic disorder hotline)
888-8-ANXIETY (anxiety disorders hotline)
www.nimh.nih.gov
Some publications available include:

- ★ *A Consumers Guide to Mental Health Services*
- ★ *Medications*
- ★ *Plain Talk About Handling Stress*

★ *Understanding Panic Disorders*
★ and many more.

Diabetes

National Diabetes Information Clearinghouse
1 Information Way
Bethesda, MD 20892
301-654-3327
www.niddk.nih.gov/health/ diabetes/ndic.htm
Some publications available include:
★ *Kidney Disease of Diabetes*
★ *Alternative Ways To Take Insulin*
★ *Financial Help for Diabetes Care*
★ *Joint and Bone Conditions Related to Diabetes*
★ *Insulin Dependent Diabetes*
★ and many more.

American Diabetes Association
1660 Duke Street
Alexandria, VA 22314
800-232-3472
www.diabetes.org
Local chapters
Some publications available include:
★ *Diabetes Diagnosis and Understanding Lab Tests*
★ *Medical Treatment of Diabetes*
★ *1999 Buyers Guide to Diabetes Supplies*
★ *Complications and Related Concerns*
★ and many more

Juvenile Diabetes Foundation International
120 Wall Street, 19th Floor

New York, NY 10005
212-785-9500
800-223-1138
www.jdfcure.org
Local chapters
Some publications available include:
- ★ *Diabetes Facts*
- ★ *COUNTDOWN for Kids*
- ★ *Diabetes Glossary*
- ★ and more.

Digestive Disorders

National Digestive Diseases Information Clearinghouse
2 Information Way
Bethesda, MD 20892
301-654-3810
www.niddk.nih.gov/health/digest/nddic.htm
Some publications available include:
- ★ *Facts and Fallacies About Digestive Diseases*
- ★ *Your Digestive System and How It Works*
- ★ *Bleeding in the Digestive Tract*
- ★ *Digestive Diseases Dictionary*
- ★ *Constipation*
- ★ *Gallstones*
- ★ and many more.

Disabilities

National Rehabilitation Information Center
National Institute on Disabilities and Rehabilitation
    Research
8455 Colesville Road, Suite 935

Silver Spring, MD 20910
301-558-9284
TTY: 301-495-5626
800-346-2742
www.cais.com/naric
Some publications available include:
*   ★ *Income and Program Participation of People with Work Disabilities*
*   ★ *Vocational Rehabilitation in the United States*
*   ★ *Health Conditions and Impairments Causing Disabilities*
*   ★ *Need for Assistance in the Activities of Daily Living*
*   ★ and many more.

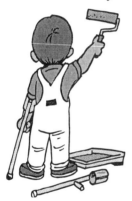

National Information Center for Children and Youth with Disabilities
P.O. Box 1492
Washington, DC 20013
800-695-0285
www.nichcy.org
Some publications available include:
*   ★ *Options After High School*
*   ★ *State Resources Sheet*
*   ★ *Parents Guide to Accessing Programs for Infants, Toddlers and Preschoolers with Disabilities*
*   ★ *Vocational Assessment*
*   ★ and many more.

PAWS With a Cause
4646 South Division
Wayland, MI 49348

616-877-0248
TDD/Voice: 800-253-PAWS
www.pawscause.org
Trains Assistance Dogs nationally
Publishes *Dogs for Dignity* Newsletter

Domestic Violence

National Domestic Violence Hotline
P.O. Box 161810
Austin, TX 78716
512-453-8117
800-799-SAFE
www.ndvh.org

Down Syndrome

National Down Syndrome Society
666 Broadway, 8th Floor
New York, NY 10012-2317
212-460-9660
800-221-4602
Fax: 212-979-2873
www.ndss.org
Local affiliate groups
Pamphlets on issues related to Down Syndrome which
include:
 ★ general
 ★ heart
 ★ speech
 ★ life planning
 ★ and more.

Eating Disorders

Overeaters Anonymous, Inc.
Public Information Director
P.O. Box 44020
Rio Rancho, NM 87174-4020
505-891-2664
Fax: 505-891-4320
www.overeatersanonymous.org/
About 9,000 groups in 50 countries worldwide
Some publications available include:
- ★ *A Program of Recovery*
- ★ *The Newcomer's Packet*
- ★ *Think First*
- ★ *Recovery Checklist*
- ★ and many more.

American Anorexia Bulimia Association
165 West 46 Street, #1108
New York, NY 10036
212-575-6200
www.aabainc.org
Local chapters in 4 states

Endometriosis

Endometriosis Research Center
751 Park of Commerce Drive, Suite 130
Boca Raton, FL 33487
561-988-0767
800-239-7200
Fax: 561-995-7121
www.endocenter.org

Some publications available include:
*   ★ *Endometriosis FAQ*
*   ★ *Endo and Infertility*
*   ★ *Laparoscopy*
*   ★ *Alternative Therapies/Diet*
*   ★ and many more.

Environmental Health

Children's Environmental Health Network
5900 Hollis Street, Suite R3
Emeryville, CA 94608
510-597-1393
Fax: 510-597-1399
www.cehn.org/cehn/index.html
Some publications available include:
*   ★ *Chronology of Children's Environmental Health*
*   ★ *Preventing Child Exposures to Environmental Hazards*
*   ★ *Children's Environmental Health and Cancer in Children*
*   ★ *Child Health and Asthma*
*   ★ and many more.

National Institute of Environmental Health Sciences
P.O. Box 12233
Mail Drop 32-05
Research Triangle Park, NC 27709
800-643-4794
919-541-3345
Fax: 919-541-4395
www.niehs.nih.gov

Some local centers
Some publications available include:
* ★ *Medicine for the Layman—Environment and Disease*
* ★ *Questions and Answers About EMF*
* ★ *Questions and Answers—EMF in the Workplace*
* ★ *Asthma and Allergy Prevention*
* ★ and many more.

Epilepsy

Epilepsy Foundation
4315 Garden City Drive
Landover, MD 20785
301-459-3700
800-EFA-1000
Fax: 301-557-4941
www.epilepsyfoundation.org
Local affiliates
Some publications available include:
* ★ *Epilepsy Facts and Figures*
* ★ *The Workbook: A Self-Study Guide for Job Seekers with Epilepsy*
* ★ *Parenting and You: A Guide for Parents with Seizure Disorders*
* ★ and many more.

Eye Problems

National Eye Institute
Bldg. 31, Room 6A32
Bethesda, MD 20892
301-496-5248
www.nei.nih.gov

Some publications available include:
- ★ *Don't Lose Sight Of Glaucoma*
- ★ *Don't Lose Sight of Cataract*

Food and Drug Information

Food and Drug Administration
Office of Consumer Affairs
5600 Fishers Lane, HFE-88
Rockville, MD 20857
888-463-6332
www.fda.gov
Some publications available
include:

- ★ *New Animal Drug for Increasing Milk Production*
- ★ *Olestra and Other Fat Substitutes*
- ★ *Questions to Ask Your Pharmacist*
- ★ *Homeopathy: Real Medicine or Empty Promise*
- ★ and many more.

Food Safety and Nutrition Information

International Food Information Council Foundation
1100 Connecticut Avenue, NW, Suite 430
Washington, DC 20036
202-296-6540
Fax: 202-296-6547
http://ificinfo.health.org
Some publications available include:
- ★ *A Consumers Guide to Pesticides*
- ★ *Everything You Need to Know About Asthma and Food*

* *Everything You Need to Know About Glutamate and Monosodium Glutamate*
* *Understanding Food Allergy*
* and many more

Center for Food Safety and Applied Nutrition
200 C Street, SW
Washington, DC 20204
800-FDA-4010
202-205-5004
http://vm.cfsan.fda.gov/
Some publications available include:
* *Foodborne Illness: What Consumers Need To Know*
* *All About Cooking Thermometers*
* *Can Your Kitchen Pass the Food Safety Test?*
* *Safer Eggs: Laying the Groundwork*
* and many more.

Gastroesophageal Reflux Disease

Pediatric/Adolescent Gastroesophageal Reflux Association
P.O. Box 1153
Germantown, MD 20875-1153
301-601-9541
www.reflux.org
Some local support chapters
Some publications available include:
* *About Pediatric GER*
* *Reflux Digest: Focus on Medication*
* *Reflux Digest: Focus on Surgery*
* *Breastfeeding*
* and more.

Head Injury

Brain Injury Association, Inc.
105 North Alfred Street
Alexandria, VA 22314:
703-236-6000
800-444-6443
Fax: 703-236-6001
www.biausa.org/
State affiliates
Some publications available include:
- ★ *Sports and Concussion*
- ★ *The Road To Rehabilitation: Cognition and Memory*
- ★ *Firearms Safety Fact Sheet*
- ★ *Living Life After Brain Injury*
- ★ and many more.

American Association of Neurological Surgeons/Congress
   of Neurological Surgeons
22 South Washington Street
Park Ridge, IL 60068
847-692-9500
Fax: 847-692-2589
www.aans.org/splash.html
Some publications available include:
- ★ *Head Injury Brochure*
- ★ *Sports-related Head Injury FAQ*
- ★ *Head Injury — Questions to Ask!*
- ★ *Questions and Answers — Head Injury*
- ★ and more.

Hearing Problems

National Institute On Deafness and Other Communication
    Disorders
1 Communication Way
Bethesda, MD 20892
800-241-1044
www.nih.gov/nidcd
Some publications available include:
- ★ *Cochlear Implants*
- ★ *Stuttering Fact Sheet*
- ★ *Silence Isn't Always Golden*

Heart Disease

American Heart Association
7272 Greenville Avenue
Dallas, TX 75231
214-706-1200
800-242-8721
www.americanheart.org
Local chapters
Some publications available include:
- ★ *Congestive Heart Failure*

★ *Implantable Defibrillators*
★ *What is Heart Disease?*
★ *Cardiac Rehabilitation*
★ and many more.

National Heart, Lung, and Blood Institute
Information Center
P.O. Box 30105
301-251-1222
800-575-WELL
www.nhlbi.nih.gov/
Some publications available include:
★ *Controlling High Blood Pressure: A Guide for Older Women*
★ *Healthy Heart Handbook for Women*
★ *Facts About Angina*
★ *Fact About Coronary Heart Disease*
★ and many more.

High Blood Pressure

National Heart Lung, and Blood Institute Information
    Center
P.O. Box 30105
Bethsda, MD 20824
301-529-8573
www.nhlbi.nih.gov/
Some publications available include:
★ *Protect Your Heat! Prevent High Blood Pressure*
★ *Controlling High Blood Pressure: A Woman's Guide*
★ *How To Prevent High Blood Pressure*

Immunizations

Centers for Disease Control and Prevention
Mail Stop D25
1600 Clifton Road, NE
Atlanta, GA 30333
800-CDC-SHOT
www.cdc.gov
Facilities in 10 states
Some publications available include:
- ★ *6 Common Misconceptions about Vaccination*
- ★ *Vaccine Safety: What You Need to Know*
- ★ *Adult Immunizations: Strategies That Work*
- ★ *Immunizations Factsheets*
- ★ and many more.

Impotence

National Kidney and Urologic Diseases Information
      Clearinghouse
3 Information Way
Bethesda, MD 20892
301-654-4415
www.niddk.nih.gov
Some publications available include:
- ★ *Impotence*

Incontinence

National Kidney and Urologic Diseases Information
      Clearinghouse
3 Information Way
Bethesda, MD 20892
301-654-4415
www.niddk.nih.gov

Some publications available include:
* ★ *Urinary Incontinence In Children*
* ★ *Urinary Tract Infections In Children*

Kidney Disease

National Kidney and Urologic Diseases Information
    Clearinghouse
3 Information Way
Bethesda, MD 20892
301-654-4415
www.niddk.nih.gov/health/kidney/nkudic.htm
Some publications available include:
* ★ *Kidney Disease of Diabetics*
* ★ *Polycystic Kidney Disease*
* ★ *Your Kidneys and How They Work*
* ★ *Kidney Transplantation*
* ★ and many more.

Lead

National Lead Information Center
8601 Georgia Avenue, Suite 503
Silver Springs, MD 20910
800-424-LEAD (clearinghouse)
800-LEAD-FYI (hotline)
www.epa.gov/lead/nlic.htm
Some publications available include:
* ★ *Lead in Your Drinking Water*
* ★ *Lead in Your Home: A Parents Reference Guide*
* ★ *Lead Poisoning and Your Children*
* ★ *Occupational Exposure to Lead: Final Standard*
* ★ and many more.

Learning Disabilities

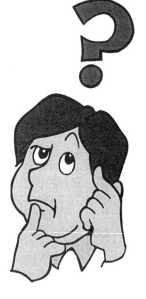

Learning Disabilities Association of
America
4156 Library Road
Pittsburgh, PA 15234-1349
412-341-1515
Fax: 412-344-0224
www.ldanatl.org
Local chapters
Some publications available include:
* ★ *Central Auditory Processing Problems in Children*
* ★ *Speech-Language Disorders, Early Identification of*
* ★ *Learning Disabilities and Educational Standards*
* ★ *Early Childhood*
* ★ and many more.

National Center for Learning Disabilities Inc.
381 Park Avenue South, Suite 1401
New York, NY 10016
212-545-7510
Toll Free and Referral: 888-575-7373
Some publications available include:
* ★ *The Evaluation Process*
* ★ *General Information Packet on Learning Disabilities*
* ★ *NCLD TIPS*
* ★ *JD/LD Link (Juvenile Delinquency and Learning Disabilities)*
* ★ and many more.

Liver Disease

American Liver Foundation
75 Maiden Lane
Suite 603
New York, NY 10038
800-GO-LIVER (465-4837)
973-256-2550
www.liverfoundation.org
Local chapters
Some publications available include:
* ★ *Hepatitis C*
* ★ *Other Diseases and Forms of Liver Injury*
* ★ *Pediatric Liver Disease*
* ★ *Diagnosis and Prevention*
* ★ and many more.

Leukemia

Leukemia Society of America
Marketing Department
600 Third Avenue, 4th Floor
New York, NY 10016
212-573-8484
800-955-4LSA
www.leukemia.org
Local chapters
Some publications available include:
* ★ *What Everyone Should Know About Leukemia*
* ★ *Emotional Aspects of Childhood Leukemia*
* ★ *Bone Marrow Transplantation*
* ★ *Making Intelligent Choices About Therapy*
* ★ and many more.

National Children's Leukemia Foundation
250 East 63rd Street
New York, NY 10021
212-644-8822
24 hour hotline: 800-GIVE HOPE (440-3467)
Fax: 212-644-8826
www.leukemiafoundation.org/home/1found/index.html

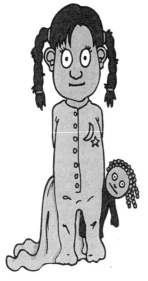

Children With Leukemia
JLS Foundation
14160 Dallas Parkway #300
Dallas, TX 75240
972-308-8383
Fax: 972-770-5666
www.jlsfoundation.org
Some publications available
include:
- ★ *What to Expect—Your Child*
- ★ *What to Expect—Parents*
- ★ *Treatments—Alternative/*
  Homeopathy
- ★ *Treatments—Chemotherapy*
- ★ and more.

National Marrow Donor Program
3433 Broadway Street, NE
Suite 500
Minneapolis, MN 55413
800-MARROW2 (800-627-7692)
www.marrow.org/
Donor centers in most states
Publication topics include:

★ explanation of marrow transplantation
★ search process
★ financing
★ other treatment options
★ and more.

Medicare

Medicare Hotline
Health Care Financing Administration
6325 Security Boulevard
Baltimore, MD 21207
800-638-6833
www.medicare.gov
Some publications available include:
★ *Medicare and You*
★ *Guide to Choosing a Nursing Home*
★ *Advance Directives*
★ *Handbookette—Understanding Your Medicare Choices*
★ and many more.

Mental Health

National Institute of Mental Health
5600 Fishers Lane, Room 7C02
Rockville, MD 20857
301-443-4513
www.nimh.nih.gov
Some publications available include:
★ *Attention Deficit Hyperactivity Disorder*
★ *Getting Treatment for Panic Disorder*

★ *Plain Talk About Depression*
★ *Anorexia Nervosa*

Multiple Sclerosis

Multiple Sclerosis Association
706 Haddonfield Road
Cherry Hill, NJ 08002-2652
609-488-4500
800-LEARN-MS
Fax: 609-661-9797
www.msaa.com/
Local support groups
Some publications available include:
★ *What is MS?*
★ *Multiple Sclerosis: The Process and Medical Treatment*
★ *Multiple Sclerosis: Managing Symptoms*
★ *Family Relationships and Multiple Sclerosis*
★ and many more.

MedSupport FSF International
3132 Timberview Drive
Dunedin, FL 34698
800-793-0766
www.medsupport.org
Some publications available include:
★ *Problems Diagnosing MS*
★ *Multiple Sclerosis Symptoms Explained*
★ *"A Journey Through Life with MS"*
★ *Finding the Right Doctor for YOU*
★ and many more.

Neurological Conditions

National Institute of Neurological Disorders and Stroke
P.O. Box 5801
Bethesda, MD 20824
800-352-9424
www.ninds.nih.gov
Some publications available include:
- ★ *Autism*
- ★ *Parkinson's*
- ★ *Stroke*

Nutrition

Food and Nutrition Information Center
U.S. Department of Agriculture
10301 Baltimore Ave., Room 304
Beltsville, MD 20705
301-504-5719
www.nal.usda.gov/fnic
Some publications available
include:
- ★ *Child Nutrition and Health*
- ★ *Dietary Guidelines for Americans*
- ★ *Nutrition and Learning/Behavior*
- ★ *Nutrition Education*
- ★ and many more.

American Dietetic Association
216 West Jackson Boulevard, Suite 800
Chicago, IL 60606
312-899-0040
800-366-1655

www.eatright.org
Affiliate (state) associations
Some publications available include:
- ★ *Nutrition for You and Your Family*
- ★ *Dieting/Low-fat Lifestyle*
- ★ *Shopping for Food*
- ★ *Women's Nutrition*
- ★ and many more.

Weight-Control Information Network
National Institute of Diabetes and Digestive and Kidney
    Diseases
1 Win Way
Bethesda, MD 20892
301-984-7378
800-WIN-8098
www.niddk.nih.gov/health/nutrit/win.htm
Some publications available include:
- ★ *Choosing a Safe and Successful Weight-Loss Program*
- ★ *Do You Know the Health Risks of Being Overweight?*
- ★ *Helping Your Overweight Child*
- ★ *Weight Loss For Life*
- ★ and many more.

Oral Health

National Oral Health Information Clearinghouse
1 NOTICE Way
Bethesda, MD 20892
301-402-7364
www.aerie.com/nohicweb
Some publications available include:

★ *What You Need to Know About Oral Cancer*
★ *Periodontal Disease and Diabetes*
★ *Temporomandibular Disorders (TMD)*
★ *NOHIC: A Resource for Special Care Patients*
★ and many more.

Academy of General Dentistry
Suite 1200, 211 East Chicago Avenue
Chicago, IL 60611-2670
312-440-4300
www.agd.org
Some publications available include:
★ *Child's First Visit*
★ *Gum Disease*
★ *Oral Cancer*
★ *Composite Fillings*
★ and many more.

Osteoporosis

Osteoporosis and Related Bone Diseases National Resource
    Center
1150 17th Street, NW, Suite 500
Washington, DC 20036
800-624-BONE
202-223-0344
www.osteo.org
Some publications available include:
★ *Osteoporosis Overview*
★ *Psychosocial Issues*
★ *Juvenile Osteoporosis*
★ *Osteoporosis and African-American Women*
★ and more.

Pregnancy

International Childbirth Education Association
P.O. Box 20048
Minneapolis, MN 55420
800-624-4934
www.icea.org
Some publications available include:
- ★ *Elisabeth Bing's Guide to Moving Through Pregnancy*
- ★ *Six Practical Lessons for an Easier Childbirth*
- ★ *Your Pregnancy Questions and Answers*
- ★ *Which Tests for My Unborn Baby?*
- ★ and many more.

National Maternal and Child Health Clearinghouse
Health Resources and Services Administration
2070 Chain Bridge Road, Suite 450
Vienna, VA 22182
703-356-1964
www.nmchc.org
Some publications available include:
- ★ *Reproductive Health*
- ★ *Perinatal Health General*
- ★ *Prenatal Care*
- ★ *Reducing Infant Mortality and Morbidity*
- ★ and many more.

Postpartum Support International
927 North Kellogg Avenue
Santa Barbara, CA 93111

805-967-7636
www.iup.edu/an/postpartum
Local chapters
Some publications available include:
*   ★ *An Introduction to Postpartum Illness*

La Leche League International
1400 North Meacham Road
P.O. Box 4079
Schaumburg, IL 60168
800-LALECHE
www.lalecheleague.org
Local support groups
Some publications available include:
*   ★ *Nursing Your Baby*
*   ★ *The Nursing Mothers' Guide to Weaning*
*   ★ *Breastfeeding the Adopted Baby*
*   ★ *Medications and Mother's Milk*
*   ★ and many more

Premature Babies

For Parents of Preemies
Meriter Hospital
Neonatology 6C, 202 South Park Street
Madison, WI 53715
{ww2.medsch.wisc.edu/chilrenshosp/
parents_of_preemie_index.html.
(Address for ordering their book only.)
Website is made up of the book, which includes these
topics:
*   ★ *Introduction to the Neonatal Intensive Care Unit*
*   ★ *Apnea and Bradycardia of Prematurity*

★ *Understanding Preemie Development*
★ *Later Problems of Former Preemies*
★ and many more.

Product Safety

U.S. Consumer Product Safety Hotline
Washington, DC 20207
800-638-2772
www.cpsc.gov
Some publications available include:
★ *Bunk Beds Safety Warning*
★ *Home Playground Safety Tips Fact Sheet*
★ *CPSC Guide to Home Wiring Hazards*
★ *Upholstered Furniture Fact Sheet*
★ and many more.

Rare Diseases

National Organization for Rare Disorder, Inc.
Fairwood Professional Building
100 Route 37
P.O. Box 8923
New Fairfield, CT 06812-8923
Voice-TDD: 203-746-6518
800-999-6673
Fax: 203-746-6481
www.rarediseases.org
Some local chapters
Some publications available include:
★ *Carcinoma, Renal Cell*
★ *Bell's Palsy*
★ *Prader-Willi Syndrome*

★ *Myopathy, Congenial, Batten-Turner Type*
★ and many more.

National Parent to Parent Support and Information System, Inc.
P.O. Box 907
Blue Ridge, GA 30513
Voice-TDD: 706-374-3822
800-651-1151
Fax: 706-374-3826
www.nppsis.org
Links families nationally

Rural Information

Rural Information Center
    Health Service
National Agricultural Library
Room 304, 1031 Baltimore
    Boulevard
Beltsville, MD 20705
800-633-7701
www.nal.usda.gov/ric/richs
Some publications available
include:

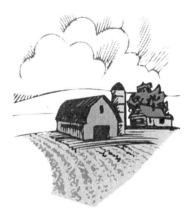

★ *Rural Entrepreneurship
    and Small Business
    Development*
★ *Rural Youth Employment*
★ *Health Care in Rural America*
★ *Arts and Humanities Programs in Rural America*
★ and many more.

Skin Disease

National Psoriasis Foundation
6600 SW 92nd Avenue, Suite 300
Portland, OR 97223-7195
503-244-7404
800-723-9166
Fax: 503-245-0626
www.psoriasis.org
Some publications available include:
* ★ *Overview of Psoriasis Treatments*
* ★ *Psoriatic Arthritis*
* ★ *Skin Cancer Risks From Psoriasis Treatments*
* ★ *Steroids*
* ★ and many more.

Foundation for Ichthyosis and Related Skin Types, Inc.
P.O. Box 669
Ardmore, PA 19003
610-789-3995
610-789-4366
www.libertynet.org/ichthyos/index.html
Regional support network
Some publications available include:
* ★ *Ichthyosis: An Overview*
* ★ *Release the Butterfly: A Handbook for Parents and Caregivers of Children with Ichthyosis*
* ★ *Ichthyosis: The Genetics of Its Inheritance*
* ★ and more.

DebRA of America, Inc.
40 Rector Street, Suite 1403
New York, NY 10006
212-513-4090

Fax: 212-513-4099
www.debra.org/welcome.htm
Some state chapters
Some publications available include:
- ★ *The Thin Skinned Kids*
- ★ *EB and the Eyes*
- ★ *Coping With Epidermolysis Bullosa in the Classroom: An Informed and Sensitive Home/School*
- ★ *Partnership Makes The Difference*
- ★ *Hope Through Research*
- ★ and many more.

Skin Cancer

Cancer Care
1180 Avenue of the Americas, 2nd Floor
New York, NY 10036
800-813-HOPE
212-221-3300
www.cancercare.org
Local chapters
Some publications available include:
- ★ *Conquering Melanoma*
- ★ *Treatment Options*
- ★ *Risk Factor and Reducing Your Risks*
- ★ *Coping with Treatment Side Effects*
- ★ and many more.

American Academy of Dermatology
930 North Meacham Road
P.O. Box 4014
Schaumburg, IL 60168-4014
847-330-0230

888-462-DERM
Fax: 847-330-0050
www.aad.org
Some publications available include:
- ★ *The ABCD's of Melanoma*
- ★ *How Skin Cancer Is Treated*
- ★ *How to Perform a Self-Examination*
- ★ *Skin Cancer Risk Profile*
- ★ and many more.

Sleep Disorders

National Center on Sleep Disorders Research
2 Rockledge Center
6701 Rockledge Drive, MSC 7920
Bethesda, MD 20892
301-435-0199
www.nhlbi.nih.gov/
Some publications available include:
- ★ *Facts About Sleep Apnea*
- ★ *Fact About Narcolepsy*
- ★ *Facts About Insomnia*
- ★ *Facts About Restless Legs Syndrome (RLS)*
- ★ and many more.

Smoking

Office on Smoking and Health
National Center for Chronic Disease
   Prevention and Health Promotion
Centers For Disease Control and
   Prevention
Mail Stop K-50

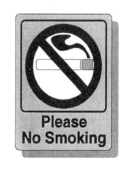

4770 Buford Highway, NE
Atlanta, GA 30341
770-488-5705
800-CDC-1311
www.cdc.gov/nccdphp/osh
Some publications available include:
- ★ *Smokeless Tobacco: A Dangerous Alternative*
- ★ *"I Quit" — What to Do When You're Sick of Smoking, Chewing, or Dipping*
- ★ *What You Can Do About Secondhand Smoke*
- ★ *Is Your Baby Smoking?*
- ★ *Clearing the Air*
- ★ *Out of the Ashes*
- ★ *Chew or Snuff Is Real Bad Stuff*
- ★ and many more.

Spina Bifida

Spina Bifida Association of America
4590 MacArthur Boulevard, NW, Suite 250
Washington, DC 20007-4226
202-944-3285
800-621-3141
Fax: 202-944-3295
www.sbaa.org/
Local chapters
Some publications available include:
- ★ *SBAA General Information Brochure*
- ★ *Answers to Your Questions About Spina Bifida*
- ★ *Learning Disabilities and the Person With Spina Bifida*
- ★ *A Cost Effective Guide in a Legal Framework*
- ★ and many more.

Spinal Cord Injury

National Spinal Cord Injury Association
8300 Colesville Road, Suite 551
Silver Spring, MD 20910
301-588-6959
800-962-9629
Fax: 301-588-9414
www.spinalcord.org
State affiliates and support groups
Some publications available include:
- ★ *Resources for Pediatric Spinal Cord Injury*
- ★ *Choosing a Spinal Cord Injury Rehabilitation Facility*
- ★ *Common Questions on Spinal Cord Injury*
- ★ *Functional Electrical Stimulation*
- ★ and many more.

Paralysis Society of America
801 18th Street, NW
Washington, DC 20006-3517
202-973-8420
SPI Hotline: 800-526-3456,
    M-F, 9am-5pm, 24 hours for new injuries
888-772-1711
TTY: 202-973-8422
Fax: 202-973-8421
www.psa.org
Some publications available include:
- ★ *PN/Paraplegia News*
- ★ *A Guide to Wheelchair Sports and Recreation*
- ★ *In Touch with Kids*

★ *An Introduction to Spinal Cord Injury:*
  Understanding the Changes
★ and many more.

Substance Abuse

National Clearinghouse for Alcohol and Drug Information
P.O. Box 2345
Rockville, MD 20847
800-729-6686
www.health.org

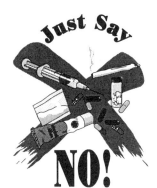

Some publications available include:
  ★ *Prevention Alert—The*
    Changing Face of Heroine:
    Teenagers at Increased Risk
  ★ *Physical and Psychological*
    Risks of Anabolic Steroid
    Use
  ★ *"Making Prevention Work"*
  ★ and many more.

PRIDE
National Parent's Resource Institute for Drug Education
3610 Dekalb Technology Parkway, Suite 105
Atlanta, GA 30340
770-458-9900
800-853-7433
www.prideusa.org
Some publications available include:
  ★ *Adolescent Health and Social Consequences of*
    Alcohol Use
  ★ *Marijuana—Accumulation in the Body*
  ★ *Drug Fads*

★ *"The Home That PRIDE Built"*
★ and many more.

National Substance Abuse Helplines
164 West 74th Street
New York, NY 10023
800-COCAINE
800-DRUGHELP
800-RELAPSE
www.drughelp.org
Some publications available include:
★ *A Guide For Parents Concerned About Drug Abuse*
★ *General Signs and Symptoms of Drug Use*
★ *Inhalants: A Household Danger*
★ *intervention information*
★ and many more.

Tay-Sachs Disease

National Tay-Sachs and Allied Diseases Association, Inc.
2001 Beacon Street, Suite 204
Brighton, MA 02135
800-906-8723
Fax: 617-277-0134
http://mcrcr2.med.nyu.edu/murphp01/taysachs.htm
Parent Peer Group
Some publications available include:
★ *What Every Family Should Know*
★ *Services To Families*
★ *Home Care Manual*
★ *Late Onset Tay-Sachs*
★ and many more

Thyroid Disease

The MAGIC Foundation for Children's Growth
1327 North Harlem Avenue
Oak Park, IL 60302-1376
708-383-0808
800-3MAGIC3
Fax: 708-383-0899
www.magicfoundation.org
National networking
Some publications available include:
  ★ *Underlying Conditions of Growth Abnormalities*
  ★ *Most Frequently Asked Questions When Beginning Growth Hormone Therapy*
  ★ *Dental Problems Associated With Growth*
  ★ *Thyroid Disorders*
  ★ and many more.

The Thyroid Society
7515 South Main Street, Suite 545
Houston, TX 77030
800-THYROID (849-7643)
713-799-9909
www.the-thyroid-society.org/
Some publications available include:
  ★ *Facts for People Given Radiation (X-ray) Treatments as Children*
  ★ *What About Tests and Treatment?*
  ★ *What Is Thyroid Disease?*
  ★ *Depression and Thyroid Disease*
  ★ and many more.

Transportation Services

The Air Care Alliance
4620 Haygood Road, Suite 8
Virginia Beach, VA 23455
888-662-6794
www.aircareall.org
Member groups in all regions

Visual Impairment

National Federation of the Blind
1800 Johnson Street
Baltimore, MD 21230
410-659-9314
www.nfb.org
Local chapters
Some publications available include:
- ★ *The Blind Child in the Regular Preschool Program*
- ★ *Focus on Success: The Dream, the Desire, and the Strategy*
- ★ *Independent Travel for the Blind*
- ★ *Of Dog Guides and White Canes*
- ★ and many more.

APPENDIX

Don't know who to call or where to turn for assistance? Never fear; the Appendix is here! This is a state-by-state listing of starting places for any problem, concern, or issue you may have. We have included address, phone number and website wherever possible. Each listing should be able to either answer your question or direct you to an office near you. Happy hunting!

The *Federal Information Center* can connect you with the appropriate federal government agency that handles your topic of interest.

The *State Information Operator* can connect you to the correct state government office that can answer your question.

State Departments on Aging focus on issues and concerns of the senior population. If you are looking for nutrition, transportation, housing, financial assistance, nursing home resources, or anything else having to do with seniors, then contact this office. They will direct you to local services and resources, as well as tell you about programs offered by the state.

State Departments of Education are responsible for the elementary and secondary schools in the state. They can provide you with the amount spent per child, student-teacher ratio, test scores, experiences, and more concerning the different school districts.

The ***Health Departments*** are in charge of various health programs offered by the state. They can direct you to local community services, and can answer questions regarding health statistics and other health information. If you cannot afford health insurance, this office can direct you to resources your state may have to provide coverage.

Insurance Commissioners enforce the laws and regulations for all kinds of insurance, and they also handle complaints from consumers. If you have a complaint about your insurance company's policies, and the company won't help you, contact the Insurance Commission in the state. This office can also let you know what insurance companies can do business in the state, and most have informative booklets to help you learn how to choose the best insurance coverage for you.

Licensing Offices can provide you with information concerning various licensed professionals, and can direct you to the appropriate office for those professions covered by other agencies or boards. If you are having trouble with your beautician, contractor, veterinarian, or other professional, call this office.

Social Services Offices are the ones in charge of child care programs, welfare, Medicaid, and other programs designed to help individuals and families get back on their feet. If you are struggling to make ends meet, contact this office to be directed to resources and services in your area.

Temporary Assistance to Needy Families (TANF) is the new office that replaced Aid to Families With Dependent

Children (AFDC). This program helps people who need funds to pay for basic necessities as they enter job training programs, finish their education, or care for small children. Welfare-To-Work is often part of this program.

In almost every state, there are ***Women's Commissions*** and similar groups that provide direction or assistance to women. Missions and programs vary, but these groups all share the goal of working toward eliminating the inequities that affect women at home and in the workplace. Some commissions are simply advocacy groups, bringing attention to issues that affect women and working to bring about legislative changes that would improve situations that women face. Others provide information and referrals to help women and even provide direct services to help women get the training, education, and financial help they need to succeed.

ALABAMA

Federal Information Center
All locations; 800-688-9889

State Information Office
334-242-8000
http://www.state.al.us

Department on Aging
Aging Commission
770 Washington Ave.
Suite 470
Montgomery, AL 36130
334-242-5743

Department of Education
Alabama Department of Education
50 N. Ripley
Montgomery, AL 36130-2101
334-242-9700
http://www.alsde.edu/

Health Department
Alabama Department of Public Health
RSA Tower
201 Monroe Street
Montgomery, AL 36104
MAILING ADDRESS:
  RSA Tower
  P.O. Box 303017
  Montgomery, AL 36130-3017
334-206-5300
www.alapubhealth.org
E-mail: webmaster@ alapubhealth.org

Insurance Commissioner
Insurance Commissioner
201 Monroe St.
Suite 1700
Montgomery, AL 36104

334-269-3550
800-243-5463

Licensing Office
State Occupational Information
Coordinating Community (SOICC)
401 Adams Ave.
P.O. Box 5690
Montgomery, AL 36103
334-242-2990

Social Services Offices
Alabama Dept. of Human Resources
P.O. Box 304000
Montgomery, AL 36130-4000
334-242-1850
www.state.al.us/govern/dhr/
dhrmain.html

Temporary Assistance to Needy Families (TANF)
Temporary Aid to Needy Families
Joel Sander
Alabama Department of Human
Resources
Gordon Persons Bldg.
50 Ripley St.
Montgomery, AL 36130
334-242-1773
www.dhr.state.al.us

Women's Commission
Alabama Women's Commission
P.O. Box 1277
Tuscaloosa, AL 35403
205-345-7668
Jean Boutwell, elected Secretary
Bab F. Hart, Chair
www.alawomenscommission.org

ALASKA

Federal Information Center
All locations; 800-688-9889

State Information Office
907-465-2111
http://www.state.ak.us

Department on Aging
Division of Senior Services
Commission on Aging
P.O. Box 110209
Juneau, AK 99811-0209
907-465-3250

Department of Education
Alaska Department of Education
Public Information
801 W. 10th St., Suite 200
Juneau, AK 99801-1894
907-465-2851
http://www.educ.state.ak.us/
report/contents.html

Health Department
Alaska Department of Health & Social
Services
350 Main Street, Room 503
Juneau, AK 99801
MAILING ADDRESS:
    P.O. Box 110610
    Juneau, AK 99811-0610
907-465-3090
Fax: 907-586-1877
http://health.hss.state.ak.us
E-mail: petern@ health.state.ak.us

Insurance Commissioner
Director of Insurance
P.O. Box 110805
Juneau, AK 99811-0805

907-465-2515
http://www.commerce.state.ak.
us/insurance

Licensing Office
Division of Occupational Licensing
Department of Commerce and
Economic Development
State of Alaska
P.O. Box 110806
Juneau, AK 99811
907-465-2534
www.commerce.state.ak.us/
occ.home.htm

Social Services Offices
Alaska Department of Health and
Social Services
3601 "C" Street, Suite 578
P.O. Box 240249
Anchorage, AK 99524
907-269-2680
www.hss.state.ak.us

**Temporary Assistance to Needy
Families (TANF)**
Temporary Aid to Needy Families
Jim Nordlund
Alaska Department of Health and
Social Services
P.O. Box 110640
Juneau, AK 99811
907-465-3347
www.hss.state.ak.us/htmlstuf/
pubassis/atap.htm

Women's Commission
Anchorage Women's Commission
P.O. Box 196650
Anchorage, AK 99519-6650

907-343-6310
Fax: 907-343-6730
www.ci.anchorage.ak.us

ARIZONA

Federal Information Center
All Locations; 800-688-9889

State Information Office
602-542-4900
http://www.state.az.us

Department on Aging
Aging and Adult Administration
Economic Security Department
1789 W. Jefferson
Phoenix, AZ 85007
602-542-4446

Department of Education
Arizona Department of Education
Research and Evaluation Division
1535 W. Jefferson
Phoenix, AZ 85007
602-542-5022
http://www.ade.state.az.us/

Health Department
Arizona Department of Health
Services
Office of Women's & Children's Health
411 North 24th Street
Phoenix, AZ 85008
602-220-6550
Fax: 602-220-6551
TDD: 602-256-7577
www.hs.state.az.us

Insurance Commissioner
Director of Insurance
2910 N. 44th St., Suite 210
Phoenix, AZ 85018
602-912-8400
800-325-2548
http://www.state.az.us/id/

Licensing Office
Registrar of Contractors
800 W. Washington
Phoenix, AZ 85007
602-542-1525 ext. 7605
www.rc.state.az.us

Social Services Offices
Arizona Dept. of Economic Security
1717 West Jefferson
Phoenix, AZ 85007
602-542-4296
www.de.state.az.us

Temporary Assistance to Needy Families (TANF)
Temporary Aid to Needy Families
Social Services Block Grant
Linda Blessing
Arizona Dept. of Economic Security
1717 West Jefferson St.
Phoenix, AZ 85007
602-542-5678
www.de.state.az.us

Women's Commissions
Phoenix Women's Commission
Equal Opportunity Department
251 West Washington, 7th Floor
Phoenix, AZ 85003-6211
602-261-8242
Fax: 602-256-3389

Tucson Women's Commission
240 North Court Ave.
Tucson, AZ 85701
520-624-8318
Fax: 520-624-5599
E-mail: tctwc@starnet.com
Neema Caughran, Executive Director
Louisa Hernandez, Chair

ARKANSAS

Federal Information Center
All Locations; 800-688-9889

State Information Office
501-682-3000
http://www.state.ar.us

Department on Aging
Aging and Adult Services Division
Box 1437, Slot 1412
Little Rock, AR 72203
501-682-2441
http://www.state.ar.us/
dhs.index2.html

Department of Education
Arkansas Department of Education
Office of Accountability
4 State Capitol Mall, 204-B
Little Rock, AR 72201
501-682-4330
http://arkedu.state.ar.us

Health Department
Arkansas Department of Health
4815 West Markham
Little Rock, AR 72201
501-661-2000
800-482-5400
http://health.state.ar.us
E-mail: wbankson@ mail.doh.state.
ar.us

Insurance Commissioner
Insurance Commissioner
1200 W. 3rd St.

Little Rock, AR 72201
501-371-2600
800-852-5494

Licensing Office
Boards and Commissions
Governor's Office
State Capitol Building
Little Rock, AR 72201
501-682-3570

Social Services Offices
Arkansas Department of Human
Services
Donaghey Plaza West
Slot 3430
P.O. Box 1437
Little Rock, AR 72203
501-682-8650
www.state.ar.us/dhs/

Temporary Assistance to Needy Families (TANF)
Temporary Aid to Needy Families
Gordon Page
Division of County Operations
Arkansas Department of Human
Services
101 East Capitol
Little Rock, AR 72203
501-682-6728
www.state.ar.us/dhs/tea/plan/

Women's Commission
Closed 96-99

CALIFORNIA

Federal Information Center
All Locations; 800-688-9889

State Information Office
916-322-9900
http://www.state.ca.us

Department on Aging
California Department of Aging
1600 K St.
Sacramento, CA 95814
916-322-5290
http://www.aging.state.ca.us

Department of Education
California Department of Education
721 Capitol Mall
P.O. Box 944272
Sacramento, CA 94244-2720
916-657-2676
http://goldmine.cde.ca.gov/

Health Department
California Department of Health
Services
Office of Women's Health
714 P Street, Room 792
Sacramento, CA 95814
906-653-3330
Fax: 916-653-3535
www.dhs.ca.gov

Insurance Commissioner
Commissioner of Insurance
300 S. Spring St., 13th Floor
Los Angeles, CA 90013
916-492-3500 (Sacramento)
213-346-6400 (Los Angeles)
800-927-HELP (complaints)

http://www.insurance.ca.gov/
docs/index.html

Licensing Office
State of California
Department of Consumer Affairs
400 R St.
Sacramento, CA 95814
916-445-1254
800-952-5210
www.dca.ca.gov

Social Services Offices
California Department of Social
Services
Office of Community Relations
744 P Street, M.S. 17-02
Sacramento, CA 95814
916-657-3661
www.dss.cahwnet.gov

Temporary Assistance to Needy Families (TANF)
Temporary Aid to Needy Families
Eloise Anderson
California Department of Social
Services
744 P Street
Mail Station 17-11
Sacramento, CA 95814
916-657-2598
www.dss.cahwnet.gov/getser/
afdc.html

Women's Commission
California Commission on the Status of
Women
1303 J St., Suite 400
Sacramento, CA 95814-2900

916-445-3173
Fax: 916-322-9466
E-mail: csw@sna.com
www.statusofwomen.ca.gov
Eileen Padberg, Chair

COLORADO

Federal Information Center
All Locations; 800-688-9889

State Information Office
303-866-5000
http://www.state.co.us

Department on Aging
Commission For Aging and Adult
Services
Social Services Department
110 16th St., Suite 200
Denver, CO 80202
303-620-4147
http://www.aclin.org/
~sherlock/colodaas.htm

Department of Education
Colorado Department of Education
Planning and Evaluation Unit
201 E. Colfax
Denver, CO 80203
303-866-6600
http://www.cde.state.co.us/

Health Department
Colorado Department of Public Health
& Environment
4300 Cherry Creek Drive South
Denver, CO 80246-1530
303-692-1000
www.state.co.us/gov_dir/ cdphe_dir/

Insurance Commissioner
Commissioner of Insurance
1560 Broadway, Suite 850
Denver, CO 80202
303-894-7499
800-544-9181

http://www.state.co.us/gov_dir/
regulatory_dir/insurance_reg. html

Licensing Office
Department of Regulatory Agencies
State Services Building
1560 Broadway, Suite 1550
Denver, CO 80303
404-894-7855
www.dora.state.co.us

Social Services Offices
Colorado Department of Human
Services
1575 Sherman Street
Denver, CO 80203-1714
303-866-5922
www.cdhs.state.co.us

**Temporary Assistance to Needy
Families (TANF)**
Temporary Aid to Needy Families
Sue Tuffin
Colorado Department of Human
Services
1575 Sherman St.
Denver, CO 80203
303-866-4630
www.cdhs.state.co.us/cdhs/
oss/Self_Sufficiency.html

Women's Commission
Denver Women's Commission
303 West Colfax, Suite 1600
Denver, CO 80204
303-640-5826
Fax: 303-640-4627
www.denvergov.org/
Marilyn Ferran, Chair

Fort Collins City Commission on the
Status of Women
c/o Human Resources
City of Ft. Collins
P.O. Box 580
Fort Collins, CO 80522
970-221-6871
970-224-6050
www.ci.fort-collins.co.us
Laurie Fonken-Joseph, Chair

CONNECTICUT

Federal Information Center
All Locations; 800-688-9889

State Information Office
860-240-0222
http://www.state.ct.us

Department on Aging
Elderly Services
Division of Social Services
25 Sigourney St.
Hartford, CT 06106
860-424-5277
http://www.dss.state.ct.us/

Department of Education
Connecticut Department of Education
Public Information Office
P.O. Box 2219
Hartford, CT 06145
860-566-5677
http://www.state.ct.us/sde/

Health Department
Connecticut Dept. of Public Health
410 Capitol Avenue
P.O. Box 340308
Hartford, CT 06134-0308
860-509-8000
TDD: 860-509-7191
www.state.ct.us'dph/
E-mail: donna.winiarski@
po.state.ct.us

Insurance Commissioner
Insurance Commissioner
P.O. Box 816
Hartford, CT 06142-0816
860-297-3802
800-203-3447
http://www.state.ct.us/cid/

Licensing Office
Occupational Licensing Division
Department of Consumer Protection
165 Capitol Ave.
Hartford, CT 06106
860-566-2825
www.dcp.state.ct.us/licensing

Social Services Offices
Connecticut Department of Social
Services
25 Siqourney Street
Hartford, CT 06106
860-424-5010
www.dss.state.ct.us

Temporary Assistance to Needy Families (TANF)
Temporary Aid To Needy Families
Joyce Thomas
Connecticut Department of Social
Services
25 Sigourney St.
Hartford, CT 06106
860-424-5008
800-842-1508
www.dss.state.ct.us/svcs/
financial.htm

Women's Commission
Connecticut Permanent Commission of
the Status of Women
18-20 Trinity St.
Hartford, CT 06106
860-240-8300
Fax: 860-240-8314
E-mail: pcsw@po.state.ct.us
www.cga.state.ct.us/pcswl/
Leslie Brett, Ph.D, Executive Director
Barbara DeBaptiste, Chair

DELAWARE

Federal Information Center
All Locations; 800-688-9889

State Information Office
302-739-4000
http://www.state.de.us

Department on Aging
Aging Division
Health and Social Services
Department
1901 N. Dupont Hwy.
New Castle, DE 19720
302-577-4791
http://kidshealth.org/
nhc/divage/index.html

Department of Education
Delaware Department of Education
Federal and Lockerman Sts.
P.O. Box 1402
Dover, DE 19903-1402
302-739-4601
http://www.doe.state.de.us/reports/
reports.html

Health Department
Delaware Division of Public Health
P.O. Box 637
Federal & Water Streets
Dover, DE 19903
302-739-4701
Fax: 302-739-6657
www.state.de.us/govern/agencies/
dhss/irm/dph/ dphhome.htm

Insurance Commissioner
Insurance Commissioner
841 Silver Lake Blvd.
Rodney Bldg.

Dover, DE 19903
302-739-4251
800-282-8611
http://www.state.de.us/govern/elecoffl/
inscom.htm

Licensing Office
Division of Professional Regulation
P.O. Box 1401
O'Neil Building
Dover, DE 19903
302-739-4522

Social Services Offices
Delaware Department of Health and
Social Services
Health and Social Service Campus
1901 North DuPont Highway
Main Building
New Castle, DE 19720
302-577-4501
www.state.de.us/govern/
agencies/dhss/irm/dhss.htm

**Temporary Assistance to Needy
Families (TANF)**
Temporary Aid to Needy Families
Nina Licht
Delaware Social Services
Lewis Bldg.
1901 North Dupont Highway
New Castle, DE 19720
302-577-4880, ext. 273
www.state.de.us/govern/
agencies/dhss/irm/dss/ dsshome.htm

Women's Commission
Delaware Commission for Women
4425 N. Market St.
Wilmington, DE 19802

302-761-8005
Fax: 302-761-6652
E-mail: cgomez@state.de.us
Romona S. Fullman, Esq., Director

DISTRICT OF COLUMBIA

Federal Information Center
All Locations; 800-688-9889

District of Columbia Information Office
202-727-6161
http://www.ci.washington.dc.us

Department on Aging
Aging Office
441 4th St., NW
Suite 900
Washington, DC 20001
202-724-5622
http://www.ci.washington.
dc.us/aging/aghome.htm

Department of Education
Public Schools
825 North Capitol Street, NE
Washington, DC 20002-4232
202-442-4289
www.K12.dc.us

Health Department
District of Columbia Department of
Health
800 9th Street, SW, 3rd Floor
Washington, DC 20024
202-645-5556

Insurance Commissioner
Commissioner of Insurance
441 4th St., NW
8th Floor N.
Washington, DC 20001
202-727-8000

Licensing Office
Department of Consumer and
Regulatory Affairs
614 H St., NW, Room 108
Washington, DC 20001
202-727-7080

Social Services Offices
Department of Human Services
Martin Luther King Ave., SE
Building 801E
Washington, DC 20032
202-279-6000
http://dhs.washington.dc.us

Temporary Assistance to Needy Families (TANF)
Welfare Reform
Patricia Handy
Washington DC Department of
Human Services
33 N St., NE
Washington, DC 20002
202-727-3444
www.dhs.washington.dc.us/
PublicInfo/WelfareReform/
REFORM.HTM

Women's Commission
Women's Bureau
U.S. Department of Labor
200 Constitution Ave., NW
Washington, DC 20210
800-827-5335
202-219-6631
Fax: 202-219-5529
www.dol.gov/dol.wb
Delores L. Crockett, Acting Director
Lillian M. Long, Chair

FLORIDA

Federal Information Center
All Locations; 800-688-9889

State Information Office
850-488-1234
http://www.state.fl.us

Department on Aging
Department of Elder Affairs
4040 Esplanade Way
Tallahassee, FL 32399-0700
850-414-2108
Elder Helpline: 800-96-ELDER (in FL)
http://www.state.fl.us/doea/ doea.html

Department of Education
Florida Department of Education
Education Information and
Accountability Services
325 W. Gaines St., Room 852
Tallahassee, FL 32399-0400
850-487-2280
http://www.firn.edu/doe/index.html

Health Department
Florida Department of Health
2020 Capital Circle SE
Tallahassee, FL 32399-1700
850-487-2945
www.doh.state.fl.us
E-mail: Dorothy_Bruce@
doh.state.fl.us
E-mail: JoAnn_Steele@doh.state.fl.us

Insurance Commissioner
Insurance Commissioner
200 E. Gaines St.
Tallahassee, FL 32399-0300
850-922-3100
800-342-2762
http://www.doi.state.fl.us/

Licensing Office
Florida Department of business and
Professional Regulation
1940 N. Monroe St.
Tallahassee, FL 32399
850-488-6602
www.state.fl.us/dbpr

Social Services Offices
Florida Dept. of Children and Families
1317 Winewood Boulevard
Building 1, Room 206
Tallahassee, FL 32399-0770
904-488-4855
www.state.fl.us\cs_web

Temporary Assistance to Needy Families (TANF)
Temporary Aid to Needy Families
Christy Moore
Florida Department of Health and
Rehabilitation Services
1317 Winewood Blvd.
Tallahassee, FL 32399
850-921-0193
http://fcn.state.fl.us/index.html

Women's Commission
Florida Commission on the Status of
Women
Office of the Attorney General, The
Capitol
Tallahassee, FL 32399-1050
850-414-3300
Fax: 850-921-4131
E-mail: Michele-Manning@
oag.state.fl.us
http://legal.firn.edu/units/fcsw
Kate Gooderham, Chair
Susan Gilbert, Vice Chair

Georgia

Federal Information Center
All Locations; 800-688-9889

State Information Office
404-656-2000
http://www.state.ga.us

Department on Aging
Aging Services Office
2 Peachtree St., NW
Atlanta, GA 30303
404-657-5258
http://www.state.ga.us/
departments/dhr/aging/html

Department of Education
Georgia Department of Education
205 Butler St.
Twin Towers East, Suite 1654
Atlanta, GA 30334
404-656-2400
http://www.doe.k12.ga.us/

Health Department
Georgia Division of Public Health
Two Peachtree Street, NW
Atlanta, GA 30303-3186
404-657-2700
www.ph.dhr.state.ga.us/
E-mail: gdphinfo@ dhr.state.ga.us

Insurance Commissioner
Insurance Commissioner
7th Floor West Tower, Floyd Bldg.
2 Martin Luther King, Jr. Dr.
Atlanta, GA 30334
404-656-2070
800-656-2298
http://www2.state.ga.us/gains.
commission/

Licensing Office
Examining Board Division
Secretary of State
166 Pryor St., SW
Atlanta, GA 30303
404-656-3900
www.sos.state.ga.us/ebd/ default.htm

Social Services Offices
Georgia Department of Human
Resources
200 Piedmont Avenue
Suite 1504, West Tower
Atlanta, GA 30303
404-656-4937
www.state.ga.us/Departments/ DHR

Temporary Assistance to Needy Families (TANF)
Temporary Aid to Needy Families
Tommy Olmstead
Georgia Department of Human
Resources
2 Peachtree St., NW, Suite 16-200
Atlanta, GA 30303
404-656-5680
www2.state.ga.us/
departments/dhr/tanf.html

Women's Commission
GA State Commission of Women
148 International Blvd., NE
Atlanta, GA 30303
404-657-9260
Fax: 404-657-2963
E-mail: gawomen@manspring.com
www.manspring.com/~gawomen
Nellie Duke, Chair
Juliana McConnell, Vice Chair

Hawaii

Federal Information Center
All Locations; 800-688-9889

State Information Office
808-548-6222
http://www.state.hi.us

Department on Aging
Aging Office
205 S. Hotel St.
Suite 107
Honolulu, HI 96813-2831
808-586-0100

Department of Education
Hawaii Department of Education
Information Branch
P.O. Box 2360
Honolulu, HI 96804
808-832-5880
http://www.k12.hi.us/

Health Department
Hawaii Department of Health
1250 Punchbowl Street
Honolulu, HI 96813
808-586-4400
Fax: 808-586-4444
www.state.hi.us/health/
E-mail: pijohnst@ health. state.hi.us

Insurance Commissioner
Insurance Commissioner
250 S. King Street, 5th Floor
Honolulu, HI 96813
808-586-2790
http://www.state.hi.us/insurance

Licensing Office
Office of the Director
Department of Commerce and
Consumer Affairs
P.O. Box 3469
Honolulu, HI 96801
808-586-2850
www.hawaii.gov/dcca/dcca.html

Social Services Offices
Hawaii Dept. of Human Services
P.O. Box 339
Honolulu, HW 96809
808-586-4888
www.hawaii.gov/csd/dhs/dhs.html

Temporary Assistance to Needy Families (TANF)
Temporary Aid to Needy Families
Kathleen Stanley
Hawaii Department of Human
Services
P.O. Box 339
Honolulu, HI 96809
808-586-4999
www.state.hi.us/dhs/index.html

Women's Commission
Hawaii State Commission on the Status
of Women
235 S. Beretaniast, Suite 401
Honolulu, HI 96813
808-586-5757
Fax: 808-586-5756
E-mail: hscsw@pixi.com
www.state.hi.us/hscsw
Alicynttikida Tasaka, Executive Director

Idaho

Federal Information Center
All Locations; 800-688-9889

State Information Office
208-334-2411
http://www.state.id.us

Department on Aging
Aging Office
P.O. Box 83720
Boise, ID 83720-0007
208-334-3833
http://www.state.id.us/icoa/

Department of Education
Idaho Department of Education
P.O. Box 83720
Boise, ID 83720-0027
208-332-6800
http://www.sde.state.id.us/dept/

Health Department
Idaho Department of Health & Welfare
450 W. State St., 10th Floor
P.O. Box 83720
Boise, ID 83720-0036
208-334-5500
Fax: 208-334-6558
TDD: 208-334-4921
www.state.id.us/dhw/
hwgd_www/home.html

Insurance Commissioner
Director of Insurance
P.O. Box 83720
Boise, ID 83720-0043
208-334-2250
http://www.doi.state.id.us/

Licensing Office
State of Idaho

Department of Self-Governing
Agencies
Bureau of Occupational Licenses
Owyhee Plaza
1109 Main, #220
Boise, ID 83720
208-334-3233

Social Services Offices
Idaho Department of Health and
Welfare
450 West State Street
Boise, ID 83720-0036
208-334-5500
www.state.id.us/dhw/
hwgd_www.home.html

**Temporary Assistance to Needy
Families (TANF)**
Temporary Aid to Needy Families
Social Services Block Grant
Linda Caballero
Idaho Department of Health and
Welfare
P.O. Box 83720
Boise, ID 83720
208-334-5500
www.state.id.us/dhw/
hwgd_www/home.html

Women's Commission
Idaho Commission on the Women's
Program
P.O. Box 83720
Boise, ID 83720-0036
208-334-4673
Fax: 208-334-4646
E_mail: ehurlbudt@ women.state.id.us
www.state.id.us/women
Linda Hurlbudt, Director
Cindy Agidius, Chair

Illinois

Federal Information Center
All Locations; 800-688-9889

State Information Office
217-782-2000
http://www.state.il.us

Department on Aging
Aging Department
421 E. Capitol Ave. #100
Springfield, IL 62701-1789
217-785-2870
http://www.state.il.us/aging/

Department of Education
Illinois State Board of Education
100 N. First St.
Springfield, IL 62777-0001
217-782-3950
http://www.isbe.state.il.us/

Health Department
Illinois Department of Public Health
535 West Jefferson Street
Springfield, IL 62761
217-782-4977
Fax: 217-782-3987
TTY: 800-547-0466
www.idph.state.il.us

Insurance Commissioner
Director of Insurance
320 W. Washington St., 4th Floor
Springfield, IL 62767-0001
217-782-4515
800-548-9034
http://www.state.il.us/ins/

Licensing Office
State of Illinois
Department of Professional
Regulations
320 W. Washington, Third Floor
Springfield, IL 62786
217-785-0800
www.state.il.us/dpr

Social Services Offices
Illinois Department of Human Services
Office of Communications
401 South Clinton, 7th Floor
Chicago, IL 60607
312-793-2343
www.state.il.us/agency/dhs

**Temporary Assistance to Needy
Families (TANF)**
Temporary Aid to Needy Families
Howard Peters
Illinois Department of Human Services
Harris Bldg.
100 South Grand Ave.
Springfield, IL 62762
217-557-1601
www.state.il.us/agency/
dhs/TANF.HTM

Women's Commission
Governor's Commission on the Status
of Women
100 W. Randolph, Suite 16-100
Chicago, IL 60601
312-814-5743
Fax: 312-814-3823
Ellen Solomon, Executive Director

Indiana

Federal Information Center
All Locations; 800-688-9889

State Information Office
317-232-1000
http://www.state.in.us

Department on Aging
Aging and Rehabilitative Services
Division
Family and Social Services
Administration
402 W. Washington St.
Room W454
Indianapolis, IN 46207
317-232-7020

Department of Education
Indiana Department of Education
Education Information Systems
Room 229, State House
Indianapolis, IN 46204-2798
317-232-0808
http://www.doe.state.in.us/

Health Department
Indiana State Department of Health
2 North Meridian Street
Indianapolis, IN 46204
317-233-1325
www.ai.org/doh/index.html
E-mail: OPA@isdh.state.in.us

Insurance Commissioner
Commissioner of Insurance
311 W. Washington St., Suite 300
Indianapolis, IN 46204-2787
317-232-2385
800-622-4461
http://www.ai.org/idoi/index.html

Licensing Office
Indiana Professional Licensing
Agency
Indiana Government Center S.
302 W. Washington St.
Room E-034
Indianapolis, IN 46204
317-232-2980
www.state.in.us/pla

Social Services Offices
Indiana Family and Social Services
Administration
402 West Washington Street
Indianapolis, IN 46204
317-232-4453
www.in.org/fssa/index.html

**Temporary Assistance to Needy
Families (TANF)**
Temporary Aid to Needy Families
James Hmurovich
Indiana Division of Family and
Children
402 West Washington St.
Room W392
Indianapolis, IN 46204
317-232-4705
www.state.in.us/fssa/HTML/
PROGRAMS/dfcfamily.html

Women's Commission
Indiana State Commission for Women
100 N. Senate Ave., N103
Indianapolis, IN 46204
317-233-6303
Fax: 317-232-6580
E-mail: icw@state.in.us
www.state.in.us/icw

Iowa

Federal Information Center
All Locations; 800-688-9889

State Information Office
515-281-5011
http://www.state.ia.us

Department on Aging
Elder Affairs Department
Clemens Building
200 W. 10th St., Third Floor
Des Moines, IA 50309
515-281-5188
http://www.sos.state.ia.us/
register/r4/r4eldaf.htm

Department of Education
Iowa Department of Education
Grimes State Office Bldg.
Des Moines, IA 50319-0146
515-281-5294
http://www.state.ia.us/educate/
depteduc/

Health Department
Iowa Department of Public Health
Lucas Building
321 East 12th Street
DesMoines, IA 50319
517-281-5787
www.idph.state.ia.us

Insurance Commissioner
Insurance Commissioner
330 E. Maple St.
Des Moines, IA 50319
515-281-5705
800-351-4664
http://www.state.ia.us/ government/com/
ins/ins.htm

Licensing Office
Bureau of Professional Licensing
Iowa Department of Health
Lucas State Office Building
Des Moines, IA 50319
515-281-4401

Social Services Offices
Iowa Dept. of Human Services
Hoover Street Office Building
5th Floor NW
1305 East Walnut
DesMoine, IA 50319
515-281-4847
www.dhs.state.ia/us

Temporary Assistance to Needy Families (TANF)
Temporary Aid to Needy Families
Chuck Palmer
Iowa Department of Human Services
Hoover State Office
Building E
13th and Walnut
Des Moines, IA 50319
515-281-5452
www.dhs.state.ia.us/HomePages/
DHS/serving.htm

Women's Commission
Iowa Commission on the Status of Women
Lucas State Office Building
Des Moines, IA 50319
515-281-4461
Fax: 515-242-6119
E-mail: icsw@compuserve.com
www.state.ia.us/dhr/sw
Charlotte Nelson, Executive Director
Kathryn Burt, Chair

Kansas

Federal Information Center
All Locations; 800-688-9889

State Information Office
913-296-0111
http://www.state.ks.us

Department on Aging
Aging Department
915 SW Harrison St., Room 150
Docking State Office Bldg.
Topeka, KS 66612-1500
913-296-4986
http://www.k4s.org/ kdoa/default.htm

Department of Education
Kansas State Department of Education
120 SE 10th Ave.
Topeka, KS 66612
785-296-3201
http://www.ksbe.state.ks.us/

Health Department
Kansas Division of Health &
Environment
Capitol Tower
400 Eighth Avenue, Suite 200
Topeka, KS 66603-3930
785-296-1500
Fax: 785-368-6368
www.kdhe.state.ks.us

Insurance Commissioner
Commissioner of Insurance
420 SW 9th St.
Topeka, KS 66612-1678
785-296-3071
800-432-2484
http://www.ink.org/public/kid/

Licensing Office
Governor's Office
State Capitol, 2nd Floor
Topeka, KS 66612
785-296-3232

Social Services Offices
Kansas Department of Social and
Rehabilitation Services
915 Harrison Street, 6th Floor
Docking State Office Building
Topeka, KS 66612
785-296-3271
www.ink.org/public/srs

**Temporary Assistance to Needy
Families (TANF)**
Temporary Aid to Needy Families
Rochelle Chronister
Kansas Department of Social and
Rehabilitation Services
Docking State Office Bldg.
915 Harrison St.
Topeka, KS 66612
785-296-3271
http://www.ink.org/public/srs/
srseescomm.html

Women's Commission
Wichita Commission on the Status of
Women
Human Services Dept., 2nd Floor
455 North Main St.
Wichita, KS 67202
316-268-4691
Fax: 316-268-4219
Shirley Mast, Contact Person

Kentucky

Federal Information Center
All Locations; 800-688-9889

State Information Office
502-564-3130
http://www.state.ky.us

Department on Aging
Aging Services Division
Cabinet for Families and Children
275 E. Main St., 5th Floor
Frankfort, KY 40621
502-564-6930

Department of Education
Kentucky Department of Education
Education Technology Assistance
Center
15 Fountain Place
Frankfort, KY 40601
502-564-2020
http://www.kde.state.ky.us/

Health Department
Kentucky Cabinet for Health Services
275 East Main Street
Frankfort, KY 40621
502-564-3970
Fax: 502-564-6533
http://cfc-chs.chr.state.ky.us

Insurance Commissioner
Insurance Commissioner
215 W. Main St.
P.O. Box 517
Frankfort, KY 40602
502-564-3630
800-595-6053
http://www.state.ky.us/agencies/insur/
default.htm

Licensing Office
Division of Occupations and
Professions
P.O. Box 456
Frankfort, KY 40602
502-564-3296

Social Services Offices
Kentucky Cabinet for Families and
Children
275 East Main Street
Frankfort, KY 40621
502-564-6786
http://cfs-chs.chr.state.ky.us/
cfachome.htm

**Temporary Assistance to Needy
Families (TANF)**
Temporary Aid to Needy Families
John Clayton
Department of Social Insurance
275 East Main St.
Third Floor, West
Frankfort, KY 40621
502-564-3703
http://cfc-chs.chr.state.ky.us/ prog.htm

Women's Commission
Kentucky Commission on Women
614A Shelby St.
Frankfort, KY 40601
502-564-6643
Fax: 502-564-2315
E-mail: gpotter@mail.state.ky.us
www.state.ky.us/agencies/
women/index.html
Genie Potter, Executive Director

Louisiana

Federal Information Center
All Locations; 800-688-9889

State Information Office
504-342-6600
http://www.state.la.us

Department on Aging
Elderly Affairs
412 N. 4th St.
Baton Rouge, LA 70802
504-342-1700

Department of Education
Louisiana Department of Education
P.O. Box 94064
Baton Rouge, LA 70804
504-342-8841
http://www.doe.state.la.us/

Health Department
Louisiana Department of Health and
Hospitals
1201 Capitol Access Road
P.O. Box 629
Baton Rouge, LA 70821-0629
225-342-9500
Fax: 225-342-5568
www.dhh.state.la.us
E-mail: Webmaster@
dhhmail.dhh.state.la.us

Insurance Commissioner
Commissioner of Insurance
P.O. Box 94214
Baton Rouge, LA 70804-9214
504-342-5900
800-259-5300
http://wwwldi.ldi.state.la.us/

Licensing Office
First Stop Shop
Secretary of State
P.O. Box 94125
Baton Rouge, LA 70804
504-922-2675
800-259-0001
www.sec.la.us

Social Services Offices
Louisiana Department of Human
Services
P.O. Box 3776
Baton Rouge, LA 70821
504-342-6729
www.dss.state.la.us

**Temporary Assistance to Needy
Families (TANF)**
Temporary Aid to Needy Families
Madlyn Bagneris
Louisiana Department of Social
Services
P.O. Box 3776
Baton Rouge, LA 70821
504-342-0286
http://www.dss.state.la.us/
offofs/html/family_independence_
temporary_.html

Women's Commission
LA Office of Women's Services
1885 Woodale Blvd., 9th Floor
Baton Rouge, LA 70806
225-922-0960
Fax: 225-922-0959
E-mail: owsbradm@ows.state.la.us
www.ows.state.la.us/
Vera Clay, Executive Director

Maine

Federal Information Center
All Locations; 800-688-9889

State Information Office
207-582-9500
http://www.state.maine.us

Department on Aging
Elder and Adult Services
Human Services Department
11 State House Station
35 Anthony Ave.
Augusta, ME 04333-0011
207-624-5335
http://www.state.me.us/
beas/dhs_beas.htm

Department of Education
Maine Department of Education
Educational Bldg.
Station No. 23
Augusta, ME 04333
207-287-5841
http://www.state.me.us/education/
homepage.htm

Health Department
Maine Department of Human Services
221 State Street
Augusta, ME 04333
207-287-3707
Fax: 207-626-5555
TTY: 207-287-4479
www.state.me.us/dhs/main/
welcome.htm

Insurance Commissioner
Superintendent of Insurance

34 State House Station
Augusta, ME 04333
207-624-8475
800-750-5353
http://www.state.me.us/pfr/ins/
inshome2.htm

Licensing Office
Department of Professional and
Financial Regulation
State House Station 35
August, ME 04333
207-624-8700
www.state.me.us/pfr/ pfrhome.htm

Social Services Offices
Maine Dept. of Human Services
221 State Street
Augusta, ME 04333
207-287-2546
www.state.me.us/dhs/main/
welcome.htm

Temporary Assistance to Needy
Families (TANF)
Temporary Aid to Needy Families
Kevin Concannon
Maine Department of Human Services
11 Statehouse Station
Augusta, ME 04333
207-287-2736
www.state.me.us/dhs/main/
welome.htm

Women's Commission
Abolished

Maryland

Federal Information Center
All Locations; 800-688-9889

State Information Office
800-449-4347
http://www.state.md.us

Department on Aging
Aging Office
301 W. Preston St., Room 1004
Baltimore, MD 21201-2374
410-767-1100
http://www.inform.umd.edu:8080/
umststate/md_resources/ooa

Department of Education
Maryland Department of Education
Office of Planning
Results and Information Management
200 W. Baltimore St.
Baltimore, MD 21201
410-767-0073
888-246-0016
http://www.mdse.state.md.us/

Health Department
Maryland Department of Health &
Mental Hygiene
State Office Building Complex
201 West Preston Street
Baltimore, MD 21201-2399
410-767-6860
TDD: 800-735-2258
www.dhmh.state.md.us/index.html

Insurance Commissioner
Insurance Commissioner
525 St. Paul Place
Baltimore, MD 21202
410-486-2090

800-492-6116
http://www.gacc.com/mia/

Licensing Office
Division of Occupational and
Professional Licensing
Department of Labor, Licensing and
Regulation
500 N. Calvert St.
Baltimore, MD 21202
410-230-6000
www.dllr.state.md.us/occprof/
index.html

Social Services Offices
Maryland Department of Human
Resources
Saratoga State Center
311 West Saratoga Street
Baltimore, MD 21201-1000
410-767-7758
www.dhr.state.md.us/dhr

**Temporary Assistance to Needy
Families (TANF)**
Temporary Aid to Needy Families
Alvin Collins
Maryland Department of Human
Resources
311 West Saratoga St., Room 1045
Baltimore, MD 21201
410-767-7000
www.dhr.state.md.us/dhr/
services.htm

Women's Commission
Maryland Commission for Women
311 West Saratoga St., Room 232
Baltimore, MD 21201
410-767-7137

Information USA, Inc.

Fax: 410-333-0079
E-mail: lsajardo@dhr.state.md.us
www.dhr.state.md.us/mcw/ index.html
Dr. Carl A. Silberg, Executive Director
Dr. Fran V. Tracy-Mumsford, Chair

Massachusetts

Federal Information Center
All Locations; 800-688-9889

State Information Office
617-722-2000
http://www.state.ma.us

Department on Aging
Elder Affairs Department
1 Ashburton Place
5th Floor, Room 506
Boston, MA 02108
617-727-7750

Department of Education
Massachusetts Department of
Education
Information and Outreach
350 Main St.
Malden, MA 02148
781-388-3300
http://info.doe.mass.edu/

Health Department
Massachusetts Department of Public
Health
250 Washington Street
Boston, MA 02108-4619
617-624-5700
Fax: 617-624-5206
www.magnet.state.ma.us/dph/
dphhome.htm

Insurance Commissioner
Commissioner of Insurance
470 Atlantic Ave., 6th Floor
Boston, MA 02210-2223
617-521-7794
800-882-2003

Licensing Office
Division of Registration
100 Cambridge St.
Boston, MA 02202
617-727-3074
www.state.ma.us/reg

Social Services Offices
Massachusetts Health and Human
Services
1 Ashburton Place, Room 1109
Boston, MA 02108
617-727-7600
www.magnet.state.ma.us/
eohhs/eohhs.htm

**Temporary Assistance to Needy
Families (TANF)**
Temporary Aid to Needy Families
Claire McIntire
Massachusetts Department of
Transitional Assistance
600 Washington St.
Boston, MA 02111
617-348-8500
www.state.ma.us/eohhs/agencies/dta.
htm

Women's Commission
Massachusetts Governor's Advisory
Committee on Women's Issues
Statehouse Governor's Office
Room 360
Boston, MA 02133
617-727-3600
Fax: 617-727-9725
Jennifer Davis Carey, Contact
Joanne Thompson, Chair

Michigan

Federal Information Center
All Locations; 800-688-9889

State Information Office
517-373-1837
http://www.state.mi.us

Department on Aging
Aging Office
P.O. Box 30026
Lansing, MI 48909
517-373-8230
http://mass.iog.wayne.edu/
masshome.html

Department of Education
Michigan Department of Education
Information Center Data Services
P.O. Box 30008
Lansing, MI 48909
517-373-3324
http://www.mde.state.mi.us/

Health Department
Michigan Department of Community
Health
Lewis Cass Building
Sixth Floor
320 South Walnut Street
Lansing, MI 48913
517-373-3500
www.mdch.state.mi.us/
E-mail: arias@state.mi.us

Insurance Commissioner
Commissioner of Insurance
Insurance Bureau
P.O. Box 30220
Lansing, MI 48909-7720
517-373-9273

800-803-7174
http://www.commerce.state.mi.us/ins/

Licensing Office
Michigan Department of Consumer
and Industry Services
P.O. Box 30650
Lansing, MI 48909
517-373-1820
www.cis.state.mi.us

Social Services Offices
Michigan Family Independence
Agency
235 South Grand Avenue
Lansing, MI 48933
517-373-7394
www.mfia.state.mi.us

**Temporary Assistance to Needy
Families (TANF)**
Temporary Aid to Needy Families
Marva Livingston Hammons
Michigan Family Independence
Agency
P.O. Box 30037
235 South Grand Ave.
Lansing, MI 48909
517-373-2000
http://www.mfia.state.mi.us/
1997fact.htm

Women's Commission
Michigan Women's Commission
741 N. Cedar St., Suite 102
Lansing, MI 48913
517-334-8622
Fax: 517-334-8641
www.mdcr.com
Patti Garrett, Chair

Minnesota

Federal Information Center
All Locations; 800-688-9889

State Information Office
612-296-6013
http://www.state.mn.us

Department on Aging
Aging Program Division
Social Services Department
444 LaFayette Rd.
St. Paul, MN 55155-3843
612-296-2770

Department of Education
Minnesota Department of Education
Information and Technology Unit
550 Cedar St.
Capitol Square Bldg.
St. Paul, MN 55101
612-296-2751
http://children.state.mn.us/

Health Department
Minnesota Department of Health
717 Delaware Street Southeast
Minneapolis, MN 55440-9441
612-676-5000
www.health.state.mn.us
E-mail: webmaster@
health.state.mn.us

Insurance Commissioner
Commissioner of Commerce
133 E. 7th St.
St. Paul, MN 55101-2362
612-297-7161
800-657-3602
800-657-3978
http://www.commerce.state.mn.us/
mainin.htm

Licensing Office
Office of Consumer Services
Office of Attorney General
1400 NCL Tower
445 Minnesota St.
St. Paul, MN 55101
651-296-2331
www.ag.state.mn.us

Social Services Offices
Minnesota Department of Human
Services
444 Lafayette Road
St.Paul, MN 555155
651-296-4416
www.dhs.state.mn.us

**Temporary Assistance to Needy
Families (TANF)**
Temporary Aid to Needy Families
David Doth
Minnesota Dept. of Human Services
444 Lafayette Rd. North
St. Paul, MN 55155
612-296-6117
http://www.dhs.state.mn.us/
ecs/Welfare/default.htm

Women's Commission
Minnesota Commission on the
Economic Status of Women
85 State Office Building
St. Paul, MN 55155
651-296-8590
Fax: 651-297-3697
E-mail: lcesw@commissions.
leg.state.mn.us
www.commissions.leg.state.mn.us/
Aviva Breen, Executive Director
Becky Lourey, Chair

Mississippi

Federal Information Center
All Locations; 800-688-9889

State Information Office
601-359-1000
http://www.state.ms.us

Department on Aging
Aging and Adult Services Division
Human Services Department
P.O. Box 352
Jackson, MS 39205-0352
601-359-4925
http://www.mdhs.state.
ms.us/aas.html

Department of Education
Mississippi Dept. of Education
P.O. Box 771
Jackson, MS 39205-0771
601-359-5615
http://mdek12.state.ms.us/

Health Department
Mississippi State Dept of Health
2423 North State Street
P.O. Box 1700
Jackson, MS 39215-1700
601-576-7400
Fax: 601-576-7364
www.msdh.state.ms.us/
msdhhome.htm
E-mail: info@msdh.state.ms.us

Insurance Commissioner
Commissioner of Insurance

1804 Walter Sillers Bldg.
P.O. Box 79
Jackson, MS 39205
601-359-3569
800-562-2957
http://www.doi.state.ms.us

Licensing Office
Secretary of State
P.O. Box 136
Jackson, MS 39205
601-359-3123
www.sos.state.ms.us

Social Services Offices
Mississippi Department of Human
Services
750 North State Street
Jackson, MS 39202
601-359-4480
www.mdhs.state.ms.us

Temporary Assistance to Needy Families (TANF)
Temporary Aid To Needy Families
Sherry Jackson
Department of Human Services
P.O. Box 352
750 State St.
Jackson, MS 39202
601-359-4688
www.mdhs.state.ms.us/ ea_tanf.html

Women's Commission
Inactive

Missouri

Federal Information Center
All Locations; 800-688-9889

State Information Office
573-751-2000
http://www.state.mo.us

Department on Aging
Aging Division
P.O. Box 1337
Jefferson City, MO 65102
573-751-3082
http://www.state.mo.us/ dss/da/da.htm

Department of Education
Missouri Department of Education
School Data Section
P.O. Box 480
Jefferson City, MO 65102-0480
573-751-2569
http://services.dese.state.mo.us/

Health Department
Missouri Department of Health
930 Wildwood
P.O. Box 570
Jefferson, MO 65102-0570
573-751-6001
Fax: 573-751-6041
www.health.state.mo.us
E-mail: info@mail.health. state.mo.us

Insurance Commissioner
Director of Insurance
301 W. High St., Room 630
P.O. Box 690
Jefferson City, MO 65102-0690
573-751-4126
800-726-7390
http://services.state.mo.us/insurance/
mohmepg.htm

Licensing Office
Division of Professional Registration
Department of Economic
Development
3605 Missouri Blvd.
Jefferson City, MO 65109
314-751-0293
www.ecodev.state.mo.us/pr

Social Services Offices
Missouri Department of Social
Services
221 West High Street
P.O. Box 1527
Jefferson City, MO 65102-1527
573-751-4815
www.dss.state.mo.us

Temporary Assistance to Needy Families (TANF)
Temporary Aid to Needy Families
Gary Stangler
Missouri Department of Social
Services
P.O. Box 1527
Jefferson City, MO 65102
573-751-4815
www.dss.state.mo.us.dfs.pap.htm

Women's Commission
Missouri Women's Council
P.O. Box 1684
Jefferson City, MO 65102
573-751-0810
Fax: 573-751-8835
E-mail: wcouncil@mail.state.mo.us
www.womenscouncil.org
Sue P. McDaniel, Executive Director
Deborah Borchers-Ausmus, Chair

Montana

Federal Information Center
All Locations; 800-688-9889

State Information Office
406-444-2511
http://www.state.mt.us

Department on Aging
Senior and Long Term Care Division
Department of Public Health and
Human Services
Box 4210
Helena, MT 59604
406-444-5900
http://www.dphhs.mt.gov/
whowhat/sltc.htm

Department of Education
Montana Office of Public Instruction
Capitol Station
Helena, MT 59620-2501
406-444-3656
http://www.opi.mt.gov/

Health Department
Montana Department of Public Health
& Human Services
111 North Sanders
Helena, MT 59620
MAILING ADDRESS:
    P.O. Box 4210
    Helena, MT 59604-4210
406-444-2596
Fax: 406-444-1970
www.dphhs.mt.gov
E-mail: kpekoc@mt.gov

Insurance Commissioner
Commissioner of Insurance
P.O. Box 4009

Helena, MT 59604-4009
406-444-2040
800-332-6148

Licensing Office
Professional and Occupational
Licensing, Business Regulation
Department of Commerce
111 N. Jackson St.
Helena, MT 59620
406-444-37373
www.com.state.mt.us/License/
POL/index.htm

Social Services Offices
Montana Department of Public Health
and Human Services
111 North Sanders
Helena, MT 59620
406-444-2596
www.dphs.mt.gov

Temporary Assistance to Needy
Families (TANF)
Temporary Aid to Needy Families
Laurie Ekanger
Montana Department of Public Health
and Human Services
111 North Sanders St.
P.O. Box 4210
Helena, MT 59604
406-444-5622
www.dphhs.mt.gov/faq/afdc.htm

Women's Commission
Interdepartmental Coordinating
Committee for Women (ICCW)
P.O. Box 1728
Helena, MT 59624
406-444-1520

E-mail: jbranscum@state.mt.us
www.mdt.state.mt.us/iccw
Jean Branscum, Chair
Jeanne Wolf, Vice Chair

Nebraska

Federal Information Center
All Locations; 800-688-9889

State Information Office
402-471-2311
http://www.state.ne.us

Department on Aging
Aging Department
P.O. Box 95044
Lincoln, NE 68509-5044
402-471-2308
http://www.hhs.state.ne.
us/ags/agsindex.htm

Department of Education
Nebraska Department of Education
Data Center
P.O. Box 94987
Lincoln, NE 68509
402-471-2295
http://www.nde.state.ne.us/

Health Department
Nebraska Health & Human Services
System
Department of Services
P.O. Box 95044
Lincoln, NE 68509-5044
402-471-2306
www.hhs.state.ne.us/index.htm
E-mail: hhsinfo@ www.hhs.
state.ne.us

Insurance Commissioner
Director of Insurance
941 O St., Suite 400
Lincoln, NE 68508-3690
402-471-2201
800-833-0920
http://www.nol.org/home/ndoi/

Licensing Office
Bureau of Examining Boards
Nebraska Department of Health
P.O. Box 95007
Lincoln, NE 68509
402-471-2115

Social Services Offices
Nebraska Health and Human Services
System
Department of Services
P.O. Box 95044
Lincoln, NE 68509-5044
402-471-9108
www.hhs.state.ne.us

**Temporary Assistance to Needy
Families (TANF)**
Temporary Aid to Needy Families
Deb Thomas
Nebraska Department of Health and
Human Services
P.O. Box 95026
Lincoln, NE 68509
402-471-3121
http://www.hhs.state.ne.us/
fia/adc.htm

Women's Commission
Nebraska Commission on the Status of
Women
301 Centennial Mall South
Box 94985
Lincoln, NE 65809
402-471-2039
Fax: 402-471-5655
E-mail: ncswmail@mail.state.ne.us
www.ncsw.org
Toni Gray, Executive Director

Nevada

Federal Information Center
All Locations; 800-688-9889

State Information Office
702-687-5000
http://www.state.nv.us

Department on Aging
Aging Services Division
Human Resources Dept.
340 N. 11th St.
Howard Cannon Center
Las Vegas, NV 89101
702-486-3545
http://www.state.nv.us/ hr/aging/

Department of Education
Nevada Department of Education
Planning Research and Evaluation
Division
400 W. King St.
Carson City, NV 89710
702-687-3130
http://www.nsn.k12.nv.us/nvdoe/

Health Department
Nevada State Health Division
505 East King Street
Room 201
Carson City, NV 89710
775-687-3786
Fax: 775-687-3859
www.state.nv.us/health/

Insurance Commissioner
Commissioner of Insurance
1665 Hot Springs Rd.
Capitol Complex 152

Carson City, NV 89706-0646
702-687-4270
800-992-0900
http://www.state.nv.us/b&i/id/

Licensing Office
Consumer Affairs Division
Department of Commerce
4600 Kietezke Lane
Bldg. B, Suite 113
Reno, NV 89502
702-688-1800
800-326-5202

Social Services Offices
Nevada Department of Human
Resources
505 East King Street
Carson City, NV 89701-3708
702-687-4356
www.state.nv.us/hr

Temporary Assistance to Needy Families (TANF)
Temporary Aid to Needy Families
Rota Rosaschi
New Employers of Nevada
2527 North Carson St.
Capitol Complex
Carson City, NV 89710
702-687-4143
www.state.nv.us/hr/mission.htm

Women's Commission
Nevada Women's Fund
201 W. Liberty
Reno, NV 89501
775-786-2335

New Hampshire

Federal Information Center
All Locations; 800-688-9889

State Information Office
603-271-1110
http://www.state.nh.us

Department on Aging
Elderly and Adult Services Division
State Office Park South
115 Pleasant St., Annex Bldg. 1
Concord, NH 03301-3843
603-271-4680
http://www.state.nh.us/
dhhs/ofs/ofscstlc.htm

Department of Education
New Hampshire Dept. of Education
Office of Information Services
State Office Park South
101 Pleasant St.
Concord, NH 03301-3860
603-271-2778
http://www.state.nh.us/doe/
education.html

Health Department
New Hampshire Department of Health
& Human Services
6 Hazen Drive
Concord, NH 03301-6505
603-271-4939
www.dhs.state.nh.us/index.htm

Insurance Commissioner
Insurance Commissioner
169 Manchester St.
Concord, NH 03301-5151
603-271-2261
800-852-3416
http://www.state.nh.us/insurance/

Licensing Office
SOICC of New Hampshire
64 B Old Sun Cook Rd.
Concord, NH 03301
603-228-3349
www.state.nh.us/soiccnh

Social Services Offices
New Hampshire Department of Health
and Human Services
6th Hazen Drive
Concord, NH 03301
603-271-4415
www.dhhs.state.nh.us/

Temporary Assistance to Needy Families (TANF)
Temporary Aid to Needy Families
Mary Anne Broschek
New Hampshire Department of Health
and Human Services
6 Hazen Dr.
Concord, NH 03301
603-271-4442
www.state.nh.us/dhhs/ofs/
ofs_ind.htm

Women's Commission
New Hampshire Commission on the
Status of Women
State House Annex, Room 334
25 Capitol St.
Concord, NH 03301-6312
603-271-2660
Fax: 603-271-2361
E-mail: kfrey@admin.state.nh.us
www.state.nh.us/csw
Katheryn Frey, Executive Director
Molly Kelly, Chair

New Jersey

Federal Information Center
All Locations; 800-688-9889

State Information Office
609-292-2121
http://www.state.nj.us

Department on Aging
Aging Division
Community Affairs Dept.
101 S. Broad St., CN 807
Trenton, NJ 08625
609-292-3766
800-792-8820
http://www.state.nj.us/
health/senior/sraffair.htm

Department of Education
New Jersey Dept. of Education
Publications Office
CN 500, 225 E. State St.
Trenton, NJ 08625
609-984-0905
http://www.state.nj.us/education/

Health Department
New Jersey Department of Health &
Senior Services
P.O. Box 360
John Fitch Plaza
Trenton, NJ 08625-0360
609-292-7836
Fax: 609-633-9601
www.state.nj.us/health/

Insurance Commissioner
Commissioner
Department of Insurance
20 W. State St.
P.O. Box 325
Trenton, NJ 08625-0325

609-292-5316
800-792-8820
http://www.naic.org/nj/div_ins.htm

Licensing Office
Division of Consumer Affairs
124 Halsey St.
Newark, NJ 07102
973-504-6200
www.state.nj.us/lps/ca/home.html

Social Services Offices
New Jersey Department of Human
Services
P.O. Box 700
Trenton, NJ 08625
609-292-3703
www.state.nj.us/humanservices/
DHSHome.html

**Temporary Assistance to Needy
Families (TANF)**
Temporary Aid to Needy Families
William Waldman
New Jersey Department of Human
Services
P.O. Box 700
Trenton, NJ 08625
609-292-3717
http://www.state.nj.us/
humanservices/W&W.html

Women's Commission
New Jersey Dept. of Community Affairs
Division of Women
101 South Broad St., CN 808
Trenton, NJ 08625-0801
609-292-8840
Fax: 609-633-6821
Elizabeth L. Cox

New Mexico

Federal Information Center
All Locations; 800-688-9889

State Information Office
505-827-4011
http://www.state.nm.us

Department on Aging
State Agency on Aging
224 E. Palance Ave.
Santa Fe, NM 87501
505-827-7640

Department of Education
New Mexico Department of Education
Education Bldg.
Data Management
300 Don Gaspar Ave.
Santa Fe, NM 87501-2786
505-827-7354
http://sde.state.nm.us/

Health Department
New Mexico Department of Health
1190 St. Francis Drive
Harold Runnels Building
Sante Fe, NM 87504
505-827-2619
Fax: 505-827-2530
www.state.nm.us/state/doh.html

Insurance Commissioner
Superintendent of Insurance
P.O. Drawer 1269
Santa Fe, NM 87504-1269
505-827-4601
800-947-4722

Licensing Office
Regulation and Licensing Department
2055 Pacheco St., Suite 300
Santa Fe, NM 87504
505-476-6200
www.state.nm.us/rld/rld_mstr.html

Social Services Offices
New Mexico Human Services
Department
P.O. Box 2348
Santa Fe, NM 87504
505-827-7750
www.state.nm.us/hsd/home.htm

Temporary Assistance to Needy Families (TANF)
Temporary Aid to Needy Families
Tom Clayton
New Mexico Department of Human
Services
P.O. Box 2348
Santa Fe, NM 87504
505-827-1323
www.state.nm.us/hsd/isd.html

Women's Commission
New Mexico Commission on the Status
of Women
2401 12th St. NW
Albuquerque, NM 87104-2302
505-841-8920
Fax: 505-841-8926
E-mail: rdakota@nm.us.
campuscwix.net
Yolanda Garcia, Info. Officer
Darlene B. Herrera, Vice Chair

New York

Federal Information Center
All Locations; 800-688-9889

State Information Office
518-474-2121
http://www.state.ny.us

Department on Aging
Aging Office
Bldg. 2
Empire State Plaza
Albany, NY 12223-001
518-474-5731
800-342-9871 (NY only)
http://aging.state.ny. us/nysofa/

Department of Education
New York Department of Education
Information Center on Education Annex,
Room 309EB
Albany, NY 12234
518-474-8073
http://www.nysed.gov/

Health Department
New York Department of Health
Corning Tower Building
Empire State Plaza
Albany, NY 12237
518-486-9002
www.health.state.ny.us
E-mail: ljr06@health.state.ny.us

Insurance Commissioner
Superintendent of Insurance
25 Beaver St.
New York, NY 10004
212-480-6400
800-342-3736 (in NY)
http://www.ins.state.ny.us

Licensing Office
New York State Education
Department
Division of Professional Licensing
Cultural Education Center
Empire State Plaza
Albany, NY 12230
518-474-3817
800-442-8106
www.nysed.gov/prof/ profhome.htm

Social Services Offices
New York State Department of Family
Assistance
40 North Pearl Street
Albany, NY 12243
518-486-7545
www.dfa.state.ny.us

Temporary Assistance to Needy Families (TANF)
Temporary Aid to Needy Families
John Johnson
Office of Children and Family Services
52 Washington St.
Rensselaer, NY 12144
518-473-8437
www.dfa.state.ny.us/tanf/

Women's Commission
New York State Division for Women
633 Third Ave.
New York, NY 10017
212-681-4547
Fax: 212-681-7626
E-mail: women@women. state.ny.us
www.women.state.ny.us
Elaine Wingate Conway, Director

North Carolina

Federal Information Center
All Locations; 800-688-9889

State Information Office
919-733-1110
http://www.state.nc.us

Department on Aging
Aging Division
Human Resources Dept.
693 Palmer Dr.
Raleigh, NC 27603
919-733-3983
http://www.state.nc.us/
dhr/doa/home.htm

Department of Education
North Carolina Department of Public
Instruction
Information Center
301 N. Wilmington St.
Raleigh, NC 27601-2825
919-715-1018
800-665-1250
http://www.dpi.state.nc.us/

Health Department
North Carolina State Center for Health
Statistics
Cotton Classing Building
222 North Dawson Street
Raleigh, NC 27603-1392
MAILING ADDRESS:
  P.O. Box 29538
  Raleigh, NC 27626-0538
919-733-4728
Fax: 919-733-8485
http://hermes.sches.chnr.state.
nc.us/SCHS/main.html

Insurance Commissioner
Commissioner of Insurance
Dobbs Bldg.
P.O. Box 26387
Raleigh, NC 27611
919-733-7349
800-662-7777 (in NC)
http://www.doi.state.nc.us/

Licensing Office
Secretary of State
Business License Information Office
110 S. Blount St.
Raleigh, NC 27601
800-228-8443
www.state.nc.us/secstate

Social Services Offices
North Carolina Department of Health
and Human Services
Adams Building, Dix Campus
101 Blair Drive
Raleigh, NC 27603-2041
919-733-9190
www.dhr.state.nc.us/DHR

Temporary Assistance to Needy Families (TANF)
Temporary Aid to Needy Families
Pheon Beal
Division of Social Services
325 North Salisbury St.
Raleigh, NC 27603
919-733-3055
www.dhhs.state.nc.us/dss/
servfami.htm

Women's Commission
North Carolina Council for Women

526 North Wilmington St.
Raleigh, NC 27604-1199
919-733-2455
Fax: 919-733-2464
www.doa.state.nc.us/doa/ cfw/cfw.htm
Juanita Bryant, Executive Director
Jane Carver, Chair

North Dakota

Federal Information Center
All Locations; 800-688-9889

State Information Office
701-224-2000
http://www.state.nd.us

Department on Aging
Aging Services Division
Human Services Dept.
600 South 2nd St.
Suite 1-C
Bismarck, ND 58504-5729
701-328-8910

Department of Education
North Dakota Department of Education
Department of Public Instruction
600 E. Boulevard Ave.
Bismarck, ND 58505-0440
701-328-2268
http://www.dpi.state.nd.us/

Health Department
North Dakota Department of Health
600 East Boulevard Avenue
Bismarck, ND 58505-0200
701-328-2372
Fax: 701-328-4727
www.ehs.health.state.nd.us/ndhd/
E-mail: rfrank@state.nd.us

Insurance Commissioner
Commissioner of Insurance
Capitol Bldg., 5th Floor
600 E. Boulevard Ave.
Bismarck, ND 58505-0320
701-328-2440
800-247-0560 (in ND)

Licensing Office
Consumer Fraud Division
Office of the Attorney General
600 East Boulevard
Bismarck, ND 58505
701-328-3404
800-472-2000
www.state.nd.us/ndag/

Social Services Offices
Department of Human Services
State Capitol, Judicial Wing
600 E. Boulevard Ave.
Department 325
Bismarck, ND 58505-0250
701-328-2310
www1.state.nd.us/hms/dhs.htm

Temporary Assistance to Needy Families (TANF)
Temporary Aid to Needy Families
John Opp
North Dakota Department of
Economic Assistance
600 East Boulevard Ave.
Bismarck, ND 58505
701-328-2310
http://207.108.104.74/dhs/
dhsweb.nsf/ServicePages/
PublicAssistance

Women's Commission
North Dakota Governor's Commission
on the Status of Women
600 East Boulevard
Bismarck, ND 58501-0250
701-328-5300
Fax: 701-328-5320
Carol Reed, Chairman

Ohio

Federal Information Center
All Locations; 800-688-9889

State Information Office
614-466-2000
http://www.state.oh.us

Department on Aging
Aging Department
50 W. Broad St., 9th Floor
Columbus, OH 43215-5928
614-466-5500

Department of Education
Ohio Department of Education
Information Management Services
65 S. Front St.
Columbus, OH 43215-4183
614-466-7000
http://www.ode.ohio.gov/

Health Department
Ohio Department of Health
246 North High Street
P.O. Box 118
Columbus, OH 43266-0118
614-466-3543
www.odh.state.oh.us
E-mail: questions@
gw.odh.state.oh.us

Insurance Commissioner
Director of Insurance
2100 Stella Court
Columbus, OH 43215-1067
614-644-2651
800-686-1526 (consumer)
800-686-1527 (fraud)

800-686-1578 (senior health)
http://www.state.oh.us/ins/

Licensing Office
State of Ohio
State Information Office
30 East Broad St., 40th Floor
Columbus, OH 43215
614-466-2000

Social Services Offices
Ohio Department of Human Services
30 East Broad Street, 32nd Floor
Columbus, OH 43266-0423
614-466-6650
www.state.oh.us/odhs

Temporary Assistance to Needy Families (TANF)
Temporary Aid to Needy Families
Welfare Reform
Issac Palmer
Office of Workforce Development
30 East Broad St., 32nd Floor
Columbus, OH 43266
614-466-4909
http://www.state.oh.us/odhs/
owf/index.htm

Women's Commission
Ohio Women's Commission
77 S. High St., 24th Floor
Columbus, OH 43266-0920
614-466-5580
Fax: 614-466-5434
Sally Farran Bulford, Executive Director
Dr. Suzanne Crawford, Chair

Oklahoma

Federal Information Center
All Locations; 800-688-9889

State Information Office
405-521-2011
http://www.state.ok.us

Department on Aging
Aging Services Division
Human Services Dept.
P.O. Box 25352
Oklahoma City, OK 73125
405-521-2327

Department of Education
Oklahoma State Department of
Education
Documents
2500 N. Lincoln Blvd.
Oklahoma City, OK 73105-4599
405-521-2293
http://www.sde.state.ok.us/

Health Department
Oklahoma State Department of Health
1000 NE 10th Street
Oklahoma City, OK 73117
405-271-5600
800-522-0203
www.health.state.ok.us
E-mail: webmaster@
health.state.ok.us

Insurance Commissioner
Insurance Commissioner
P.O. Box 53408
Oklahoma City, OK 73152-3408
405-521-2828
800-522-0071
http://www.oid.state.ok.us

Licensing Office
Governor's Office
State Capitol
Oklahoma City, OK 73105
405-521-2342

Social Services Offices
Oklahoma Department of Human
Services
2400 North Lincoln Boulevard
P.O. Box 25352
Oklahoma City, OK 73125
405-521-3027
www.onenet.net/okdhs

Temporary Assistance to Needy Families (TANF)
Temporary Aid to Needy Families
Mary Stalnakger
Oklahoma Department of Human
Service
P.O. Box 25352
Oklahoma City, OK 73125
405-521-4415
www.onenet.net/okdhs/programs/
programs.htm#tanf

Women's Commission
Oklahoma Governor's Commission on
the Status of Women
101 State Capitol Bldg.
2300 North Lincoln Blvd.
Oklahoma City, OK 73105-4897
918-492-4492
Fax: 918-492-4472
Claudia Tarrington, Chair
Kathi Goebel, Senior Vice Chair

Lawton Mayor's Commission on the
Status of Women

102 SW 5th St.
Lawton, OK 73501
405-581-3260
Janet Childress, Chair
Emma Crowder, Vice Chair

Tulsa Mayor's Commission on the
Status of Women
c/o Department of Human Rights
200 Civic Center
Tulsa, OK 74103
918-582-0558
918-592-7818

Oregon

Federal Information Center
All Locations; 800-688-9889

State Information Office
503-378-3111
http://www.state.or.us

Department on Aging
Senior and Disabled Services
500 Summer St., NE
Salem, OR 97310-1015
503-945-5811
http://www.sdsd.hr.state.or.us/

Department of Education
Oregon Department of Education
Data Information Service
Public Service Bldg.
255 Capitol St., NE
Salem, OR 97310-0230
503-378-3310
http://www.ode.state.or.us/

Health Department
Oregon Health Division
800 NE Oregon Street
Portland, OR 97232
503-731-4000
www.ohd.hr.state.or.us
E-mail: ohd.info@state.or.us

Insurance Commissioner
Insurance Commissioner
440 Labor and Industries Bldg.
330 Winter St., NE
Salem, OR 97310
503-378-4271
800-722-4134
http://www.state.or.us/agencies.ns/4400
0/ 00070/index.html

Licensing Office
Business Information Center
Corporations Division
255 Capitol St., NW
Suite 151
Salem, OR 97310
503-986-2222
www.sos.state.or.us/corporation/
bic/bic.htm

Social Services Offices
Oregon Department of Human
Resources
500 Summer Street, NE
Salem, OR 97310-1012
503-945-5738
www.hr.state.or.us/

Temporary Assistance to Needy Families (TANF)
Temporary Aid to Needy Families
Sandie Hoback
Oregon Department of Human
Resources
500 Summer St., NE
Salem, OR 97310
503-945-6116
http://www.afs.hr.state.or.us/
overview.html

Women's Commission
Oregon Commission for Women
Portland State University
Smith Center, Room M315
Portland, OR 97207
503-725-5889
Tracy Davis, Contact

Pennsylvania

Federal Information Center
All Locations; 800-688-9889

State Information Office
717-787-2121
http://www.state.pa.us

Department on Aging
Aging Department
400 Market St.
State Office Bldg., 6th Floor
Harrisburg, PA 17101-2301
717-783-1550
http://164.156.7.66/pa_exec/
aging/overview.html

Department of Education
Pennsylvania Dept. of Education
Office of Data Services
333 Market St.
Harrisburg, PA 17126-0333
717-787-2644
http://www.cas.psu.edu/pde.html

Health Department
Pennsylvania Department of Health
P.O. Box 90
Health & Welfare Building
Harrisburg, PA 17108
800-692-7254
www.health.state.pa.us
E-mail: webmaster@
heath.state.pa.us

Insurance Commissioner
Insurance Commissioner
1326 Strawberry Square
Harrisburg, PA 17120
717-787-2317
800-783-7067

http://www.state.pa.us/pa_exec/
insurance/ overview.html

Licensing Office
Bureau of Professional and
Occupational Affairs
618 Transportation and Safety Bldg.
Harrisburg, PA 17120
717-783-4854
800-822-2113
www.dos.state.pa.us/bpoa/ poa.htm

Social Services Offices
Pennsylvania Department of Public
Welfare
333 Health and Welfare Building
Harrisburg, PA 17105
717-787-4592
www.state.pa.us/PA_Exec/
Public_Welfare/overview.html

Temporary Assistance to Needy Families (TANF)
Temporary Aid to Needy Families
Feather Houston
Pennsylvania Dept. of Public Welfare
33 Health and Welfare Building
Harrisburg, PA 17105
717-787-3600
www.state.pa.us/PA_Exec/
Public_Welfare/secletter.html

Women's Commission
Pennsylvania Commission for Women
Finance Building, Room 205
Harrisburg, PA 17120
888-615-7477
Fax: 717-772-0653
E-mail: lesbn@oa.state.pa.us
Loida Esbri, Executive Director

Rhode Island

Federal Information Center
All Locations; 800-688-9889

State Information Office
401-222-2000
http://www.state.ri.us

Department on Aging
Elderly Affairs Department
160 Pine St.
Providence, RI 02903
401-222-2858
http://www.sec.state.ri.
us/stdept/sd23.htm

Department of Education
Management Information Services
Rhode Island Department of Education
255 Westminster St.
Providence, RI 02903-3400
401-222-4600, ext. 6
http://instruct.ride.ri.net/ride_
home_page.html

Health Department
Rhode Island Department of Health
3 Capitol Hill
Providence, RI 02908
401-222-2231
Fax: 401-222-6548
TTY: 800-745-5555
www.health.state.ri.us/
E-mail: library@health.state.ri.us

Insurance Commissioner
Insurance Commissioner
233 Richmond St., Suite 233
Providence, RI 02903
401-277-2223
800-322-2880

Licensing Office
Rhode Island Occupational
Information Coordinating Commission
101 Friendship St.
Providence, RI 02903
401-272-0830
www.dlt.state.ri.us/webdev/lmi/
rioicc/rioicchm.html

Social Services Offices
Rhode Island Department of Human
Services
600 New London Avenue
Cranston, RI 02920
401-464-2121
www.athena.state.ri.us/info/
human.htm

Temporary Assistance to Needy Families (TANF)
Temporary Aid to Needy Families
Edward Sneesby
Field Operations
Aimy Forand Bldg.
Cranston, RI 02920
401-464-2424
www.dhs.state.ri.us

Women's Commission
Rhode Island Advisory Commission on
Women
260 W. Exchange St., Suite 4
Providence, RI 02093
401-222-6105
E-mail: tayers@doa.state.ri.us
Toby Ayers, Ph.D., Director
James M. Anthony, Chair

South Carolina

Federal Information Center
All Locations; 800-688-9889

State Information Office
803-734-1000
http://www.state.sc.us

Department on Aging
Office on Aging
South Carolina Department of Health
and Human Services
P.O. Box 8206
Columbia, SC 29201
803-253-6177

Department of Education
South Carolina Dept. of Education
Management Information Section
1206 Rutledge Bldg.
1429 Senate St.
Columbia, SC 29201
803-734-8262
http://www.state.sc.us/sde/

Health Department
South Carolina Department of Health
and Environmental Control
2600 Bull Street
Columbia, SC 29201
803-898-3432
www.state.sc.us/dhec/
E-mail: menchima@
columb29.dhec.state.sc.us

Insurance Commissioner
Chief Insurance Commissioner
P.O. Box 100105
Columbia, SC 29202-3105
803-737-6150

800-768-3467
http://www.state.sc.us/doi/

Licensing Office
South Carolina Department of Labor,
Licensing, and Regulation
P.O. Box 11329
Columbia, SC 29211
803-896-4363
www.llr.state.sc.us/boards.htm

Social Services Offices
South Carolina Department of Social
Services
P.O. Box 1520
Columbia, SC 29202-1520
803-734-6180
www.state.sc.us/dss

**Temporary Assistance to Needy
Families (TANF)**
Temporary Aid to Needy Families
James Clark
South Carolina Department of Social
Services
P.O. Box 1520
Columbia, SC 29202
803-734-5760
www.state.sc.us/dss/ programs.htm

Women's Commission
Governor's Office Commission on
Women
1205 Pendleton St., Suite 306
Columbia, SC 29201
803-734-1609
Fax: 803-734-0241
Rebecca Collier, Executive Director

South Dakota

Federal Information Center
All Locations; 800-688-9889

State Information Office
605-773-3011
http://www.state.sd.us

Department on Aging
Adult Services on Aging Office.
Social Services Department
700 Governors Dr.
Pierre, SD 57501
605-773-3656
http://www.state.sd.us/state/
executive/social/asa/asa.htm

Department of Education
South Dakota Department of Education
and Cultural Affairs
Office of Finance Management
700 Governors Dr.
Pierre, SD 57501-2291
605-773-3248
605-773-4748
http://www.state.sd.us/state/
executive/deca/

Health Department
South Dakota Dept. of Health
Health Building
600 East Capitol
Pierre, SD 57501-2563
800-738-2301
Fax: 605-773-5683
www.state.sd.us/state/executive/
doh/doh.html
E-mail: Info@doh.state.sd.us

Insurance Commissioner
Director of Insurance
Insurance Building
118 W. Capitol St.
Pierre, SD 57501
605-773-3563
800-822-8804
http://www.state.sd.us/insurance/

Licensing Office
Dept. of Commerce and Regulation
118 E. Capitol Ave.
Pierre, SD 57501
605-773-3178
www.state.sd.us/dcr/dcr.html

Social Services Offices
South Dakota Department of Social
Services
700 Governors Drive
Pierre, SD 57501-2291
605-773-3165
www.state.sd.us/state/executive/
social/social.html

**Temporary Assistance to Needy
Families (TANF)**
Temporary Aid to Needy Families
Judy Thompson
South Dakota Department of Social
Services
700 Governors Dr.
Pierre, SD 57501
605-773-3493
http://www.state.sd.us/state/
executive/social/TANF/tanf.htm

Women's Commission
Abolished

Tennessee

Federal Information Center
All Locations; 800-688-9889

State Information Office
615-741-3011
http://www.state.tn.us

Department on Aging
Aging Commission
500 Deaderick St., 9th Floor
Nashville, TN 37243-0860
615-741-2056

Department of Education
Tennessee Dept. of Education
Office of Accountability
Gateway Plaza
710 James Robertson Parkway
Nashville, TN 37243-0381
615-532-4703
http://www.state.tn.us/education

Health Department
Tennessee Department of Health
425 5th Avenue North
Nashville, TN 37247
615-741-3111
www.state.tn.us/health
E-mail: DDenton@mail.state.tn.us

Insurance Commissioner
Commissioner of Insurance
500 James Robertson Parkway
Nashville, TN 37243-0565
615-741-2241

800-342-4029
http://www.state.tn.us/commerce

Licensing Office
Division of Regulatory Boards
Department of Commerce and
Insurance
500 James Robertson Parkway
Nashville, TN 37243
615-741-3449
www.state.tn.us/commerce

Social Services Offices
Tennessee Department of Human
Services
Citizens Plaza Building
400 Deaderick Street
Nashville, TN 37248-0001
615-313-4707
www.state.tn.us/humanserv

Temporary Assistance to Needy Families (TANF)
Temporary Aid to Needy Families
Wanda Moore
Tennessee Department of Human
Services
400 Deaderick St., 12th Floor
Nashville, TN 37248
615-313-4867
www.state.tn.us/humanserv/
fmfirst.htm

Women's Commission
Abolished

Texas

Federal Information Center
All Locations; 800-688-9889

State Information Office
512-463-4630
http://www.state.tx.us

Department on Aging
Aging Department
Box 12786
Austin, TX 78711
512-424-6840
http://www.texas.gov/ agency/
340.html

Department of Education
Texas Education Agency
Division of Public Information
1701 N. Congress
Austin, TX 78701-1494
MAILING ADDRESS:
  P.O. Box 13817
  Austin, TX 78711-3817
512-463-9734
http://www.tea.state.tx.us/

Health Department
Texas Department of Health
1100 West 49th Street
Austin, TX 78756-3199
512-458-7111
www.tdh.texas.gov/

Insurance Commissioner
Director
Claims and Compliance Division
State Board of Insurance
P.O. Box 149104
Austin, TX 78714-9104
512-463-6464

800-252-3439
http://www.tdi.state.tx.us

Licensing Office
Department of Licensing and
Regulation
P.O. Box 12157
Austin, TX 78711
512-463-6599
800-803-9202
www.license.state.tx.us

Social Services Offices
Texas Department of Human Services
701 West 51st Street
Austin, TX 78751
512-438-3045
www.dhs.texas.gov

Temporary Assistance to Needy Families (TANF)
Temporary Aid to Needy Families
Eric Bost
Texas Department of Human Services
P.O. Box 149030
Austin, TX 78714
512-438-3280
http://www.dhs.state.tx.us/dhs/
cssind.htm

Women's Commission
Texas Governor's Commission for
Women
P.O. Box 12428
Austin, TX 78711
512-463-1782
512-475-2615
Fax: 512-463-1832
www.governor.state.tx.us/women/
Ashley Horton, Executive Director

Utah

Federal Information Center
All Locations; 800-688-9889

State Information Office
801-538-3000
http://www.state.ut.us

Department on Aging
Aging and Adult Services Division
Human Services Dept.
120 North, 200 West
Salt Lake City, UT 84107
801-538-3910
http://www.dhs.state.ut.us/
agency/daas/homeage.htm

Department of Education
Utah Board of Education
Department of Finance
250 E. 500 S.
Salt Lake City, UT 84111
801-538-7660
http://www.usoe.k12.ut.us/

Health Department
Utah Department of Health
P.O. Box 1010
Salt Lake City, UT 84114-1010
801-538-5101
http://hlunix.ex.state.ut.us/
E-mail: pwightma@doh.state.ut.us

Insurance Commissioner
Commissioner of Insurance
3110 State Office Bldg.
Salt Lake City, UT 84114
801-538-3805
800-439-3805
http://www.ins-dept.state.ut.us/

Licensing Office
Division of Occupational and
Professional Licensing
Department of Commerce
160 East 300 South
P.O. Box 45802
Salt Lake City, UT 84145
801-530-6628
www.commerce.state.ut.us

Social Services Offices
Utah Department of Human Services
P.O. Box 45500
120 North 200 West
Salt Lake City, UT 84145-0500
801-538-3991
www.dhs.state.ut.us

Temporary Assistance to Needy Families (TANF)
Temporary Aid to Needy Families
Robin Arnold Williams
Utah Department of Human Services
120 North 200 West, Suite 319
Salt Lake City, UT 84103
801-538-3998
http://www.dws.state.ut.us

Women's Commission
Utah Governor's Commission for
Women and Families
1160 State Office Bldg.
Salt Lake City, UT 84114
801-538-1736
Fax: 801-538-3027
E-mail: women&families@
gov.state.ut.us
www.governor.state.ut.us/women/
Michael Neider, Chair

Vermont

Federal Information Center
All Locations; 800-688-9889

State Information Office
802-828-1110
http://www.state.vt.us

Department on Aging
Vermont Department of Aging and
Disabilities
103 S. Main St.
Waterbury, VT 05676
802-241-2400
http://www.state.vt.us/ dad/busdir.htm

Department of Education
Vermont Department of Education
School Finance Department
State Office Bldg.
120 State St.
Montpelier, VT 05620-2501
802-828-3147
http://www.state.vt.us/educ/

Health Department
Vermont Department of Health
108 Cherry Street
Burlington, VT 05402-0070
800-464-4343
Fax: 802-863-7475
www.state.vt.us/health

Insurance Commissioner
Commissioner of Banking and
Insurance
89 Main St., Drawer 20
Montpelier, VT 05620-3101
802-828-3301
800-642-5119
http://www.state.vt.us/bis/

Licensing Office
Office of Professional Regulation
Secretary of State
Pavilion Office Building
Montpelier, VT 05609
802-828-2363
http://vtprofessionals.org

Social Services Offices
Vermont Agency of Human Services
103 South Main Street
Waterbury, VT 05671-2401
802-241-2220
www.ahs.state.vt.us

**Temporary Assistance to Needy
Families (TANF)**
Temporary Aid to Needy Families
Jane Kitchel
Vermont Department of Social
Welfare
103 South Main St.
Waterbury, VT 05671
802-241-2853
http://www.dsw.state.vt.us/
wrp/tanf_stp.htm

Women's Commission
Vermont Governor's Commission on the
Status of Women
126 State St.
Drawer 33
Montpelier, VT 05602
802-828-2851
Fax: 802-828-2930
E-mail: info@women.state.vt.us
www.state.vt.us/wom
Judith Sutphen, Executive Director

Virginia

Federal Information Center
All Locations; 800-688-9889

State Information Office
804-786-0000
http://www.state.va.us

Department on Aging
Aging Department
1600 Forest Ave., Suite 102
Richmond, VA 23229
804-662-9333
http://www.aging.state. va.us/

Department of Education
Virginia Department of Education
Management Information Office
101 N. 14th St., 22nd Floor
Richmond, VA 23219
804-225-2540
800-292-3820
http://www.pen.k12.va.us/
Anthology/VDOE/

Health Department
Virginia Department of Health
Main Street Station
Richmond, VA 23219
804-786-5916
Fax: 804-371-4110
www.vdh.state.va.us/
E-mail: rnash@vdh.state.va.us

Insurance Commissioner
Commissioner of Insurance
1300 E. Main St.
P.O. Box 1157
Richmond, VA 23218
804-371-9741

800-552-7945
http://dit1.state.va.us/scc/division/
boi/index.htm

Licensing Office
Virginia Department of Professional
and Occupational Regulation
3600 W. Broad St.
Richmond, VA 23230
804-367-8500
www.state.va.us/dpor/indexie.html

Social Services Offices
Virginia Department of Social Services
730 East Broad Street
Richmond, VA 23219
804-692-1906

**Temporary Assistance to Needy
Families (TANF)**
Temporary Aid to Needy Families
Marsha Sharpe
Department of Social Services
730 East Broad St., 7th Floor
Richmond, VA 23229
804-692-1730
www.dss.state.va.us/tempasst. html

Women's Commission
Alexandria Council on the Status of
Women
110 North Royal St., Suite 201
Alexandria, VA 22314
703-838-5030
Fax: 703-838-4976
http://ci.alexandria.va.us/
alexandria.html
Norma Gattsek, Executive Director
Tara Hardiman, Chair

Arlington Commission on the Status of
Women
2100 Clarendon Blvd., Suite 310
Arlington, VA 22201
703-228-3257
Fax: 703-228-3295
E-mail: publicaffairs@co. arlington.va.us
www.co.arlington.va.us/cmo
Katherine Hoffman

Fairfax City Commission for Women
10455 Armstrong St.
Fairfax, VA 22030
703-385-7894
Fax: 703-385-7811
www.ci.fairfax.va.us
Louise Armitage, Director

Fairfax County Commission for Women
12000 Government Center Pkwy.
Suite 318
Fairfax, VA 22035
703-324-5720
Fax: 703-324-3959
TTY: 703-222-3504
Leia Francisco, Executive Director

Richmond Mayor's Committee on the
Concerns of Women
City Hall
900 East Marshall St., Room 302
Richmond, VA 23219
804-646-5987
Nancy Ownes, Admin. Assistant
Caroline Adams, Chair

Washington

Federal Information Center
All Locations; 800-688-9889

State Information Office
360-753-5000
http://www.state.wa.us

Department on Aging
Aging and Adult Services
P.O. Box 45050
Olympia, WA 98504-5600
360-586-8753

Department of Education
Washington Superintendent of Public
Instruction
47200 Old Capitol Bldg.
Olympia, WA 98504-7200
360-753-1700
http://www.ospi.wednet.edu/

Health Department
Washington State Department of
Health
1112 SE Quince Street
P.O. Box 47890
Olympia, WA 98504-7890
360-236-4010
www.doh.wa.gov/
E-mail: gkm0303@doh.wa.gov

Insurance Commissioner
Insurance Commissioner
Insurance Bldg. AQ21
P.O. Box 40255
Olympia, WA 98504-0255
360-753-7301
800-562-6900
http://www.wa.gov/ins/

Licensing Office
Department of Licensing
Department of Health
P.O. Box 9020
Olympia, WA 98507
360-644-1400
www.wa.gov/dol/main.htm

Social Services Offices
Washington Department of Social and
Health Services
DSHS Constituent Services
P.O. Box 45130
Olympia, WA 98504-5130
360-902-7892
www.wa.gov/dshs

**Temporary Assistance to Needy
Families (TANF)**
Temporary Aid to Needy Families
Roxane Lowe
Department of Social and Health
Services
1009 College St., SE
P.O. Box 45400
Olympia, WA 98504
360-413-3010
www.wa.gov/dshs/workfirst/ tanf.html

Women's Commission
Seattle Women's Commission
c/o Seattle Office for Civil Rights
700 Third Ave, Suite 250
Seattle WA 98104
206-684-4500
Fax: 206-684-0332
E-mail: diane.pina@ci.seattle.wa.us
www.ci.seattle.wa.us/seattle/
civil/swc.htm

West Virginia

Federal Information Center
All Locations; 800-688-9889

State Information Office
304-558-3456
http://www.state.wv.us

Department on Aging
Aging Commission
1900 Kanawha Blvd.
State Capitol, Holly Grove
Charleston, WV 25305
304-558-3317
http://www.wvdhhr.org/
pages/bcs/aging.htm

Department of Education
West Virginia Dept. of Education
Department of Statistical Information
Bldg. 6, Room B-346
1900 Kanawha Blvd. E.
Charleston, WV 25305-0330
304-558-8869
http://wvde.state.wv.us/

Health Department
West Virginia Bureau for Public Health
Building 3, Room 518
State Capitol Complex
Charelston, WV 25305
304-228-2971
Fax: 304-558-1035
http://wvbph.marshall.edu

Insurance Commissioner
Insurance Commissioner
2019 Washington St., E.
P.O. Box 50540
Charleston, WV 25305-0540
304-558-3394
800-642-9004

Licensing Office
Secretary of State
State Capitol
Charleston, WV 25305
304-558-6000

Social Services Offices
West Virginia Department of Health
and Human Resources
State Capital Complex
Building 3, Room 218
Charleston, WV 25305
304-558-8886
www.wvdhhr.org

Temporary Assistance to Needy Families (TANF)
Temporary Aid to Needy Families
Sharon Paterno
West Virginia Department of Health
and Human Resources
Building 6, Room 650
State Capitol Complex
Charleston, WV 25305
304-558-4069
www.wvdhhr.org/pages/bcf/
cf-family.htm

Women's Commission
West Virginia Women's Commission
Building 6, Room 637
Capitol Complex
Charleston, WV 25305
304-558-0070
Fax: 304-558-5767
E-mail: vrobinson@wvdhhr.org
www.state.wv.us/womenscom
Joyce M. Stover, Acting Executive
Director
Sally Riley, Chair

Wisconsin

Federal Information Center
All Locations; 800-688-9889

State Information Office
608-266-2211
http://www.state.wi.us

Department on Aging
Aging and Long Term Care Board
217 S. Hamilton St., Suite 300
Madison, WI 53703
608-266-2536

Department of Education
Wisconsin Department of Public
Instruction
Center for Education Statistics
125 S. Webster
P.O. Box 7841
Madison, WI 53707-7841
608-266-3390
800-441-4563
http://www.dpi.state.wi.us/

Health Department
Wisconsin Department of Health &
Family Services
1 West Wilson Street
Madison, WI 53702-0007
608-266-1865
TTY: 608-267-7371
www.dhfs.state.wi.us

Insurance Commissioner
Commissioner of Insurance
P.O. Box 7873
Madison, WI 53707-7873
608-266-3585
800-236-8517

http://badger.state.wi.us/agencies/oci/
oci_home.htm

Licensing Office
Department of Regulation and
Licensing
P.O. Box 8935
Madison, WI 53708
608-266-7482
http://bager.state.wi.us/ agencies/drl

Social Services Offices
Wisconsin Department of Health and
Family Services
1 West Wilson Street
Madison, WI 53702
608-266-1683
www.dhfs.state.wi.us

**Temporary Assistance to Needy
Families (TANF)**
Temporary Aid to Needy Families
Linda Stewart
Work Force Development
P.O. Box 7946
Madison, WI 53707
608-266-7553
www.dwd.state.wi.us/desw2/
W2Home.htm

Women's Commission
Wisconsin Women's Council
16 North Carroll St., Suite 720
Madison, WI 53703
608-266-2219
Fax: 608-261-2432
E-mail: Katie.Mnuk@wwc. state.wi.us
http://wwc.state.wi.us
Katie Mnuk, Executive Director

Wyoming

Federal Information Center
All Locations; 800-688-9889

State Information Office
307-777-7011
http://www.state.wy.us

Department on Aging
Division on Aging
Department of Health
117 Hathaway Bldg., Room 139
Cheyenne, WY 82002
307-777-7986
http://wdhfs.state.wy.us/
wdh/default.htm

Department of Education
Wyoming Department of Education
Statistical Department
Hathaway Bldg., 2nd Floor
2300 Capitol Ave.
Cheyenne, WY 82002-0050
307-777-7673
http://www.k12.wy.us/ wdehome.html

Health Department
Wyoming Department of Health
2300 Capitol Avenue
MAILING ADDRESS:
   117 Hathaway Building
   Cheyenne, WY 82002
307-777-7657
Fax: 307-777-7439
TTY: 307-777-5648
http://wdhfs.state.wy.us/wdh/
E-mail: wdh@missc.state.wy.us

Insurance Commissioner
Commissioner of Insurance
Herschler Bldg. 3 East
122 W. 25th St.

Cheyenne, WY 82002
307-777-7401
800-438-5768

Licensing Office
Governor's Office
State Capitol
Cheyenne, WY 82002
307-777-7434
www.state.wy.us/governor/
governor_home.html

Social Services Offices
Wyoming Department of Family
Services
Hathaway Building
Cheyenne, WY 82002-0490
307-777-3679
www.dfsweb.state.wy.us

Temporary Assistance to Needy Families (TANF)
Temporary Aid to Needy Families
Marianne Lee
Department of Family Services
2300 Capitol Ave.
Hathaway Building, 3rd Floor
Cheyenne, WY 82002
307-777-7531
http://dfsweb.state.wy.us/ updtanf.htm

Women's Commission
Wyoming State Government
Commission for Women
c/o Department of Employment
Herschler Building
122 West 25th St.
Cheyenne, WY 82002
307-777-7671
http://wydoe.state.wy.us
Amy McClure, Chair

Index

C

G

Hill-Burton free care program,
114
HIV, 28
pregnancy and, 317
support services, 65
Homeless Children's Program,
471
Hospice care, 38-39
Hotline
Medicare, 385, 394, 479
Pharmaceutical Manufacturers
Association, 72
women's health, 385

I

Idaho
dental programs, 160
health insurance assistance
programs, 388
health insurance for children,
346
insurance commissioner, 481
long term care ombudsman,
496
maternal and child health
programs, 290
Medicaid officials, 399
medical association hotline,
129
medical boards, 487
public health hotline, 118
services for children with
disabilities, 281
Illinois
dental programs, 161
health insurance assistance
programs, 388
health insurance for children,
346
insurance commissioner, 481
long term care ombudsman,
496

maternal and child health
programs, 290
Medicaid officials, 399
medical association hotline,
129
medical boards, 487
prescription drug discount
programs, 100
public health hotline, 118
services for children with
disabilities, 281
Immunizations, 558
flu shots, 376
for children, 377, 378
for travelers, 378
Impotence, 558
Incontinence, 558
Indiana
dental programs, 163
health insurance assistance
programs, 388
health insurance for children,
347
insurance commissioner, 481
long term care ombudsman,
496
maternal and child health
programs, 290
Medicaid officials, 399
medical association hotline,
129
medical boards, 487
public health hotline, 119
services for children with
disabilities, 282
Indigent patient programs
prescription drugs, 71
Infertility help line, 31
Insurance commissioners
state listing of, 480
International Childbirth
Educational Association, 312,
325

Liver disease, 561
Living will, 392
Louisiana
dental programs, 169
health insurance assistance
programs, 388
health insurance for children,
350
insurance commissioner, 482
long term care ombudsman,
497
maternal and child health
programs, 290
Medicaid officials, 400
medical association hotline,
129
medical boards, 488
public health hotline, 119
services for children with
disabilities, 282
Loving Paws Assistance Dogs, 58
Lupus, 61

M

Maine
dental programs, 170
health insurance assistance
programs, 388
health insurance for children,
351
insurance commissioner, 482
long term care ombudsman,
497
maternal and child health
programs, 291
Medicaid officials, 400
medical association hotline,
129
medical boards, 488
prescription drug discount
programs, 101
public health hotline, 119

services for children with
disabilities, 282
Mammograms, 9
low-cost, 424
regional contacts for, 431
Managed care, 391
March of Dimes Birth Defects
Foundation, 310, 320
Maryland
dental programs, 171
health insurance assistance
programs, 388
health insurance for children,
352
insurance commissioner, 482
long term care ombudsman,
497
maternal and child health
programs, 291
Medicaid officials, 401
medical association hotline,
130
medical boards, 488
prescription drug discount
programs, 102
public health hotline, 119
services for children with
disabilities, 282
Massachusetts
dental programs, 173
health insurance assistance
programs, 388
health insurance for children,
352
insurance commissioner, 482
long term care ombudsman,
497
maternal and child health
programs, 291
Medicaid officials, 401
medical association hotline,
130
medical boards, 488

health insurance for children, 355
insurance commissioner, 483
long term care ombudsman, 497
maternal and child health programs, 291
Medicaid officials, 401
medical association hotline, 130
medical boards, 489
public health hotline, 120
services for children with disabilities, 283

Missouri
dental programs, 178
health insurance assistance programs, 389
health insurance for children, 355
insurance commissioner, 483
long term care ombudsman, 498
maternal and child health programs, 291
Medicaid officials, 401
medical association hotline, 130
medical boards, 489
public health hotline, 120
services for children with disabilities, 283

Models That Work Campaign (MTW), 474

Montana
dental programs, 179
health insurance assistance programs, 389
health insurance for children, 356
insurance commissioner, 483
long term care ombudsman, 498

maternal and child health programs, 292
Medicaid officials, 402
medical association hotline, 130
medical boards, 489
public health hotline, 120
services for children with disabilities, 283

Multiple Sclerosis, 60, 564
Muscular Dystrophy, 517

N

National Action Plan on Breast Cancer, 430
National Adoption Foundation, 11
National Alliance of Breast Cancer Organizations, 426
National Association of Childbearing Centers (NACC), 330
National Breast Cancer Coalition, 430
National Cancer Institute, 427, 448
National Committee to Prevent Child Abuse, 326
National Domestic Violence Hotline, 14
National Immunization Information Hotline, 377
National Institute of Child Health and Human Development, 314
National Institutes of Health (NIH) Clinical Center, 106
eligibility requirements, 109
financial assistance, 109
patient referrals, 108
National Maternal and Child Health Clearinghouse, 316
National Organization for Women's Legal Defense Fund, 57

National Parkinson Foundation,
Inc, 44
National Women's Health
Network, 317
Nebraska
dental programs, 180
health insurance assistance
programs, 389
health insurance for children,
357
insurance commissioner, 483
long term care ombudsman,
498
maternal and child health
programs, 292
Medicaid officials, 402
medical association hotline,
130
medical boards, 489
public health hotline, 120
services for children with
disabilities, 283
Neurological disorders, 565
Neurology, 517
Nevada
dental programs, 181
health insurance assistance
programs, 389
health insurance for children,
358
insurance commissioner, 483
long term care ombudsman,
498
maternal and child health
programs, 292
Medicaid officials, 402
medical association hotline,
130
medical boards, 489
public health hotline, 120
services for children with
disabilities, 284

New Hampshire
dental programs, 182
health insurance assistance
programs, 389
health insurance for children,
358
insurance commissioner, 483
long term care ombudsman,
498
maternal and child health
programs, 292
Medicaid officials, 402
medical association hotline,
130
medical boards, 489
public health hotline, 121
services for children with
disabilities, 284
New Jersey
dental programs, 183
health insurance assistance
programs, 389
health insurance for children,
359
insurance commissioner, 483
long term care ombudsman,
499
maternal and child health
programs, 292
Medicaid officials, 402
medical association hotline,
131
medical boards, 490
prescription drug discount
programs, 102
public health hotline, 121
services for children with
disabilities, 284
New Mexico
dental programs, 184
health insurance assistance
programs, 389

O

Y